Community Pharmacy

This book is due for return not later than the
last date stamped below, unless recalled sooner.

Commissioning Editor: Pauline Graham
Development Editor: Sally Davies
Project Manager: Anne Dickie and Shereen Jameel
Designer/Design Direction: George Ajayi
Illustration Manager: Kirsteen Wright

Community Pharmacy

Symptoms, Diagnosis and Treatment

Paul Rutter BPharm MRPharmS PhD

Department of Pharmacy, University of Wolverhampton

SECOND EDITION

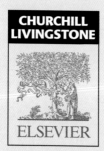

CHURCHILL
LIVINGSTONE

ELSEVIER

Edinburgh   London   New York   Oxford   Philadelphia   St Louis   Sydney   Toronto   2009

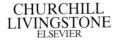

CHURCHILL
LIVINGSTONE
ELSEVIER

An imprint of Elsevier Limited

Second Edition © 2009, Elsevier Limited. All rights reserved.
First Edition © 2004, Elsevier Limited. All rights reserved.

ISBN 978 0 7020 2995 0

British Library Cataloguing in Publication Data
A catalogue record for this book is available from the British Library

Library of Congress Cataloging in Publication Data
A catalog record for this book is available from the Library of Congress

Notice
Knowledge and best practice in this field are constantly changing. As new research and experience broaden our knowledge, changes in practice, treatment and drug therapy may become necessary or appropriate. Readers are advised to check the most current information provided (i) on procedures featured or (ii) by the manufacturer of each product to be administered, to verify the recommended dose or formula, the method and duration of administration, and contraindications. It is the responsibility of the practitioner, relying on their own experience and knowledge of the patient, to make diagnoses, to determine dosages and the best treatment for each individual patient, and to take all appropriate safety precautions. To the fullest extent of the law, neither the Publisher nor the Author assumes any liability for any injury and/or damage to persons or property arising out of or related to any use of the material contained in this book.

The Publisher

Working together to grow
libraries in developing countries

www.elsevier.com | www.bookaid.org | www.sabre.org

ELSEVIER   BOOK AID International   Sabre Foundation

ELSEVIER   your source for books, journals and multimedia in the health sciences

www.elsevierhealth.com

The publisher's policy is to use paper manufactured from sustainable forests

Printed in China

Contents

Preface

Demand on healthcare professionals to deliver high-quality patient care has never been greater. A multitude of factors impinge on healthcare delivery today, including an aging population, more sophisticated medicines, high patient expectation, health service infrastructure as well as adequate and appropriate staffing levels. In primary care the medical practitioner's role is pivotal in providing this care and they remain the central member of the healthcare team, but demands on their time mean other models of service delivery are being adopted in the UK and in other developed countries that utilise other healthcare professionals.

This is leading to the traditional boundaries of care between doctors, nurses and pharmacists being broken down. In particular, certain medical practitioner responsibilities that were once seen as their sole domain are now being performed by nurses and pharmacists, for example, specialist practice nurses such as asthma and diabetes nurses, and more recently independent prescribing status allowing nurses and pharmacists to prescribe medicines. This change in responsibilities is now firmly established in UK government healthcare policy. Probably of greatest impact to community pharmacy practice is the emphasis placed on self care by Western governments. In the UK, such government strategy is evidenced by the Department of Health having a dedicated website on self care (http://www.dh.gov.uk/en/Policyandguidance/Organisationpolicy/Selfcare/index.htm).

This drive for patients to manage their own health has been facilitated by government making more medicines available over-the-counter. In the UK, between 1983 and 2007, over 80 prescription-only medicines have been reclassified as pharmacy medicines (sold under the supervision of the pharmacist). In recent years, the reclassification of medicines has included products from new therapeutic classes (e.g. anti-emetics, H_2 antagonists and triptans) allowing community pharmacists the scope to manage more conditions.

Further deregulation of medicines to treat acute illness from different therapeutic areas seems likely, especially as more than one in three GP consultations are for minor illnesses and an estimated 20 to 40% of GP time could be saved if patients exercised self care.

Since the first edition of this book, government policy now seems also to embrace chronic disease management as a self-care activity (Supporting people with long-term conditions to self care: A guide to developing local strategies and good practice, 2006). This might then well be the largest area for future growth of reclassification of medicines. The UK, in 2004, was the first country in the world to deregulate simvastatin, and this might well pave the way for further medicines to be available to manage chronic illness.

Pharmacists, now more than ever before, will have to demonstrate that they are competent practitioners to be trusted with this additional responsibility. Therefore, pharmacists will require greater levels of knowledge and understanding about commonly occurring medical conditions. They will need to be able to recognise their signs and symptoms, and use an evidence-based approach to treatment.

This was, and still is, the catalyst for this book. Although other books on diagnosis targeted at pharmacists are published, this book aims to give a more in-depth view of minor conditions and how to differentiate them from more sinister pathology that may present in a similar way. The book is intended for all pharmacists, from undergraduate students to experienced practitioners.

It is hoped that the information contained within the book is both informative and useful.

Paul Rutter

Introduction

Community pharmacists are the most accessible healthcare professionals. In the UK one report suggested that 6 million people a day visit community pharmacies. No appointment is needed to consult a pharmacist and patients can receive free, unbiased advice almost anywhere. On a typical day a pharmacist practising in an 'average' community pharmacy can realistically expect to help between 5 and 15 patients a day who present with various symptoms for which they are seeking advice, reassurance, treatment or a combination of all three. Unlike most other healthcare professionals, community pharmacists do not normally have access to the patient's medical record and thus have no idea about what the person's problem is until a conversation is initiated. This presents the community pharmacist with a great challenge to correctly differentially diagnose the patient.

Communication skills

For the most part, pharmacists will be totally dependent on their ability to question patients in order to arrive at a differential diagnosis. This is in stark contrast to the GP and to a lesser extent the nurse, who can draw on physical examination and diagnostic tests to help them arrive at a diagnosis. Opportunities for pharmacists to perform a physical examination are limited by the lack of privacy within a pharmacy and also a lack of training in correct examination technique; diagnostic testing is never employed because of the costs (which would have to be passed on to the patient) and the invasive nature of most tests (e.g. blood-taking for analysis).

Having said this, a number of studies have shown that in more than three-quarters of all cases taking a patient history alone will result in the correct diagnosis. This figure rises slightly if a history is supplemented with a physical examination and rises still further if laboratory investigations are also conducted.

It is vital, therefore, that pharmacists possess excellent communication skills to ensure the correct information is obtained from the patient. This will be drawn from a combination of good questioning technique, listening actively to the patient and picking up on non-verbal cues.

Approaches to differential diagnosis

Try to avoid using acronyms

Traditionally, the use of acronyms has been advocated to help pharmacists remember what questions to ask a patient. However, it is important that pharmacists do not solely rely on acronyms in trying to differentially diagnose a person's presenting complaint; acronyms are rigid, inflexible and often inappropriate. Every patient is different and therefore it is unlikely that an acronym can be fully applied and, more importantly, using acronyms can mean that vital information is missed, which could shape the course of action. Some of the more commonly used acronyms are discussed briefly below.

WWHAM

This is the simplest acronym to remember but it is also the worst one to use. It gives the pharmacist very limited information from which to work and it is unlikely that a correct differential diagnosis will be made. It should be used with caution, if at all, and is probably only helpful for counter assistants to use when a patient first presents, so that a general picture of the person's presenting complaint can be established.

	Meaning of the letter	Attributes of the acronym
W	Who is the patient?	**Positive points**
W	What are the symptoms?	Establishes presenting complaint
H	How long have the symptoms been present?	
A	Action taken?	**Negative points**
M	Medication being taken?	Fails to consider general appearance of patient. No social/lifestyle factors taken into account; no family history sought; not specific or in-depth enough; no history of previous symptoms

Other acronyms that have been suggested as being helpful for pharmacists in differential diagnosis are ENCORE, ASMETHOD and SIT DOWN SIR. Although, these three acronyms are more comprehensive than WWHAM, they still are limited. No one acronym takes into consideration all the factors that might impinge on the differential diagnosis. All fail to establish a full history from the patient in respect to lifestyle and social factors or the relevance of a family history. They are very much designed to establish the nature and severity of the presenting complaint. This, in many instances, will be adequate, but for intermittent conditions (e.g. irritable bowel syndrome, asthma, hay fever) they might well miss important information. Likewise, positive family history with certain conditions (e.g. psoriasis, eczema) provides useful clues to establish a diagnosis.

	Meaning of the letter	Attributes of the acronym
E	Explore	**Positive points**
N	No medication	'Observe' section suggests taking into account the appearance of the patient – does he or she look poorly?
C	Care	
O	Observe	
R	Refer	
E	Explain	
		Negative points
		Sections on 'No medication' and 'Refer' add little to the differential diagnosis process. No social/lifestyle factors taken into account; no family history sought

	Meaning of letter	Attributes of the acronym
A	Age/appearance?	**Positive points**
S	Self or someone else?	Establishes the nature of problem and if patient has suffered from previous similar episodes
M	Medication?	
E	Extra medicines?	
T	Time persisting?	
H	History?	
O	Other symptoms?	**Negative points**
D	Danger symptoms?	Exact symptoms and severity not fully established. No social/lifestyle factors taken into account; no family history sought

	Meaning of the letter	Attributes of the acronym
S	Site or location?	**Positive points**
I	Intensity or severity?	Establishes the severity and nature of problem and if the patient has suffered from previous similar episodes
T	Type or nature?	
D	Duration?	
O	Onset?	
W	With (other symptoms)?	
N	Annoyed or aggravated?	**Negative points**
S	Spread or radiation?	Fails to consider general appearance of patient. No social/lifestyle factors taken into account; no family history sought
I	Incidence or frequency pattern?	
R	Relieved by?	

Clinical reasoning

Whether we are conscious of it or not, most people will – at some level – use clinical reasoning to arrive at a differential diagnosis. Clinical reasoning relates to the decision-making processes associated with clinical practice. It is a thinking process directed towards enabling the pharmacist to take appropriate action in a specific context. It fundamentally differs from using acronyms in that it is built around clinical knowledge and skills that are applied to the individual patient. It involves recognition of cues and analysis of data. Very early in a clinical encounter, and based on limited information, a pharmacist will arrive at a small number of hypotheses. The pharmacist then sets about testing these hypotheses by asking the patient a series of questions. The answer to each question allows the pharmacist to narrow down the possible diagnosis by either eliminating particular conditions or confirming his or her suspicions of a particular condition. Once the questioning is over, the pharmacist should be in a position to differentially diagnosis the patient's condition.

In addition, clinical experience (pattern recognition) also plays a part in the process. Certain conditions have very characteristic presentations and, once seen, it is a relatively straightforward task to diagnose the next case by recalling the appearance of the rash. Therefore, much of daily practice will consist of seeing new cases that strongly resemble previous encounters.

Key steps in the process

1. Formulating a diagnosis based on the patient and the initial presenting complaint

Before any questions are asked of the patient you should think about the line of questioning you are going to take.

- What is the general appearance of the patient? Does the person look well or poorly? Is the person you are about to talk to the patient or someone acting on the patient's behalf? This will shape your thinking as to the severity of the problem.
- How old is the patient? This is very useful information. Epidemiological studies for a wide range of conditions and disease states have shown that certain age groups will suffer from certain problems. For example, it is very unlikely that a child who presents with cough will have chronic bronchitis but the probability of an elderly person having chronic bronchitis is much higher.
- What sex is the patient? As with age, sex can dramatically alter the chances of suffering from certain conditions. Migraines are five times more common in women than men, yet cluster headache is nine times more common in men than women.
- What is the presenting complaint? Some conditions are much more common than others. Therefore you could form an idea of what condition the patient is likely to be suffering from based on the laws of probability (epidemiology). For example, if a person presents with a headache then you should already know that the most common cause of headache is tension-type headache, followed by migraine and then sinusitis. Other causes of headache are rare but obviously need to be eliminated. Your line of questioning should try to confirm or refute the most likely causes of headache.

2. Asking questions

The questions you ask the patient will be specific to that patient. After establishing who the person is, how poorly he or she is and what the presenting complaint is, a number of targeted questions specific to that patient should be asked. The following scenario will illustrate this point.

A 31-year-old female asks for advice about a headache she has.

What are your initial thoughts? (Formulating a diagnosis based on the patient and the initial presenting complaint.):

- the patient is present
- the patient is female and in her early thirties
- the patient looks and sounds OK

- epidemiology states tension-type headache is most likely but women are more prone to migraine than men.

What line of questioning do you take?
Your main aim is to differentiate between tension-type and migraine headache.

Nature of the pain
Tension headache usually produces a dull ache, as opposed to the throbbing nature of migraine pain:

- Patient's response: dull ache
- Pharmacist's thoughts: suggestive of tension headache

Location of pain
Tension headache is generally bilateral; migraine is normally unilateral

- Patient's response: all over
- Pharmacist's thoughts: suggestive of tension headache

Severity of pain
Tension headache is not usually severe and disabling; migraine can be disabling

- Patient's response: bothersome more than stopping her doing things
- Pharmacist's thoughts: suggestive of tension headache

The answers so far are indicative of tension-type headache. However, further specific questions relating to lifestyle and previous and family history should be asked. It would be expected that there was no family history of migraine and there is probably some trigger factor causing the headache, for example, increased stress due to work or personal pressures. The patient might therefore have had similar headaches in the past.

Finally, even though at this stage you are confident of your differential diagnosis you should still ask a couple of questions to rule out any sinister pathology. Obviously you are expecting the answers from these questions to be negative to support your differential diagnosis. Any questions that invoke the opposite to that expected will require further investigation.

3. Confirm facts

Before making a recommendation to the patient it is always helpful to try and re-cap on the information elicited. This is especially important when you have had to ask a lot of questions. It is well known that short-term working memory is relatively small and that remembering all the pertinent facts is difficult. Summarising the information at this stage will not only help you formulate your final diagnosis but will also allow the patient to add further information or correct you on facts that you have failed to remember correctly.

The way in which one goes about establishing what is wrong with the patient will vary from practitioner to practitioner. However, it is important that whatever method is adopted it must be sufficiently robust enough to be of benefit to the patient. Using a clinical reasoning approach to differential diagnosis allows you to build a fuller picture of the patient's presenting complaint. It is both flexible and specific to each individual, unlike the use of acronyms.

How to use the book

The book is divided into 10 chapters. The first 9 chapters are systems based and structured in the format shown in Fig. 1. The final chapter is product based and has a slightly different format. A list of abbreviations and a glossary are included at the end of the book.

Key features of each chapter

At the beginning of each chapter a short section addressing basic anatomy and history taking specific to that body system is presented. A basic understanding of the anatomical location of major structures is useful when attempting to diagnose/exclude conditions from a patient's presenting complaint. It would be almost impossible to know whether to treat or refer a patient who presented with symptoms suggestive of renal colic if one does not know where the kidneys are. However, this book is not intended to replace an anatomy text and the reader is referred to the lists of further reading for anatomy texts.

Self-assessment questions

Twenty multiple choice questions and at least two case study questions are presented at the end of each chapter. These are designed to test factual recall and applied knowledge. The multiple choice questions are constructed to mimic those set in the pre-registration examination. They start with simple traditional multiple choice questions in which the right answer has to be picked from a series of five possible answers, and work up to more complex, interrelated questions.

The case studies challenge you with 'real-life' situations. All are drawn from practice and have been encountered by practising pharmacists, but have been modified for inclusion in the book.

Elements included under each condition

The same structure has been adopted for every condition. This is intended to help the reader approach differential diagnosis from the position of clinical decision making. To help summarise the information, tables and algorithms are included for many of the conditions.

Arriving at a differential diagnosis

A table summarising the key questions that should be asked for each condition is included. The relevance (i.e. the rationale for asking the question) is given for each question. This will allow pharmacists to determine what questions to ask of every patient to enable a differential diagnosis.

Primer for differential diagnosis

A 'primer for differential diagnosis' is available for a number of conditions covered. This algorithmic approach to differential diagnosis is geared towards nearly or recently qualified pharmacists. They are not intended to be solely relied upon in making a differential diagnosis but to act as an aide memoire. It is anticipated that the primers will be used in conjunction with the text, thus allowing a broader understanding of the differential diagnosis of the condition to be considered.

Trigger points indicative of referral

A summary box of trigger factors when it would be prudent to refer the patient to a medical practitioner is presented for each condition. These trigger factors are not absolute and the pharmacist will have to use their professional judgement on a case-by-case basis. For example, a person with a cough of 3 days' duration might need referral if they are visibly poorly.

Evidence-based OTC medication and Practical prescribing and product selection

These two sections present the reader, first, with an evaluation of the current literature on whether over-the-

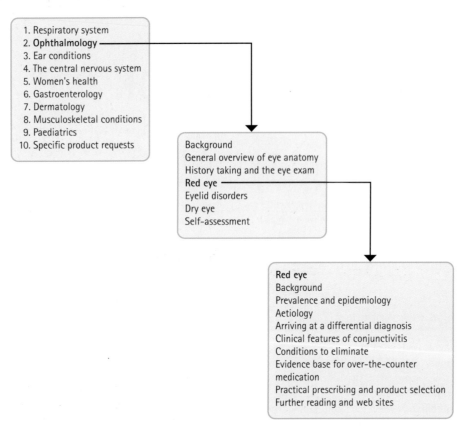

Figure 1 Structure of this book

counter medicine works and, second, with a quick reference to the dose of the medicine and when it cannot be prescribed. This does not replace standard textbooks such as *Martindale* or *Stockley's drug interactions* but it does allow the user to find basic data in one text without having to reach for three or four other texts to answer simple questions.

The pregnancy and breast-feeding recommendations in this book are based largely on those from standard texts such as Briggs' *Drugs in pregnancy and lactation* and Schaefers' *Drugs in pregnancy and lactation*. In addition, the UkMi web site has been used (http://www.ukmicentral.nhs.uk/drugpreg/qrg_p1.asp). Many manufacturers of over-the-counter medicines advise against their products being used in these groups but, where possible, in the summary tables reference is made to the recommendations made from these sources. This hopefully will provide extra information for pharmacists if faced with queries from pregnant and lactating women.

Hints and tips boxes

A summary box of useful information is provided near the end of each condition. This contains information that

does not fall readily into any of the other sections but is nonetheless useful. For example, some of the hints and tips boxes give advice on how to administer eye drops, suppositories and other forms of medicines that are not taken via the oral route.

Further reading and web sites

To supplement the text, at the end of each condition a list of selected references and reading is provided for those that wish to seek further information on the subject. Web sites are also provided, and all sites have been checked and were active and relevant at the time of writing (winter 2007).

Finally, all information presented in the book is accurate and factual as far as the author is aware. It is acknowledged that guidelines change, products become discontinued and new information becomes available over the lifetime of a book. Therefore, if any information in the book is not current or valid, the author would be grateful of any feedback, positive or negative, to ensure that the next edition is as up-to-date as possible.

Respiratory system

Background

Diseases of the respiratory tract are among the most common reasons for consulting a GP. The average GP sees approximately 700 to 1000 patients each year with respiratory disease. Although respiratory disease can cause significant morbidity and mortality, the vast majority of conditions are minor and self-limiting.

A community pharmacist is often the first health professional the patient seeks advice from and, as such, provides a filtering mechanism whereby minor self-limiting conditions can be appropriately treated with the correct medication and patients with more sinister pathology referred on to the GP for further investigation.

General overview of the anatomy of the respiratory tract

The basic requirement for all living cells to function and survive is a continuous supply of oxygen. However, a by-product of cell activity is carbon dioxide, which, if not removed, poisons and kills the cells of the body. The principal function of the respiratory system is therefore the exchange of carbon dioxide and oxygen between blood and atmospheric air. This exchange takes place in the lungs, where pulmonary capillaries are in intimate contact with the linings of the lung's terminal air spaces: the alveoli. All other structures associated with the respiratory tract serve to facilitate this gaseous exchange.

The respiratory tract is divided arbitrarily into the upper and lower respiratory tract. In addition to these structures, the respiratory system also includes the oral cavity, rib cage and diaphragm.

Upper respiratory tract

The upper respiratory tract comprises those structures located outside the thorax: the nasal cavity, pharynx and larynx.

Nasal cavity

The internal portion of the nose is classed as the nasal cavity. The nasal cavity is connected to the pharynx through two openings called the internal nares. Besides receiving olfactory stimuli (smell), the nasal cavity plays an important part in respiration because it filters out large dust particles and warms and moistens incoming air.

Pharynx

The pharynx is divided into three sections:

- nasopharynx, which exchanges air with the nasal cavity and moves particulate matter towards the mouth
- oropharynx and laryngopharynx, which serve as a common passageway for air and food
- laryngopharynx, which connects with the oesophagus and the larynx and, like the oropharynx, serves as a common pathway for the respiratory and digestive systems.

Larynx (voice box)

The larynx is a short passageway that connects the pharynx with the trachea. The glottis and epiglottis are located here and act like 'trap doors' to ensure that liquids and food are routed into the oesophagus and not the trachea.

Lower respiratory tract

The lower respiratory tract is located almost entirely within the thorax and comprises the trachea, bronchial tree and lungs.

Trachea and bronchi

The trachea connects the larynx with the bronchi. The bronchi divide and subdivide into bronchioles and these in turn divide to form terminal bronchioles, which give rise to alveoli where gaseous exchange takes place. The epithelial lining of the bronchial tree acts as a defence mechanism known as the mucociliary escalator. Cilia on the surface of cells beat upwards in organised waves of contraction thus expelling foreign bodies.

Lungs

The lungs are cone shaped and lie in the thoracic cavity. Enclosing and protecting the lungs are the pleural membranes; the inner membrane covers the lungs and the outer membrane is attached to the thoracic cavity. Between the membranes is the pleural cavity, which contains fluid and prevents friction between the membranes during breathing.

History taking and physical exam

Cough, cold, sore throat and rhinitis often coexist and an accurate history is therefore essential to differentially diagnose a patient who presents with symptoms of respiratory disease. A number of similar questions must be asked for each symptom, although symptom-specific questions are also needed (these are discussed under each heading, below). Currently, examination of the respiratory tract is outside the remit of the community pharmacist.

Cough

Background

The main function of coughing is airway clearance. Excess secretions and foreign bodies are cleared from the lungs by a combination of coughing and the mucociliary escalator (upward beating of bronchial cilia that move mucus and entrapped foreign bodies to be expectorated or swallowed). Cough is the most common respiratory symptom and one of the few ways by which abnormalities of the respiratory tract manifest themselves.

Coughs can be described as either productive (chesty) or non-productive (dry, tight, tickly). However, many patients will say that they are not producing sputum, although they go on to say that they 'can feel it on their chest'. In these cases the cough is probably productive in nature and should be treated as such.

Coughs can be either acute or chronic. Recent British Thoracic Society Guidelines (2006) recommend that:

an acute cough lasts less than 3 weeks
chronic cough lasts more than 8 weeks.

The guidelines acknowledge that a 'grey area' exists for those coughs lasting between 3 and 8 weeks as it is difficult to define their aetiological basis because all chronic coughs will have started as an acute cough. For community pharmacy practice this 'grey area' is rather academic, as any cough lasting longer than the accepted definition of acute should be referred to a medical practitioner for further investigation.

Prevalence and epidemiology

Statistics from general medical practice show that respiratory illness accounts for more GP visits than any other disease category. Acute cough is usually caused by a viral upper respiratory tract infection (URTI) and constitutes 20% of consultations. This translates to 12 million GP visits per year and represents the largest single cause of primary care consultation. In community pharmacy the figures are even higher with at least 24 million visits per year (or 2000 visits per pharmacy per year).

Young children (0 to 4 years) are four times more likely to experience an URTI than adults, and women aged 16 to 64 years are twice as likely to consult a GP than men. Acute viral URTIs exhibit seasonality, with higher incidence seen in the winter months.

Aetiology

A five-part cough reflex is responsible for cough production. Receptors located mainly in the pharynx, larynx, trachea and bifurcations of the large bronchi are stimulated via mechanical, irritant or thermal mechanisms. Neural impulses are then carried along afferent pathways of the vagal and superior laryngeal nerves, which terminate at the cough centre in the medulla. Efferent fibres of the vagus and spinal nerves carry neural activity to the muscles of the diaphragm, chest wall and abdomen. These muscles contract, followed by the sudden opening of the glottis that creates the cough.

Arriving at a differential diagnosis

The most common cause of acute cough is viral URTI in all ages. Recurrent viral bronchitis is most prevalent in preschool and young school-aged children and is the most common cause of persistent cough in children of all ages. Other causes of acute cough include allergies, bronchitis, croup and postnasal drip. It is the pharmacist's responsibility to differentiate other causes of cough from viral causes and also refer those cases of cough that might have more serious pathology. Asking symptom-specific questions will help the pharmacist to determine if referral is needed (Table 1.1).

Clinical features of acute viral cough

Viral coughs typically present with sudden onset and associated fever. Sputum production is minimal and symptoms are often worse in the evening. Associated cold symptoms are also often present; these usually last between 7 and 10 days. Duration of longer than 14 days might suggest 'postviral cough' or possibly indi-cate a bacterial secondary infection but this is clinically difficult to establish without sputum samples being analysed.

Conditions to eliminate

Acute cough

Laryngotracheobronchitis (croup)

Symptoms are triggered by a recent viral infection, with parainfluenza virus being the most commonly identified, although other viral pathogens implicated include the rhinovirus and respiratory syncytial virus. It affects infants aged between 3 months and 6 years old and affects 2 to 6% of children. The incidence is highest between 1 and 2 years of age and it occurs in boys more than girls; it is more common in autumn and winter months. It often follows on from an URTI and occurs in

Table 1.1	Specific questions to ask the patient: Cough
Question	**Relevance**
Sputum colour	• Mucoid (clear and white) is normally of little consequence and suggests that no infection is present • Yellow, green or brown sputum normally indicates infection. However, mucopurulent sputum is probably caused by a viral infection and does not require automatic referral • Haemoptysis can either be rust coloured (pneumonia), pink tinged (left ventricular failure) or dark red (carcinoma). Occasionally, patients can produce sputum with bright red blood as one-off events. This is due to the force of coughing causing a blood vessel to rupture. This is non-serious and does not require automatic referral
Nature of sputum	• Thin and frothy suggests left ventricular failure • Thick, mucoid to yellow can suggest asthma • Offensive foul-smelling sputum suggests either bronchiectasis or lung abscess
Onset of cough	• A cough that is worse in the morning may suggest postnasal drip, bronchiectasis or chronic bronchitis

Duration of cough	• URTI cough can linger for more than 3 weeks and is termed 'postviral cough'. However, coughs lasting longer than 3 weeks should be viewed with caution as the longer the cough is present the more likely serious pathology is responsible; for example, the most likely diagnoses of cough are as follows:
	  • at 3 days duration will be an URTI;
	  • at 3 weeks duration will be acute or chronic bronchitis;
	  • and at 3 months duration conditions such as chronic bronchitis, tuberculosis and carcinoma become more likely

Periodicity	• Adult patients with recurrent cough might have chronic bronchitis, especially if they smoke • Care should be exercised in children who present with recurrent cough and have a family history of eczema, asthma or hay fever. This might suggest asthma and referral would be required for further investigation
Age of the patient	• Children will most likely be suffering from an URTI but asthma and croup should be considered • With increasing age, conditions such as bronchitis, pneumonia and carcinoma become more prevalent
Smoking history	• Patients who smoke are more prone to chronic and recurrent cough. Over time this might develop into chronic bronchitis and emphysema

the late evening and night. The cough can be severe and violent and described as having a barking (seal-like) quality. In between coughing episodes the child may be breathless and struggle to breathe properly. Typically symptoms improve during the day and often recur again the following night, with the majority of children seeing symptoms resolve in 48 hours. Warm moist air as a treatment for croup has been used since the 19th century and is still advocated by some review articles for home treatment (Knutson 2004). This is either done by moving the child to a bathroom and running a hot bath or shower or by boiling a kettle in the room. Croup management is based on an assessment of severity. Advice by pharmacists should be that the parents manage only mild croup and any symptoms of stridor indicate that medical intervention is required. Standard treatment for those children with stridor is oral or intramuscular steroids (dexamethasone). A review in the Drug and Therapeutics Bulletin (2000) suggested GPs should give corticosteroids to all children with croup before referral to hospital.

Postnasal drip

Postnasal drip is characterised by a sinus or nasal discharge that flows behind the nose and into the throat. Patients should be asked if they are swallowing mucus or notice that they are clearing their throat more than usual, as these features are commonly seen in patients with postnasal drip.

Allergy-related cough

Coughs caused by allergies are often non-productive and worse at night. However, there are usually other associated symptoms, such as sneezing, nasal discharge/blockage, conjunctivitis and itching oral cavity. Cough of allergic origin may show seasonal variation, for example, hay fever.

Acute bronchitis

Most cases are seen in autumn or winter and symptoms are similar to viral URTI but patients also tend to exhibit dyspnoea and wheeze. Infection is believed to trigger acute bronchitis but this is not conclusive. Antibiotics are often prescribed but there is debate as to their effectiveness in clinical improvement.

Chronic cough

Chronic bronchitis

Chronic bronchitis (CB) is the most common cause of chronic cough in adults. Patients often present with a longstanding history of recurrent acute bronchitis in which episodes become increasingly severe and persist for increasing duration until the cough becomes continual. CB has been defined as coughing up sputum on most days for three or more consecutive months over the previous 2 years. CB is caused by chronic irritation of the airways by inhaled substances, especially tobacco smoke.

A history of smoking is the single most important factor in the aetiology of CB. In non-smokers the likely cause of CB is postnasal drip, asthma or gastro-oesophageal reflux. One study has shown that 99% of non-smokers with CB and a normal chest X-ray suffered from one of these three conditions.

CB starts with a non-productive cough that later becomes a mucopurulent productive cough. The patient should be questioned about smoking habits. If the patient is a smoker the cough will usually be worse in the morning. Secondary infections contribute to acute exacerbations seen in CB. It typically occurs in patients over the age of 40 and is more common in men. Pharmacists have an important role to play in identifying smokers with CB as this provides an excellent opportunity for health promotion advice and assessing the patient's willingness to stop smoking.

Asthma

The exact prevalence of asthma is unknown due to differing terminologies and definitions plus difficulties in correct diagnosis, especially in children, and comorbidity with chronic obstructive pulmonary disease (COPD) in the elderly. Best estimate of asthma prevalence in adults is approximately 4%, but it may be up to 10%. In children the figures are higher (10 to 15%) because a proportion of children will 'grow out' of it and be symptom-free by adulthood.

Asthma is a chronic inflammatory condition of the airways characterised by coughing, wheeze, chest tightness and shortness of breath. Classically these symptoms tend to be variable, intermittent, worse at night and provoked by triggers. In addition, possible associated features are family or personal history of atopy and worsening symptoms after taking non-steroidal anti-inflammatories (NSAIDs) or beta-blockers. However, asthma can present solely as a non-productive cough, especially in young children where the cough is often worst at night. Diagnosis should be made by a combination of a medical history, symptoms and lung function tests (e.g. using peak expiratory flow)

Pneumonia (community acquired)

Bacterial infection is usually responsible for pneumonia and most commonly caused by *Streptococcus pneumoniae* (80% of cases), although other pathogens are also responsible, e.g. *Chlamydia* and *Mycoplasma*. Initially, the cough is non-productive and painful (first 24 to 48 hours), but rapidly becomes productive, with sputum being stained red. The intensity of the redness varies depending on the causative organism. The cough tends to be worst at night. The patient will be unwell, with a high fever, malaise, headache, breathlessness and experience pleuritic pain (inflammation of pleural membranes, manifested as pain to the sides) that worsens on inspiration. Clinical findings alone are not enough for an accurate diagnosis and a chest X-ray is required.

Rare causes of chronic cough

Cough is a symptom of many other conditions, although the majority will be rarely encountered in community pharmacy. However, it is important to be aware of these rare causes of cough to ensure that appropriate referrals are made.

Productive coughs

Heart failure

Heart failure is a condition of the elderly. The prevalence of heart failure rises with increasing age; 3 to 5% of people aged over 65 are affected and this increases to approximately 10% of patients aged 80 and over. Heart failure is characterised by insidious progression and diagnosing early mild heart failure is extremely difficult because symptoms are not pronounced. Often, the first symptoms patients experience are shortness of breath, orthopnoea and dyspnoea at night. As the condition progresses from mild/moderate to severe heart failure patients might complain of a productive, frothy cough, which may have pink-tinged sputum.

Bronchiectasis

Bronchiectasis is caused by irreversible dilation of the bronchi. Characteristically, the patient has a chronic cough of very long duration, which produces copious amounts of mucopurulent sputum (green-yellow in colour) that is usually foul smelling. The cough tends to be worse in the morning and evening. In longstanding cases the sputum is said to display characteristic layering with the top being frothy, the middle clear and the bottom dense with purulent particles.

Tuberculosis

Tuberculosis (TB) is a bacterial infection caused by *Mycobacterium tuberculosis* and is transmitted primarily by inhalation. After many decades of decline, the number of new TB cases occurring in industrialised countries is now starting to increase. In 2006, UK figures showed that over 8000 cases were notified – an increase of 2% on the previous year. The incidence is higher in inner city areas, among the elderly and immigrants from developing countries. TB is characterised by its slow onset and initial mild symptoms. The cough is chronic in nature and sputum production can vary from mild to severe with associated haemoptysis. Other symptoms of the condition are malaise, fever, night sweats and weight loss. However, not all patients will experience all symptoms. A patient with a productive cough for more than 3 weeks and exhibiting one or more of the associated symptoms should be referred for further investigation, especially if they fall into one of the groups listed above. Chest X-rays and sputum smear tests can be performed to confirm the diagnosis.

Carcinoma of the lung

A number of studies have shown that between 20 and 90% of patients will develop a cough at some point during the progression of carcinoma of the lung. The possibility of carcinoma increases in long-term cigarette smokers who have had a cough for a number of months or who develop a marked change in the character of their cough. The cough produces small amounts of sputum that might be blood-streaked. Other symptoms that can be associated with the cough are dyspnoea, weight loss and fatigue.

Nocardiasis

Nocardiasis is an extremely rare bacterial infection caused by *Nocardia asteroides*; it is transmitted primarily by inhalation. It is very unlikely a pharmacist will ever encounter this condition and it is included in this text only for the sake of completeness. It has a higher incidence in the elderly population, especially men. The sputum is purulent, thick and possibly blood tinged. Fever is prominent and night sweats, pleurisy, weight loss and fatigue might also be present.

Non-productive coughs

Gastro-oesophageal reflux disease

Gastro-oesophageal reflux disease (GORD) does not usually present with cough but patients with this condition might cough when recumbent (lying down). The patient might show symptoms of reflux or heartburn. Patients with GORD have increased cough reflex sensitivity and respond well to proton pump inhibitors. It should always be considered in all cases of unexplained cough.

Lung abscess

A typical presentation is of a non-productive cough with pleuritic pain and dyspnoea. It is more common in the elderly. Signs of infection such as malaise and fever can also be present. Later the cough produces large amounts of purulent and often foul-smelling sputum.

Medicine-induced cough or wheeze

A number of medicines may cause bronchoconstriction, which presents as cough or wheeze. Angiotensin converting enzyme (ACE) inhibitors are most commonly associated with cough. Incidence might be as high as 16%; it is not dose-related and time to onset is variable, ranging from a few hours to more than 1 year after the start of treatment. Cough invariably ceases after withdrawal of the ACE inhibitor but takes 3 to 4 weeks to resolve. Other medicines that are associated with cough or wheeze are NSAIDs and beta-blockers. If an adverse drug reaction (ADR) is suspected then the pharmacist should discuss alternative medication with the prescriber, for example, almost all patients with ACE inhibitor cough can tolerate angiotensin II receptor blockers.

Spontaneous pneumothorax (collapsed lung)

Rupture of the bullae (the small air or fluid-filled sacs in the lung) can cause spontaneous pneumothorax but normally there is no underlying cause. It affects approximately 1 in 10 000 people, usually tall, thin men between 20 and 40 years old. Cigarette smoking and a family history of pneumothorax are contributing risk factors. This can be a life-threatening disorder causing a non-productive cough and severe respiratory distress. The patient experiences sudden sharp unilateral chest pain that worsens on inspiration. The symptoms often begin suddenly, and can occur during rest or sleep.

Figure 1.1 will aid the differentiation between serious and non-serious conditions of cough in adults.

 TRIGGER POINTS indicative of referral: Cough

- Chest pain
- Cough that recurs on a regular basis
- Debilitating symptoms in the elderly
- Duration longer than 3 weeks
- Haemoptysis
- Pain on inspiration
- Persistent nocturnal cough in children
- Wheeze and/or shortness of breath

Evidence base for over-the-counter medication

Cough is often trivialised by practitioners but coughing can impair quality of life and cause anxiety to parents of children with cough. Patients who exercise self-care will be confronted with a plethora of over-the-counter (OTC) medication and many will find the choice overwhelming. The pharmacist must ensure that the most appropriate medication is selected for the patient, but this must be done on an evidence-based approach.

All the active ingredients to treat cough were brought to the market many years ago when clinical trials suffered from flaws in study design compared to today's standards, thus clinical efficacy is therefore difficult to establish.

Expectorants

A number of active ingredients have been formulated to help expectoration, including guaifenesin, ammonium salts, ipecacuanha, creosote and squill. The majority of products marketed in the UK for productive cough contain guaifenesin, although products containing squill (Buttercup syrup), ipecacuanha (Galloway's cough syrup) and ammonium salts (Histalix syrup) are available. The clinical evidence available for any active ingredient is limited. Older ingredients such as ammonium salts, ipecacuanha and squill were traditionally used to induce vomiting as

it was believed that at subemetic doses they would cause gastric irritation, triggering reflex expectoration. This has never been proven and belongs in the annals of folklore. Guaifenesin is thought to stimulate secretion or respiratory tract fluid, increasing sputum volume and decreasing viscosity so assisting in removal of sputum. Guaifenesin is the only active ingredient that has any evidence of effectiveness. Two studies identified by Schroeder & Fahey (Cochrane Review 2004) found conflicting results for guaifenesin as an expectorant. In the largest study (n = 239), participants stated guaifenesin significantly reduced cough frequency and intensity compared to placebo. In the smaller trial (n = 65), guaifenesin was stated to have an antitussive not expectorant effect.

Summary

Based on studies, guaifenesin is the only expectorant with any evidence of effectiveness. However, trial results are not convincing and guaifenesin is probably little or no better than placebo. Given its proven safety record, placebo properties and the public's desire to treat productive coughs with a home remedy it would seem reasonable to supply OTC cough medicines containing guaifenesin.

Cough suppressants (antitussives)

Cough suppressants act directly on the cough centre to depress the cough reflex. Their effectiveness has been investigated in patients with acute and chronic cough as well as citric acid-induced cough. Although trials on healthy volunteers – in whom coughing was induced by citric acid – allowed reproducible conditions to assess the activity of antitussives, they are of little value because they do not represent physiological cough. Of greatest interest to OTC medication are trials investigating acute cough, because patients suffering from chronic cough should be referred to the GP.

Codeine

Codeine is generally accepted as a standard or benchmark antitussive against which all others are judged. A review by Eddy et al showed codeine to be an effective antitussive in animal models, and cough-induced studies in humans have also shown codeine to be effective. However, these findings appear to be less reproducible in acute and pathological chronic cough. More recent studies have failed to demonstrate a significant clinical effect of codeine compared with placebo in patients suffering with acute cough. Greater voluntary control of the cough reflex by patients has been suggested for the apparent lack of effect codeine has on acute cough.

Pholcodine

Pholcodine, like codeine, has been subject to limited clinical trials, with the majority being either animal

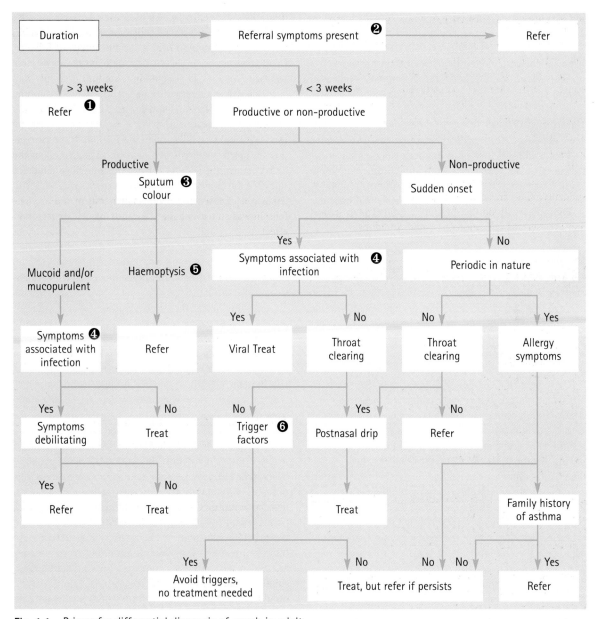

Fig. 1.1 Primer for differential diagnosis of cough in adult

❶ Duration of cough
Coughs lasting longer than 3 weeks are considered chronic in nature. Most acute, self-limiting coughs usually resolve within 3 weeks; conditions with sinister pathology are more likely the longer the cough has been present. However, not all coughs that have lasted 3 weeks have to be referred automatically. Postnasal drip and seasonal allergies (e.g. hay fever) can persist for weeks and be managed by community pharmacists.

❷ Referral symptoms
Certain symptoms warrant direct referral to the GP or even casualty. For example, shortness of breath, breathlessness (possible asthma), chest pain (possible cardiovascular cause) or pain on inspiration (pleurisy or pneumothorax).

❸ Sputum colour
Sputum colour can be helpful in deciding when to refer. However, there is a common misconception that patients who present with green-yellow or brown sputum have a bacterial infection; this is

not normally the case. If the cough has persisted for more than 7 to 10 days it is possible that an initial viral infection has become secondarily infected with a bacterial infection. This could indicate referral, especially if the symptoms are debilitating or if the patient is elderly.

❹ Symptoms associated with infection
The patient might have associated symptoms of fever, rhinorrhoea and sore throat.

❺ Haemoptysis
Blood in the sputum requires further investigation, especially if the person has had the symptoms for a period of time.

❻ Trigger factors
Certain atmospheric factors can trigger cough. These factors include air temperature changes, pollution (e.g. cigarette smoke) and dry atmospheres (e.g. air conditioning).

models or citric acid-induced cough studies in man. These studies have shown pholcodine to have antitussive activity. A review by Findlay (1988) concluded that, on balance, pholcodine appears to possess antitussive activity but advocates the need for better, well-controlled studies.

Dextromethorphan

Trial data for dextromethorphan, like that for codeine and pholcodine, is limited. It has been shown to be effective in citric acid-induced cough and chronic cough but studies assessing the efficacy of dextromethorphan in acute cough have shown it to be no better than placebo. It appears to have limited abuse potential and fewer side effects than codeine.

Antihistamines

Antihistamines have been included in cough remedies for decades. Their mechanism of action is thought to be through the anticholinergic-like drying action on the mucous membranes and not via histamine. There are numerous clinical trials involving antihistamines for the relief of cough and cold symptoms, most notably with diphenhydramine.

Citric acid-induced cough studies have demonstrated significant antitussive activity compared to placebo and results from chronic cough trials support an antitussive activity for diphenhydramine. However, trials that showed a significant reduction in cough frequency suffered from having small patient numbers, thus limiting their usefulness. Additionally, poor methodological design of trials investigating the antitussive activity of diphenhydramine in acute cough makes assessment of its effectiveness difficult. It is now generally accepted that diphenhydramine is ineffective when compared to placebo for treatment of acute cough resulting from an URTI.

Trials using non-sedating antihistamines (e.g. terfenadine – now discontinued) have also failed to demonstrate greater effectiveness than placebo.

Demulcents

Demulcents, such as simple linctus, are pharmacologically inert and are used on the theoretical basis that they reduce irritation by coating the pharynx and so prevent coughing. There is no evidence for their efficacy and they are used mainly for their placebo effect. They are a suitable recommendation for very young children who cannot take other cough suppressants.

Summary

Antitussives have been traditionally evaluated for efficacy in animal studies or cough-induced models on healthy volunteers. This presents serious problems in assessing their effectiveness because support for their antitussive activity does not come from patients with acute cough associated with URTI. Furthermore, there appear to be no comparative studies of sound design to allow judgements to be made on their comparable efficacy. Compounding these problems is the self-limiting nature of acute cough, which further hinders differentiation between clinical efficacy and normal symptom resolution.

Antitussives therefore probably have a limited role in the treatment of acute non-productive cough. Patients should be encouraged to drink more fluid and told that their symptoms will resolve in time on their own. If medication is required then any active ingredient could be recommended; side effect profile and abuse tendency rather than clinical efficacy will drive choice. On this basis, pholcodine and dextromethorphan would be first-line therapy and codeine, because of its greater side effect profile and tendency to be abused, should be reserved for second-line treatment. Antihistamines should not be used routinely, unless night-time sedation is perceived as an additional benefit to help the patient sleep.

Cough medication for children

Very few well-designed studies have been conducted in children. A review published in the Drug and Therapeutics Bulletin identified just five trials of sound methodological design. However, of these five trials, one study used illogical drug combinations (expectorant combined with suppressant) and a further three studies used combination products not available on the UK market. This left one study, involving Dimotapp elixir, that could be evaluated. The results from this study showed no significant differences between the active ingredients, placebo or no medication. It therefore appears, from the limited data available, that cough medication for children is no better than placebo. However, many parents will insist on treatment for their children and in such cases, as long as no contraindications are present, supplying a suitable 'theoretical' cough medication would not be unjustified as adverse events from cough medication are rare.

The latest Cochrane Review (Schroeder & Fahey 2004) looking at OTC medicines for acute cough in children and adults concluded that there was no good evidence for or against the effectiveness of OTC medicines in acute cough. In addition, a report published in *Respiratory Physiology and Neurobiology* (Eccles 2005) proposes that the sweet taste of cough medicines as well as their placebo effect accounts for any activity they might have.

Practical prescribing and product selection

Prescribing information relating to the cough medicines reviewed in the section 'Evidence base for over-the-counter medication' is discussed and summarised in Table 1.2; useful tips relating to patients presenting with cough are given in Hints and Tips Box 1.1.

Table 1.2
Practical prescribing: Summary of cough medicines

Name of medicine	Use in children	Likely side effects	Drug interactions of note	Patients in whom care should be exercised	Pregnancy and breast-feeding
Cough expectorants					
Guaifenesin	>1 year	None	None	None	OK
Cough suppressants*					
Codeine	>1 year	Sedation, constipation	Increased sedation with alcohol, opioid analgesics, anxiolytics, hypnotics and antidepressants	Asthmatics	Best avoided in 3rd trimester
Pholcodine	>1 year	Possible sedation			Short periods OK in breast-feeding
Dextromethorphan	>1 year				
Antihistamines					
Chlorphenamine	>1 years	Dry mouth, sedation and constipation	Increased sedation with alcohol, opioid analgesics, anxiolytics, hypnotics and antidepressants	Glaucoma, prostate enlargement	Standard references state OK, although some manufacturers advise avoidance
Diphenhydramine	>6 years**				
Promethazine	>1 year***				
Triprolidine	>1 year				
Demulcents					
Simple linctus	>3 months, (paediatric version)	None	None	None	OK

*Cough suppressants generally not recommended in children (BNF guidance), but some product licences of OTC medicines do allow them to be given to children.
**Most products licensed for children over 6 years, however Benylin Children's Night Coughs has a product licence stating it can be given from 1 year upwards.
***Normally not recommended under 2 years of age, however Tixylix Night Cough has a product licence stating it can be given from 1 year upwards.

HINTS AND TIPS BOX 1.1: COUGH

Insulin-dependent diabetics	People with insulin-dependent diabetes should be asked to monitor their blood glucose more frequently because insulin requirements increase during acute infections
Avoid theophylline	Theophylline is available in OTC products but it is best avoided because patients requiring medication to help with shortness of breath or wheeze are best referred
Alternative delivery routes	Dextromethorphan is available as a lozenge (Robitussin Soft Pastilles for Dry Coughs). This is a useful alternative for those patients who find carrying a bottle of liquid around with them difficult
Avoid illogical combinations	Very few cough remedies now have illogical medicine combinations. However, there are still a few on the market and these are best avoided. For example, combinations of expectorants and suppressants (e.g. Pulmo Bailey) and expectorant antihistamine combinations (e.g. Histalix)

Cough expectorants

Guaifenesin

A number of manufacturers include guaifenesin in their cough product ranges, including Benylin, Robitussin and Vicks. It can be given to children over 1 year old (e.g. Robitussin for Chesty Coughs and Benylin Children's Chesty Coughs – 50 mg (5 mL) four times a day); children aged between 6 and 12 years should take 100 mg four times a day and the dose for adults, if it is going to work, must be 200 mg four times a day. Some products deliver suboptimal doses or the quantity taken in a single dose would be so large that the product only lasts 1 or 2 days. It is therefore advisable to always check the label of any branded guaifenesin product before recommendation to ensure the patient is receiving appropriate treatment. Guaifenesin-based products have no cautions in their use and no side effects; they are also free from clinically significant drug interactions so can be given safely with prescribed medication. Sugar-free versions (e.g. Robitussin range) are available.

Cough suppressants (codeine, pholcodine, dextromethorphan)

Codeine, pholcodine and dextromethorphan are all opiate derivatives and therefore – broadly – have the same interactions, cautions in use and side effect profile. They do interact with prescription-only medications (POMs) and also with OTC medications, especially those that cross the blood–brain barrier. Their combined effect is to potentiate sedation and it is important to warn the patient of this, although short-term use of cough suppressants with the interacting medication is unlikely to warrant dosage modification. Care should be exercised when giving cough suppressants to asthmatics because, in theory, they can cause respiratory depression. However, in practice this is very rarely observed and does not preclude the use of cough suppressants in asthmatic patients. However, other side effects can occur (e.g. constipation), especially with codeine. If a cough suppressant is unsuitable, for example in late pregnancy and children, then a demulcent can be offered.

Codeine

Children from 1 year upwards can be treated (e.g. codeine linctus paediatric BP, 5 mL (3 mg) three or four times a day) although codeine is generally not recommended for children. The maximum dose should not exceed 5 mL because doses higher than this change the legal status of codeine to a POM. Codeine is still available in a number of proprietary brands but the majority of pharmacies restrict sales due to the abuse potential of codeine. Sugar-free versions (e.g. Galen range) are available.

Pholcodine

Pholcodine can also be given for children aged over 1 year old (e.g. Tixylix Dry Cough, 2.5 mL (2 mg) four times a day or Benylin Childen's Dry Cough, 5 ml (2 mg) three times a day) but, like codeine, treatment in children is generally not recommended and most marketed products recommend it should not be used under the age of 6 years. The adult dose is 5 to 10 mL (5 to 10 mg) three or four times a day, and half the adult dose is suitable for children. Sugar-free versions (e.g. Pavacol-D) are available.

Dextromethorphan

Dextromethorphan can also be given in children over the age of 6 years. The dose is 5 mL (7.5 mg) four times a day (e.g. Covonia Original Bronchial Balsam and Benylin Dry Cough Non-drowsy), and is doubled in adults and children over 6 years (10 mL (15 mg) four times a day).

Antihistamines

Routine use of antihistamines is unjustified in treating non-productive cough. However, the sedative side effects from antihistamines can, on occasion, be useful to allow the patient an uninterrupted night's sleep.

All antihistamines included in cough remedies are first-generation antihistamines and associated with sedation. They interact with other sedating medication, resulting in potentiation of the sedative properties of the interacting medicines. They also possess antimuscarinic side effects, which commonly result in dry mouth and possibly constipation. It is these antimuscarinic properties that mean patients with glaucoma and prostate enlargement should ideally avoid their use, because it could lead to increased intraocular pressure and precipitation of urinary retention.

Demulcents

Demulcents, for example simple linctus, provide a safe alternative for at-risk patient groups such as the elderly, pregnant women, young children and those taking multiple medication. They can act as useful placebos when the patient insists on a cough mixture and will not take no for an answer. If recommended they should be given three or four times a day.

Further reading

Anon. Corticosteroids for croup. Drug Ther Bull 2000;38:22–4.

Anon. Cough medications in children. Drug Ther Bull 1999;37:19–21.

Eccles R. Respiratory Physiology and Neurobiology, 2005. Online first doi:10.1016/j.resp.2005.10.004.

Eddy NB, Friebel H, Hahn KJ, et al. Codeine and its alternatives for pain and cough relief. Geneva: World Health Organisation; 1970:1–253.

Findlay JWA. Review articles: pholcodine. J Clin Pharmacol Ther 1988;13:5–17.

Knutson D, Aring A. Viral croup. Am Fam Physician 2004;69:535–40, 541–2.

Morice AH, McGarvey L, Pavord I. Recommendations for the management of cough in adults. Thorax 2006;61:S1–24.

Schroeder K, Fahey T. Over-the-counter medications for acute cough in children and adults in ambulatory settings. Cochrane Database of Systematic Reviews 2004, issue 4.

Web sites

British Lung Foundation: http://www.lunguk.org

National Asthma Campaign: http://www.asthma.org.uk

Action on Smoking and Health (ASH): http://www.newash. org.uk/ash_home.htm

British Thoracic Society: http://www.brit-thoracic.org.uk

Guidance from NICE on tuberculosis: http://www.nice.org.uk/ pdf/cg033niceguideline.pdf

Health Protection Agency (Tuberculosis): http://www.hpa.org. uk/infections/topics_az/tb/menu.htm

The common cold

Background

Colds, along with coughs, represent the largest caseload for primary healthcare workers. Because the condition has no specific cure and is self-limiting with two-thirds of sufferers recovering within a week, it would be easy to dismiss the condition as unimportant. However, because of the very high number of cases seen it is essential that pharmacists have a thorough understanding of the condition so that severe symptoms or symptoms suggestive of influenza are identified.

Prevalence and epidemiology

The common cold is extremely prevalent and like cough is caused by viral upper respiratory tract infection. Children contract colds more frequently than adults with on average five to six colds per year compared to two to four colds in adults, although in children this can be as high as 12 colds per year. Children aged between 4 and 8 years are most likely to contract a cold and it can appear to a child's parents that one cold follows another with no respite. By the age of 10 the number of colds contracted is half that observed in preschool children. In the UK, colds peak in December and January.

Aetiology

A number of different virus types can produce symptoms of the common cold, including rhinoviruses (accounting for 30 to 50% of all cases), coronaviruses, parainfluenza virus, respiratory syncytial virus and adenovirus. Transmission is primarily by the virus coming into contact with the hands (direct contact transmission). Droplets shed from the nose coat surfaces such as door handles and telephones. Cold viruses can remain viable on these surfaces for several hours and when an uninfected person touches the contaminated surface transmission occurs. Transmission by coughing and sneezing infected mucous particles does occur, although it is a secondary mechanism.

The virus then invades the nasal and bronchial epithelia, attaching to specific receptors and causing damage to the ciliated cells. This results in the release of inflammatory mediators, which in turn leads to inflammation of the tissues lining the nose. Permeability of capillary cell walls increases, resulting in oedema, which is experienced by the patient as nasal congestion and sneezing. Fluid might drip down the back of the throat, spreading the virus to the throat and upper chest causing cough and sore throat.

Arriving at a differential diagnosis

It is extremely likely that someone presenting with cold symptoms will have a viral infection. Most people will accurately self-diagnose a common cold and it is the pharmacist's role to confirm this self-diagnosis and assess the severity of the symptoms as some patients, for example the elderly, infirm and those with existing medical conditions, might need greater support and care. In the first instance, the pharmacist should make an overall assessment of the person's general state of health. Anyone with debilitating symptoms that effectively prevents him or her from doing their normal day-to-day routine should be managed more carefully. While it is likely that a patient will have a common cold, severe colds can mimic the symptoms of flu, which is the main condition of any real significance that has to be eliminated before treatment can be given. Asking symptom-specific questions will help the pharmacist to determine if referral is needed (Table 1.3).

Clinical features of the common cold

Symptoms of the common cold are well known. However, the nature and severity of symptoms will be influenced by factors such as the causative agent, patient age and underlying medical conditions. Following an incubation period of between 1 and 3 days, the patient develops a sore throat and sneezing, followed by profuse nasal discharge and congestion. Cough and postnasal drip commonly follow. In addition, headache, mild to moderate fever (< 102°F, 38.9°C) and general malaise might be present. Most colds resolve in 1 week, but up to a quarter of people will have symptoms lasting 14 days or more.

Table 1.3
**Specific questions to ask the patient:
The common cold**

Question	Relevance
Onset of symptoms	• Peak incidence of flu is in the winter months; the common cold occurs any time throughout the year • Flu symptoms tend to have a more abrupt onset than the common cold – a matter of hours rather than 1 or 2 days • Summer colds are common but they must be differentiated from seasonal allergic rhinitis (hay fever)
Nature of symptoms	• Marked myalgia, chills and malaise are more prominent in flu than the common cold. Loss of appetite is also common with flu
Aggravating factors	• Headache/pain that is worsened by sneezing, coughing and bending over suggests sinus complications. If ear pain is present, especially in children, middle ear involvement is likely

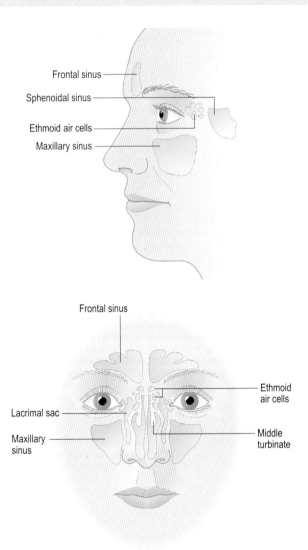

Fig. 1.2 Location of the sinuses

Conditions to eliminate

Influenza

Patients often use the word 'flu' when describing a common cold. However, subtle differences in symptoms between the two conditions should allow differentiation. It is helpful to remember that the 'flu' season tends to be between December and March, whereas the common cold, although more common in winter months, can occur at any time. The onset of influenza is sudden and the typical symptoms are shivering, chills, malaise, marked aching of limbs, insomnia, a non-productive cough (cough in the common cold is usually productive) and loss of appetite. Influenza is therefore normally debilitating and a person with flu is much more likely to send a third party to the pharmacy for medication than present in person.

Rhinitis

A blocked or stuffy nose, whether acute or chronic in nature, is a common complaint. Rhinitis is covered in more detail on page 22 and the reader is referred to this section for differential diagnosis of rhinitis from the common cold.

Acute sinusitis

Sinusitis, now termed rhinosinusitis, is inflammation of one or more of the paranasal sinuses. Up to 2% of patients will develop acute sinusitis as a complication of the common cold. Anatomically the sinuses are described in four pairs: frontal, ethmoid, maxillary and sphenoid (Fig. 1.2). All are air-filled spaces that drain into the nasal cavity. Following a cold, sinus air spaces can become filled with nasal secretions, which stagnate because of a reduction in ciliary function of the cells lining the sinuses. Bacteria – commonly *Streptococcus* and *Haemophilus* – can then secondarily infect these stagnant secretions. It is clinically defined by at least two of the following symptoms: blockage or congestion; discharge or postnasal drip; facial pain or pressure; reduction or loss of smell. The pain in the early stages tends to be relatively mild and localised, usually unilateral and dull but becomes bilateral and more severe the longer the condition persists. Bending forwards often exacerbates the pain (moving the eyes from side to side, coughing or sneezing can also increase the pain) and sinuses will be tender when gently palpated. If the ethmoid sinuses are involved, retro-orbital pain (behind the eye) is often experienced. A loss of smell is also common. Guidelines to help with diagnosis do exist, for example, at http://www.prodigy.nhs.uk/sinusitis. Analgesics for pain relief and oral or nasal sympathomimetics can be tried, to remove the nasal secretions, but if this fails then referral is needed because antibiotic therapy (amoxicillin or cefaclor – if penicillin allergy) might be needed.

Acute otitis media

This is commonly seen in children following a common cold and results from the virus spreading to the middle ear via the eustachian tube – an accumulation of pus within the middle ear or inflammation of the tympanic membrane (eardrum) results. The overriding symptom is ear pain but the child may rub or tug at the ear and be more irritable. Referral to the GP would be appropriate for auroscopical examination, unless the pharmacist is competent to perform this procedure. Examination reveals a bulging tympanic membrane, loss of normal landmarks and a change in colour (red or yellow). Rupture of the eardrum causes purulent discharge and relieves the pain.

GPs tend to prescribe antibiotic treatment, although the importance of antibiotics in decreasing pain and speeding the resolution of otitis media has not been definitively established. The pharmacist should offer symptomatic relief of pain.

> **TRIGGER POINTS indicative of referral:**
> **The common cold**
>
> * Acute sinus involvement that fails to respond to decongestant therapy
> * Middle ear pain that fails to respond to analgesia
> * Patients with symptoms indicative of flu
> * Vulnerable patient groups, such as the very elderly

Evidence base for over-the-counter medication

Many of the active ingredients found in cold remedies are also constituents of cough products. Often they are combined and marketed as cough and cold or flu remedies. For information relating to cough ingredients the reader is referred to the sections on OTC medication for coughs (page 6).

Antihistamines

Data from a Cochrane review conducted by De Sutter et al (2003) showed that antihistamines when used as monotherapy did not have significant benefit clinically in nasal congestion, rhinorrhoea or sneezing in older children and adults. Additionally, they appeared not to influence subjective improvement. Only two trials were evaluated in young children, the results of which were conflicting. However, the larger study, which was more robustly conducted, showed no beneficial effect of antihistamines on the common cold.

Trials that used antihistamines in combination with other products such as decongestants and antitussives did show some beneficial global effects in adults and older children. Unfortunately, in most trials it was not possible to assess the clinical significance of these benefits because of insufficient data.

Sympathomimetics

Trial data specifically looking at the effects of decongestants in the common cold are limited. A Cochrane review (Taverner et al 2007) identified seven trials that met their inclusion criteria, which involved topical oxymetazoline and oral pseudoephedrine and phenylpropanolamine. Data support their use in adults when used in single doses. However, data were lacking in children under 12 years. No difference in efficacy was found between topical or systemic products.

Multi-ingredient preparations

There is no shortage of cold and flu remedies marketed. Many combine three or more ingredients. In the majority of cases either the patient will not require all the active ingredients to treat symptoms or the 'drug cocktail' administered will not contain active ingredients that have proven efficacy. A more sensible approach to medicine management would be to match symptoms with active ingredients with known evidence of efficacy. In many cases this can be achieved by providing the patient with monotherapy or a product containing two active ingredients. Preparations with multiple ingredients therefore have a very limited role to play in the management of coughs and colds. However, patients might perceive that an 'all in one' medicine is better value for money and, potentially, compliance with such preparations might be improved.

Alternative therapies

Many products are advocated to help treat cold symptoms. Three products in particular have received much attention and are widely used.

Zinc lozenges

The argument for zinc as a plausible treatment in ameliorating symptoms of the common cold can be traced back to 1984. A number of studies have investigated whether zinc lozenges can decrease the severity and duration of the common cold. A meta-analysis conducted in 2000 concluded that there was insufficient evidence to establish efficacy and any benefit would probably be modest. A further trial by Prasad et al (2000), which was published after the meta-analysis, did show zinc lozenges to significantly decrease the duration and severity of the common cold, although numbers in the study were low. This later study provides important additional evidence that zinc lozenges might have a beneficial effect. Larger studies are needed to establish the role of zinc in the common cold but if patients wanted to try a zinc supplement then it would not seem unreasonable.

Vitamin C

Vitamin C has been widely recommended as a 'cure' for the common cold by many sources both medical and non-medical. However, controversy still remains as to whether it is an effective weapon in combating the common cold. A large number of clinical trials have investigated the effect of vitamin C on the prevention and treatment of the common cold. The most recent Cochrane review (Douglas et al 2007) analysed 30 trials (n = 11 350) looking at prevention and treatment of the common cold. It concluded that vitamin C has no effect on the incidence of common cold, but it did reduce the duration and severity of symptoms – although the effects were small and probably clinical unimportant. Trials involving up to 4 g of vitamin C a day at the onset of colds were found to be of no benefit, although one trial reported benefits when given at 8 g per day.

Echinacea

The herbal remedy echinacea is marketed as a treatment for upper respiratory tract infections, including the common cold. Several reviews have reported echinacea's effect as inconsistent. This is in part due to the limited number of trials that are comparable, as different echinacea species are used as well as differing plant parts and extraction methods. A Cochrane review (Linde et al 2006) has attempted to take these factors into consideration and found some evidence that aerial parts of Echinacea purpurea (either alcoholic extract or pressed juice) might be effective in the early treatment of colds in adults. Following on from the Cochrane review, Shah et al (2007) conducted a further review, which also included experimentally induced colds. From the 14 trials that met the inclusion criteria, results drawn showed that treatment with echinacea reduced the chance of developing a cold by about half and the duration of colds was reduced by 1.4 days. The authors did, however, acknowledge various limitations of the study, including variability in product composition and plant species used, possible bias and problems with heterogeneity.

Vapour inhalation

Steam inhalation has long been advocated to aid symptoms of the common cold, usually with the addition of menthol crystals. Trial data appear to show conflicting evidence in symptom relief of the common cold (Singh 2006). However, it is cheap and does not carry any significant risks apart from minor discomfort and irritation of the nose. It appears that steam is the key to symptom resolution, and not any additional ingredient that is added to the water.

General summary

Evidence of efficacy for Western and complementary medicines in preventing and treating the common cold are weak. Decongestants used on a when needed basis probably have the strongest evidence base in treating symptoms, although recent studies suggests that echinacea might well have beneficial effects.

Practical prescribing and product selection

Prescribing information relating to the cold medicines reviewed in the section 'Evidence base for over-the-counter medication' is discussed and summarised in Table 1.4 and useful tips relating to patients presenting with a cold are given in Hints and Tips Box 1.2.

Antihistamines

Antihistamines, especially first-generation antihistamines, are included in many cough and cold remedies and further information on antihistamines can be found on page 8.

Sympathomimetics

Sympathomimetics serve to constrict dilated blood vessels and swollen nasal mucosa, easing congestion and helping breathing. Owing to concerns over illicit manufacture of methylamphetamine (crystal meth) from OTC sympathomimetics, the Medicines and Healthcare Products Regulatory Agency (MHRA) in August 2007 announced that products containing pseudoephedrine and ephedrine were to have tighter controls. The Commission on Human Medicines has recommended that large packs of pseudoephedrine and ephedrine will be replaced by smaller packs of 720 mg (the equivalent of 12 tablets or capsules of 60 mg or 24 tablets or capsules of 30 mg) and sales limited to one pack per person. This pack size restriction became law in 2008 meaning larger pack sizes reverted back to POM control. The Commission also recommends that a pharmacist should carry out the sale. Furthermore, the MHRA states that all pseudoephedrine- and ephedrine-containing products will be reclassified from pharmacy-only to prescription-only unless the risk of the misuse of these products is contained by these new measures.

Table 1.4
Practical prescribing: Summary of cold medicines

Name of medicine	Use in children	Likely side effects	Drug interactions of note	Patients in whom care should be exercised	Pregnancy and breast-feeding
Antihistamines					
Chlorphenamine	>1 years	Dry mouth, sedation and constipation	Increased sedation with alcohol, opioid analgesics, anxiolytics, hypnotics and antidepressants	Glaucoma, prostate enlargement	Standard references state OK, although some manufacturers advise avoidance
Diphenhydramine	>6 years*				
Promethazine	>1 year**				
Triprolidine	>1 year				
Systemic sympathomimetics					
Phenylephrine	>2 years	At OTC doses insomnia most likely. Possibly may cause tachycardia	Avoid concomitant use with MAOIs and moclobemide because of risk of hypertensive crisis. Avoid in patients taking beta-blockers and TCAs	Control of hypertension and diabetes may be affected, but a short treatment course is unlikely to be clinically important	Best avoided in pregnancy as mild foetal malformations have been reported
Pseudoephedrine	>2 years				Breast-feeding – lack of evidence, best avoided
Topical sympathomimetics					
Oxymetazoline	>5 years	Possible local irritation in ~5% of patients	Avoid concomitant use with MAOIs and moclobemide because of risk of hypertensive crisis	None	Not adequately studied but not yet shown to be a risk – probably OK
Xylometazoline	>2 years				

*Most products licensed for children over 6 years, however Benylin Children's Night Coughs has a product licence stating it can be given from 1 year upwards.
**Normally not recommended under 2 years of age, however Tixylix Night Cough has a product licence stating it can be given from 1 year upwards.
MAOI, monoamine oxidase inhibitor; OTC, over-the-counter; TCA, tricyclic antidepressant.

HINTS AND TIPS BOX 1.2: THE COMMON COLD

Limiting viral spread	Use disposable tissues rather than handkerchiefs Wash hands frequently, especially after nose blowing Do not share hand towels Try to avoid touching your nose
Stuffy noses in babies	Saline nose drops can be used from birth to help with congestion. This would be a more suitable and safer alternative than a topical sympathomimetic
General Sales List cold remedies	Products such as the Lemsip and Beechams ranges contain paracetamol. It is important to ensure patients are not taking excessive doses of analgesia unknowingly. Also, many products contain sub-therapeutic doses of sympathomimetics. If a sympathomimetic is needed then these products are generally best avoided
Administration of nasal drops	The best way to administer nose drops is to have the head in the downward position facing the floor. Tilting the head backward and toward the ceiling is incorrect as this facilitates swallowing of the drops. However, most patients will find the latter way of putting drops into the nose much easier than the former

Sympathomimetics interact with monoamine oxidase inhibitors (MAOIs) (e.g. phenelzine, isocarboxazid, tranylcypromine and moclobemide), which can result in a fatal hypertensive crisis. The danger of the interaction persists for up to 2 weeks after treatment with MAOIs is discontinued. In addition, systemic sympathomimetics can increase blood pressure, which might, although unlikely with short courses of treatment, alter control of blood pressure in hypertensive patients and disturb blood glucose control in diabetics. However, coadministration of medicines such as beta-blockers is probably clinically unimportant and does not preclude patients on beta-blockers from taking a sympathomimetic. A topical sympathomimetic could be given to such patients to negate this potential interaction. The most likely side effects of sympathomimetics are insomnia, restlessness and tachycardia. Patients should be advised not to take a dose just before bed-time because their mild stimulant action can disturb sleep.

Systemic sympathomimetics

Phenylephrine Phenylephrine is available in a number of proprietary cold remedies, for example Lemsip and Beechams, in doses ranging between 5 and 20 mg three or four times a day. Most products are not licensed for use in children, although phenylephrine is one of the ingredients in Beechams Powders capsules, which can be given to children over 6 years of age.

Pseudoephedrine Pseudoephedrine is widely available as either a single ingredient (e.g. Sudafed tablets) or in multi-ingredient products in cold and cough remedies (e.g. Benylin Four Flu tablets and Actifed cough range). The standard adult dose is 60 mg four times a day and half the adult dose is suitable for children between 6 and 12 years of age. It can be given to children older than 1 year of age (e.g. Tixylix Cough and Cold, 2.5 mL (10.0 mg) every 6 hours).

Phenylpropanolamine Phenylpropanolamine used to be the active ingredient of many decongestant products (e.g. Mucron and Eskornade) but, following safety concerns over phenylpropanolamine and the possible increased risk of haemorrhagic stroke, manufacturers reformulated their products with pseudoephedrine or withdrew the product.

Nasal sympathomimetics

Nasal administration of sympathomimetics represents the safest route of administration. They can be given to most patient groups, including children over 2 years of age, pregnant women after the first trimester and patients with pre-existing heart disease, diabetes, hypertension and hyperthyroidism. However, a degree of systemic absorption is possible, especially when using drops, as a small quantity might be swallowed, and therefore they should be avoided in patients taking MAOIs. All topical decongestants should not be used for longer than 5 to 7 days (British National Formulary 54 states a maximum of 7 days) otherwise rhinitis medicamentosa (rebound congestion) can occur.

Ephedrine and phenylephrine Both are short acting and need to be administered three or four times a day. Ephedrine can be given to babies from 3 months onward but phenylephrine (e.g. Fenox nasal drops/spray) is only licensed for children over 5 years old.

Oxymetazoline and xylometazoline These agents are longer acting than ephedrine and phenylephrine and require less frequent dosing, typically two or three times a day. They are made by a number of manufacturers (e.g. Afrazine nasal spray, Otrivine range, Sudafed decongestant nasal spray and Vicks Sinex decongestant nasal spray) Within the Otrivine range a paediatric drop is made that can be given to children over 2 years of age (1–2 drops into each nostril bd).

Further reading

Chadha NK, Chadha R. 10-minute consultation: sinusitis. BMJ 2007;334:1165.

De Sutter AIM, Lemiengre M, Campbell H. Antihistamines for the common cold. Cochrane Database of Systematic Reviews 2003, issue 3.

Douglas RM, Hemilä H, Chalker E, Treacy B. Vitamin C for preventing and treating the common cold. Cochrane Database of Systematic Reviews 2007, issue 3.

Glasziou PP, Del Mar CB, Sanders SL, Hayem M. Antibiotics for acute otitis media in children. Cochrane Database of Systematic Reviews 2004, issue 1.

Linde K, Barrett B, Wölkart K, et al. Echinacea for preventing and treating the common cold. Cochrane Database of Systematic Reviews 2006, issue 1.

Prasad AS, Fitzgerald JT, Bao B et al. Duration of symptoms and plasma cytokine levels in patients with the common cold treated with zinc acetate. A randomized, double-blind, placebo-controlled trial. Ann Intern Med 2000;133:245–52.

Shah S, Sander S, White CM, et al. Evaluation of echinacea for the prevention and treatment of the common cold: a meta-analysis. Lancet Infect Dis 2007;7:473–80.

Singh M. Heated, humidified air for the common cold. Cochrane Database of Systematic Reviews 2006, issue 3.

Taverner D, Latte J. Nasal decongestants for the common cold. Cochrane Database of Systematic Reviews 2007, issue 1.

Web sites

Common Cold Centre: http://www.cf.ac.uk/biosi/associates/cold/

Prodigy Guidance: http://www.prodigy.nhs.uk/common_cold

SIGN Guidelines on diagnosis and management of childhood otitis media in primary care: http://www.sign.ac.uk/guidelines/fulltext/66/index.html

Commoncold, Inc: http://www.commoncold.org

Sore throat

Background

Any part of the respiratory mucosa of the throat can give rise to symptoms of throat pain. This includes the pharynx (pharyngitis) and tonsils (tonsillitis) yet clinical distinction between pharyngitis and tonsillitis is unclear and the term sore throat is commonly used. Pain can range from scratchiness to severe pain. Sore throats are often associated with the common cold. However, in this section, people who present with sore throat as the principal symptom are considered.

Prevalence and epidemiology

Sore throats are extremely common. UK figures show that a GP with a list size of 2000 patients will see about 120 people each year with a throat infection. However, four to six times as many people will visit the pharmacy and self-treat. Figures from other countries such as New Zealand and Australia broadly support UK findings.

On average an adult will experience 2 to 3 sore throats each year. Streptococcal sore throat is more commonly associated with people under the age of 30, particularly those of school age (5 to 10 years) and young adults (15 to 25 years).

Aetiology

Viral infection accounts for between 70 and 90% of all sore throat cases. Remaining cases are nearly all bacterial; the most common cause being group A beta-haemolytic *Streptococcus* (also known as *Streptococcus pyogenes*). A fuller account of the aetiology of viral and bacterial pathogens that affect the upper respiratory tract appears on page 11.

Arriving at a differential diagnosis

The overwhelming majority of cases will be acute and self-limiting upper respiratory tract infection, whether viral or bacterial in origin. Other causes, although uncommon, include glandular fever, herpes simplex, candidiasis, medicines and carcinomas. Clinically, differentiation between viral and bacterial infection is extremely difficult, although specific symptom clusters are suggestive for sore throat of bacterial origin (see Conditions to eliminate) but these are by no means foolproof. Asking symptom-specific questions will help the pharmacist to determine the cause and whether referral is needed (Table 1.5).

After questioning, the pharmacist should inspect the mouth and cervical glands (located just below the angle of the jaw) to substantiate the differential diagnosis (Fig. 1.3). Using a good light source (e.g. pen torch) ask the patient to say 'ah'; this should allow you to see the pharynx well. When examining the mouth pay particular attention to the fauces and tonsils. Are they red and swollen? Is there any exudate present? Is there any sign of ulceration?

Clinical features of sore throat

Many studies have now shown that it is exceedingly difficult to differentiate viral and bacterial infection on patient history and clinical findings. Patients will present with a sore throat as an isolated symptom or as part of a cluster of symptoms that include rhinorrhoea, cough, malaise, fever, headache and hoarseness (laryngitis). Symptoms are relatively short-lived with 40% of people being symptom-free after 3 days and 85% of people symptom-free after 1 week.

Table 1.5
Specific questions to ask the patient: Sore throat

Question	Relevance
Age of the patient	• Although viruses are the commonest cause of sore throat there are epidemiological variances with age: • Under 3 years old *Streptococcus* is uncommon • Streptococcal infections are more prevalent in school-aged children (5 to 15 years old) • Viral causes are the commonest cause of sore throat in adults • Glandular fever is most prevalent in adolescents • Oral thrush affects the very young and very old
Tender cervical glands	• On examination, patients suffering from glandular fever and streptococcal sore throat often have markedly swollen glands. This is less so in viral sore throat
Tonsillar exudate present	• Marked tonsillar exudate is more suggestive of a bacterial cause than a viral cause
Ulceration	• Herpetiform and herpes simplex ulcers can also cause soreness in the mouth especially in the posterior part of the mouth. For further information see Chapter 6, page 125

Conditions to eliminate

Streptococcal sore throat

Patients who present with pharyngeal or tonsillar exudates, swollen anterior cervical glands, high-grade fever (over 101°F, 39.4°C) and absence of cough are more likely to have a bacterial infection. However, even if the patient exhibits all these four 'classic' symptoms, up to 40% will not have bacterial infection. To further compound the difficulty of diagnosis, the routine use of throat swabs performed by GPs is not recommended as asymptomatic carriage of *Streptococcus* affects up to 40% of people making it impossible to differentiate between infection and carriage. Table 1.6 summarises the potential distinguishing features of viral and bacterial infection

If bacterial infection is suspected then referral to the GP is appropriate. The use of antibiotics in such situations is debatable as a Cochrane review (Del Mar et al 2004) found that the absolute benefit of antibiotics was modest. The maximum benefit was seen by day 3 of treatment, with an average reduction in illness time of 1 day. The National Institute of Health and Clinical Excellence recommends a 10-day course of penicillin or erythromycin (where an allergy to penicillin exists) if the patient has a history of rheumatic fever, increased risk from acute infection, unilateral peritonsillitis and marked systemic upset.

Glandular fever (infectious mononucleosis)

Glandular fever is caused by the Epstein-Barr virus and is often called the kissing disease because transmission primarily occurs from saliva. It has a peak incidence in adolescents and young adults. The signs and symptoms of glandular fever can be difficult to distinguish from sore throat because it is characterised by pharyngitis (occasionally with exudates), fever, cervical lymphadenopathy and fatigue. The person can also suffer from general malaise prior to the start of the other symptoms. A macular rash can also occur in a small proportion of patients.

Trauma-related sore throat

Occasionally, patients develop a sore throat from direct irritation of the pharynx. This can be due to substances such as cigarette smoke, a lodged foreign body or from acid reflux.

Medicine-induced sore throat

A rare complication associated with certain medication is agranulocytosis, which can manifest as a sore throat. The patient will also probably present with signs of infection including fever and chills. Medicines known to cause this adverse event are listed in Table 1.7.

Laryngeal and tonsillar carcinoma

Both these cancers have a strong link with smoking and excessive alcohol intake, and are more common in men than women. Sore throat and dysphagia are the common presenting symptoms. In addition, patients with tonsillar cancer often develop referred ear pain. Any person, regardless of age, that presents with dysphagia should be referred.

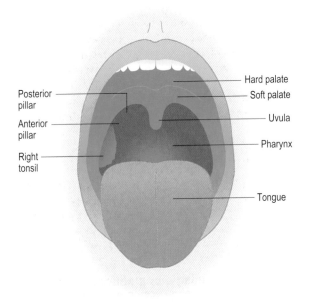

Posterior pillar
Anterior pillar
Right tonsil
Hard palate
Soft palate
Uvula
Pharynx
Tongue

Fig. 1.3 Major structures of the mouth

Table 1.6
Features of viral and bacterial sore throat

	Age	Tonsillar/pharyngeal exudate	Duration	Cervical glands	Cough present	Other symptoms
Viral infection	Any age	Possible but generally limited	3–7 days	Normal	Common	Low-grade fever, headache
Bacterial infection	School children	Often present and can be substantial	3–7 days	Swollen	Rare	High-grade fever, possible rash

Table 1.7
Examples of medication known to cause agranulocytosis

| Captopril |
| Carbimazole |
| Cytotoxics |
| Neuroleptics, e.g. clozapine |
| Penicillamine |
| Sulfasalazine |
| Sulphur-containing antibiotics |

Figure 1.4 will help in the differentiation of serious and non-serious conditions in which sore throat is a major presenting complaint.

TRIGGER POINTS indicative of referral: Sore throat

- Adverse drug reaction
- Associated skin rash
- Duration of more than 2 weeks
- Dysphagia
- Marked tonsillar exudate accompanied with a high temperature and swollen glands

Evidence base for over-the-counter medication

The majority of sore throats are viral in origin and self-limiting. Medication therefore aims to relieve symptoms and discomfort while the infection runs its course. Lozenge and spray formulations incorporating antibacterials and anaesthetics provide the mainstay of treatment for which there is no shortage on the market. In addition, systemic analgesics and antipyretics will help reduce the pain associated with sore throat.

Local anaesthetics

Lidocaine and benzocaine are included in a number of marketed products. Very few published clinical trials involving products marketed for sore throat have been conducted yet local anaesthetics have proven efficacy. It therefore appears that manufacturers are using trial data on local anaesthetic efficacy for conditions other than sore throat to substantiate their effect.

Antibacterial and antifungal agents

Antibacterial agents include chlorhexidine, tyrothricin, dequalinium chloride and benzalkonium chloride. In vitro testing has shown that many of the proprietary products do have antibacterial activity, and some inhibit *Candida albicans* growth. In vivo tests have also shown antibacterial effects. The use of antibacterial and antifungal agents should not be routinely recommended as the vast majority of sore throats are caused by viral infections, against which these agents have no action. As adverse effects are rare and stimulation of saliva from sucking the lozenge may confer symptomatic relief, the use of such products may be justified.

Anti-inflammatories

Benzydamine is available as a spray or mouthwash and one small trial involving benzydamine as a gargle resulted in significantly greater relief of pain compared to placebo (Thomas et al 2000).

Analgesia

There is good evidence to show that simple systemic analgesia, for example, paracetamol, aspirin and ibuprofen, is effective in reducing pain associated with sore throat. In trials NSAIDs were superior to paracetamol and placebo, although these benefits were short-lived. Given the tendency for NSAIDs to be associated with a greater incidence of serious adverse events than paracetamol, and aspirin's link with Reye's syndrome, it would seem wise to recommend paracetamol as the analgesic of choice.

Flurbiprofen lozenges are also available OTC and trials have shown them to be significantly more effective than placebo in reducing pain associated with sore throat.

Aspirin and salt water gargles

Gargling with aspirin or salt water is a common lay remedy for sore throat. No trials appear to have been conducted on their effectiveness and until such time that evidence becomes available they should not be recommended.

Practical prescribing and product selection

Prescribing information relating to the sore throat medicines reviewed under 'Evidence base for over-the-counter medication' is discussed and summarised in Table 1.8 and useful tips relating to patients presenting with a sore throat are given in Hints and Tips Box 1.3.

Local anaesthetics (lidocaine, benzocaine)

All local anaesthetics have a short duration of action and frequent dosing is required to maintain the anaesthetic effect whether formulated as a lozenge or spray. They appear to be free from any drug interactions, have minimal side effects and can be given to most patients, including pregnant and breast-feeding women. A small number of patients may experience a hypersensitivity reaction with either ingredient although this appears to

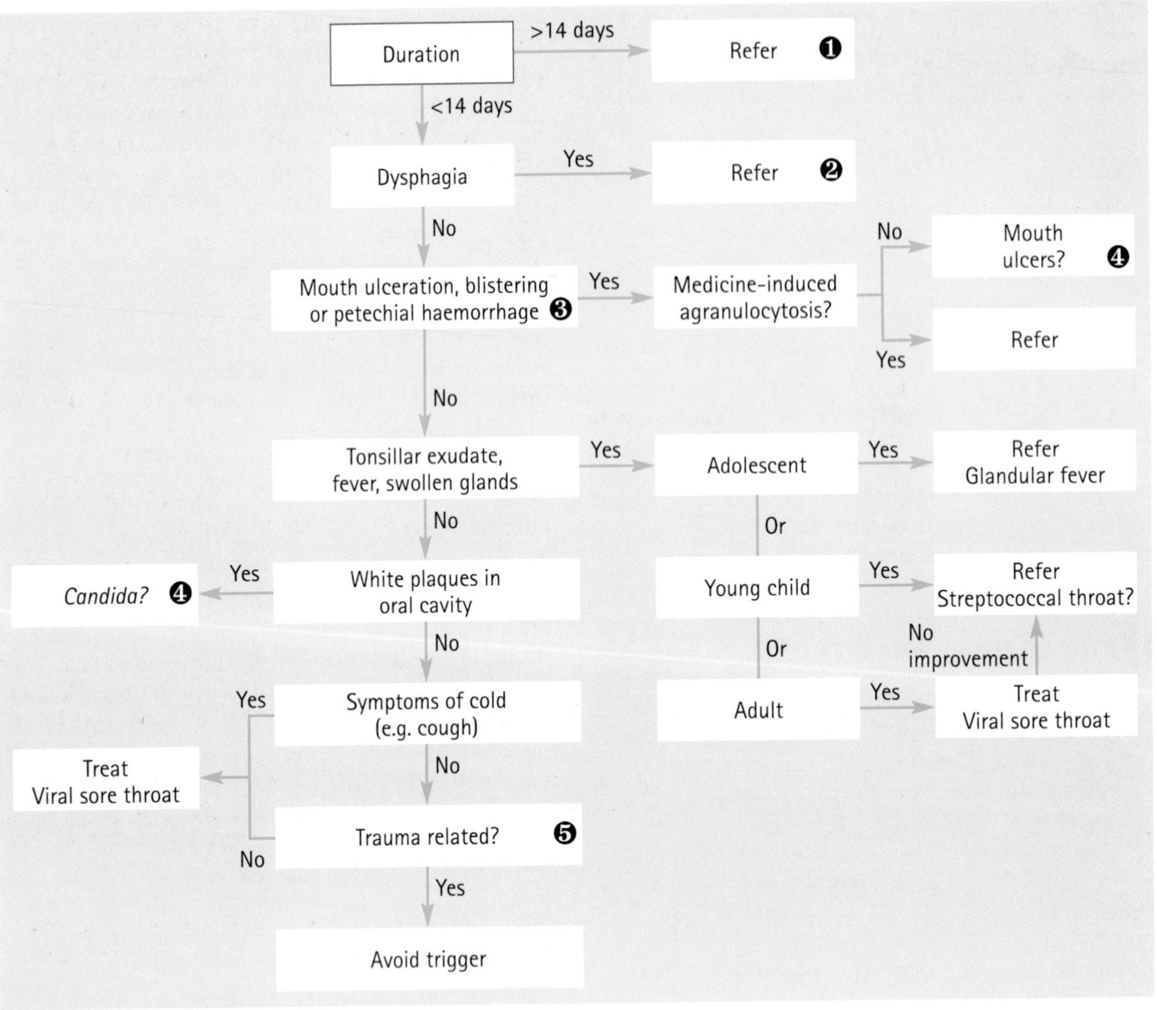

Fig. 1.4 Primer for differential diagnosis of sore throat

❶ **Duration longer than 2 weeks**
The overwhelming majority of cases resolve spontaneously in this time; it is therefore prudent to refer these cases for further investigation.

❷ **Dysphagia**
True difficulty in swallowing (i.e. not just caused by pain but by a mechanical blockage) should be referred. Most patients with sore throat will find it less easy to swallow but this has to be differentiated from actual difficulty in swallowing. Severe inflammation of the throat can cause restriction of the airways and thus hinder breathing. Additionally, rare causes of sore throat also have associated dysphagia symptoms, such as peritonsillar abscess, thyroiditis and oesophageal carcinoma.

❸ **Signs of agranulocytosis**
A severe reduction in the number of white blood cells can result in neutropenia, which is manifested as fever, sore throat, ulceration and small haemorrhages under the skin.

❹ **Mouth ulceration and *Candida* (oral thrush) primers**
See Chapter 6 and Figs 6.6 & 6.7 for further differentiation of these conditions.

❺ **Trauma related**
Simple acts of drinking fluids that are too hot can give rise to ulceration of the pharynx. It is worth asking whether any such factors could have triggered the sore throat.

be more common with benzocaine. Owing to differences in the chemical structure of these products, cross-sensitivity is unusual and therefore if a patient experiences side effects with one then the other can be tried. Most products do contain a sugar base but the amount of sugar is too small to substantially affect blood glucose control and therefore can be recommended to diabetic patients.

Lidocaine

Lidocaine is available as a spray (Covonia throat spray (0.05%) and Dequaspray (2.0%)). Lidocaine is licensed only for adults and is best taken on a when needed basis. As both proprietary products have differing strengths of lidocaine the dosing schedules differ – for Covonia the dose is 3–5 sprays between 6 and 10 times a day and for

Table 1.8
Practical prescribing: Summary of sore throat medicines

Name of medicine	Use in children	Likely side effects	Drug interactions of note	Patients in whom care should be exercised	Pregnancy and breast-feeding
Local anaesthetics					
Lidocaine	>12 years	Can cause sensitisation reactions	None	None	OK
Benzocaine	Lozenge >3 years Spray >6 years				
Anti-inflammatories					
Benzydamine	Rinse >12 years Spray >6 years	Oral rinse may cause stinging	None	None	OK, but in pregnancy limit use after 30 weeks
Flurbiprofen	>12 years	None reported	None	Avoid in patients with peptic ulcers	Avoid if possible

HINTS AND TIPS BOX 1.3: SORE THROAT

Stimulation of saliva production	Sucking a lozenge or pastille promotes saliva production, which will lubricate the throat and thus exert a soothing action
Gargles or lozenges?	Gargles have very short contact time with inflamed mucosa and therefore any effect will be short-lived. A lozenge or a pastille is preferable, as contact time will be longer

Dequaspray the dose is 3 sprays up to a maximum of 6 times per day.

Benzocaine

Unlike lidocaine, benzocaine can be given to children both in lozenge and spray formulations. Lozenges are available and can be given from age 3 years and over (Tyrozets 1 lozenge (5 mg) every 3 hours when needed, maximum of 6 in 24 hours); adults can take up to 8 in 24 hours (e.g. Merocaine, Dequacaine). Additionally, children over the age of 6 years can use a spray formulation (Ultra Chloraseptic (0.71%) or AAA spray (1.5%)), although the dosing varies between products.

Anti-inflammatories (benzydamine, Difflam Sore Throat Rinse and Difflam Spray)

The product should be used every 1½ to 3 hours for maximum benefit. It has no drug interactions of note, can be used by all patient groups and only occasionally does the rinse cause stinging, in which case it can be diluted with water. The manufacturers advise that the product should be stored in the box away from direct sunlight; however, the stability of the product is not known to be affected by sunlight. The spray can be used in children although the dose is based on mg/kg dosing for those under the age of 6 years; for 6 to 12 years the dose is four puffs and adults four to eight puffs. The rinse

is licensed for adults only. It is relatively expensive and many patients might prefer to purchase a cheaper anaesthetic-based alternative.

Flurbiprofen (Strefen)

Strefen lozenges (8.75 mg flurbiprofen) can only be given to adults and children over the age of 12 years. The dose is one lozenge to be sucked every 3 to 6 hours with a maximum of five lozenges in 24 hours. They are contraindicated in patients with peptic ulceration and those patients allergic to flurbiprofen, and must be used with caution in pregnant and breast-feeding women.

Further reading
Del Mar CB, Glasziou PP, Spinks AB. Antibiotics for sore throat. Cochrane Database of Systematic Reviews 2004, issue 2.
Middleton DB. Pharyngitis. Prim Care 1996;23:719–39.
Thomas M, Del Mar C, Glasziou P. How effective are treatments other than antibiotics for acute sore throat? Br J Gen Pract 2000;50:817–20.
Watson N, Nimmo WS, Christian J, et al. Relief of sore throat with the anti-inflammatory throat lozenge flurbiprofen 8.75 mg: a randomised, double-blind, placebo-controlled study of efficacy and safety. Int J Clin Pract 2000;54:490–6.

Web sites

Prodigy Guidelines: http://www.prodigy.nhs.uk/sore_throat_
    acute

Sinus Care Center: http://www.sinuscarecenter.com/

Rhinitis

Background

Rhinitis simply means inflammation of the nasal lining and is characterised by rhinorrhoea, nasal congestion, sneezing and itching. The majority of cases that present in a community pharmacy will be either viral infection or allergic rhinitis, which can either be seasonal (hay fever) or year round (perennial rhinitis). Allergic rhinitis is often associated with a significant reduction in quality of life and guidelines produced by the World Health Organization (ARIA – Allergic Rhinitis and its Impact on Asthma) incorporate quality of life parameters. One survey conducted by Allergy UK in May 2005 found that half of respondents reported their symptoms moderately or severely affected their performance at school/work and 85% reported symptoms that disrupted their sleep.

Prevalence and epidemiology

Allergic rhinitis is a global health problem and has dramatically increased over the last 20 years with studies suggesting the prevalence has at least doubled in that time. It is believed that improved living standards and reduced risk of childhood infections might increase susceptibility to hay fever. The UK has one of the highest levels of allergic rhinitis in the world, with estimates ranging from 10 to 25% of adults and as many as 40% of children affected (ARIA). These figures might, however, represent an underestimate as many people do not consult their doctor and choose to self-medicate. Hay fever commonly affects school-aged children with 10 to 30% of the adolescent population suffering from the condition. The mean age of onset is 10 years and the incidence peaks between the ages of 13 and 19 years. A person is also more likely to suffer from hay fever if there is a family history of asthma, eczema or hay fever. It has also been reported that patients with concurrent asthma have up to an 80% chance of developing allergic rhinitis.

Aetiology

Allergic rhinitis is a mucosal reaction in response to allergen exposure. Initially, the patient must come into contact with an allergen. The allergen (most commonly grass pollen) lodges within the mucous blanket lining the nasal membranes, and activates IgE antibodies (formed from previous pollen exposure) on the surface of mast cells. Potent chemical mediators are released, primarily histamine, but also leukotrienes, kinins and prostaglandins, which exert their action via neural and vascular mechanisms. This immediate response to an allergen is known as the early-phase allergic reaction and gives rise to nasal itch, rhinorrhoea, sneezing and nasal congestion. A late-phase reaction then occurs 4 to 12 hours after allergen exposure with nasal congestion as the main symptom.

Also of importance is the phenomenon of nasal priming. Patients, after a period of continuous allergen exposure, can find that they experience the same level of severity in symptoms with lower levels of allergen exposure. Similarly, symptoms will be worse than previously experienced when levels of the allergen are the same. This may explain why patients complain of worsening hay fever symptoms the longer the season goes on. Table 1.9 highlights the main allergens responsible for allergic rhinitis.

Arriving at a differential diagnosis

Rhinitis is not difficult to diagnose. Within the community pharmacy setting the majority of patients who present with rhinitis will be suffering from a cold or hay fever. Diagnosis is largely dependent upon the patient having a family history of atopy, clinical symptoms and worsening symptoms at a particular time of year. Asking symptom-specific questions will help the pharmacist to determine the cause and whether referral is needed (Table 1.10).

Table 1.9
Allergens responsible for rhinitis

	When	Causative allergen
Hay fever	March to May	Tree pollen
	May to August (peak in June and July)	Grass pollen
	September to October	Fungal spores
Perennial rhinitis	Year round	House dust mite, animal dander, especially cats

Table 1.10
Specific questions to ask the patient: Rhinitis

Question	Relevance
Seasonal variation	• Symptoms in the summer months suggest hay fever whereas year-round symptoms suggest perennial rhinitis
History of asthma, eczema or hay fever in the family	• If a first-degree relative suffers from atopy then hay fever is much more likely
Triggers	• When pollen counts are high symptoms of hay fever worsen • Infective rhinitis is unaffected by pollen count • Patients with perennial rhinitis might suffer from worsening symptoms when pollen counts are high but symptoms should still persist when indoors compared with hay fever sufferers who usually see improvement of symptoms when away from pollen

Clinical features of hay fever

The patient will experience a combination or all four of the classical rhinitis symptoms of nasal itch, sneeze (especially paroxysmal), watery rhinorrhoea and nasal congestion. In addition, the patient might also suffer from ocular irritation giving rise to allergic conjunctivitis. The symptoms should occur intermittently (i.e. times of pollen exposure) and tend to be worse in the morning and evening as pollen levels peak at this time, as they do when the weather is hot and humid.

Conditions to eliminate

Perennial allergic rhinitis

Perennial allergic rhinitis is 10 times less common than hay fever. As its name suggests, the problem tends to be persistent and does not exhibit seasonality. However, it must be remembered that patients suffering from perennial rhinitis might also be allergic to pollen and experience worsening symptoms in the summer months. Besides not having a seasonal cause, there are a number of other clues to look out for that aid differentiation. Nasal congestion is much more common, which often leads to hyposmia (poor sense of smell) and ocular symptoms are uncommon. Additionally, perennial allergic rhinitis sufferers tend to sneeze less frequently and experience more

episodes of chronic sinusitis. The most common allergen causing perennial rhinitis is the house dust mite but animal dander (particularly from cats, dogs and horses) is a common cause of symptoms, and so it is prudent to ask about pets that are kept.

Non-allergic rhinitis

Patients with non-allergic rhinitis present with perennial or persistent symptoms that can be attributed to a number of causes including infective rhinitis, hormonal rhinitis (e.g. pregnancy) and medicine-induced rhinitis.

Infective rhinitis

This is normally viral in origin and associated with the common cold. Nasal discharge tends to be more mucopurulent than allergic rhinitis and nasal itching is uncommon. Sneezing tends not to occur in paroxysms and the condition resolves more quickly, whereas allergic rhinitis lasts for as long as the person is exposed to the allergen. Other symptoms, such as cough and sore throat, are much more prominent in infective rhinitis than allergic rhinitis.

Vasomotor rhinitis (intrinsic rhinitis)

It is thought that vasomotor rhinitis is caused by oversensitive or excessive blood vessels in the nasal membrane. This causes an over reaction to stimuli such as changes in weather, temperature or chemical irritants. The symptoms are similar to allergic rhinitis although itching and sneezing are less common. If an allergy test is performed the result will be negative.

Rhinitis of pregnancy

This occurs due to hormonal changes and spontaneously resolves after childbirth.

Rhinitis medicamentosa and drug-induced rhinitis

Rhinitis medicamentosa is a condition induced by overuse of nasal decongestants. Prolonged use of topical decongestants (more than 5 to 7 days) causes rebound vasodilatation of the nasal arterioles leading to further nasal congestion although the exact pathophysiology is not clear. Systemic preparations have also been implicated in causing this condition and include β-adrenoceptor antagonists, phosphodiesterase type 5 inhibitors (e.g. sildenafil), antipsychotics (e.g. chlorpromazine), oral contraceptives and antihypertensives.

Nasal blockage

In the absence of rhinorrhoea, nasal itch and sneezing it is possible that the problem is mechanical or anatomical. If the blockage is continuous and unilateral this may relate to a deviated nasal septum in adults. This may develop or be a result of trauma. Referral is needed and surgery is recommended. If the obstruction is bilateral this may relate to nasal polyps in adults. Nasal obstruction is progressive and is often accompanied by hyposmia. Referral is needed for corticosteroids or surgery.

Nasal foreign body

A trapped foreign body in a nostril commonly occurs in young children, often without the parents' knowledge. Within a matter of days of the foreign body being lodged the patient experiences an offensive nasal discharge. Any unilateral discharge, particularly in a child, should be referred for nasal examination, as it is highly likely that a foreign body is responsible.

Figure 1.5 will aid in differentiating the different types of rhinitis.

TRIGGER POINTS indicative of referral: Rhinitis

- Failed medication
- Medicine-induced rhinitis
- Nasal obstruction that fails to clear
- Unilateral discharge especially in children

Evidence base for over-the-counter medication

Before medication is started it is clearly important to try and identify the causative allergen. If this can be achieved then measures to limit the exposure to the allergen will be beneficial in reducing the symptoms experienced by the patient. This is more easily accomplished in perennial rhinitis than in hay fever.

Allergen avoidance

Avoidance of pollen is almost impossible but if the patient follows a few simple rules then exposure to pollen can be reduced. Patients may choose to stay indoors when pollen counts are high. Windows should be closed (both when in the house and when travelling in cars) and 'wrap around' sunglasses worn. Air conditioning in cars fitted with a pollen filter is also beneficial. Patients should avoid walking in areas with the potential for high pollen exposure (grassy fields, parks and gardens) as well as areas such as city centres as many hay fever sufferers will have increased sensitivity to other irritants such as car exhaust fumes and cigarette smoke.

The two main causative agents of perennial rhinitis, house dust mite and animal dander, can be more easily avoided. The offending pet can be excluded from certain parts of the house such as living areas and bedrooms. Acaricidal sprays and strict bedroom cleaning regimes have shown to be of some benefit in reducing rhinitis symptoms (Sheikh & Hurwitz 2001).

Medication

Pharmacists now possess a wide range of therapeutic options to treat both hay fever and perennial rhinitis. A number of deregulated POM products enable the vast majority of sufferers to be appropriately managed without the need for referral to the GP. However, for many patients the cost of treatment may be too prohibitive to self-medicate for the entire period for which they suffer and they will seek a prescription. Management of allergic rhinitis falls broadly into two categories: systemic and topical.

Systemic therapy: antihistamines

Both sedating and non-sedating antihistamines are clinically effective in reducing the symptoms associated with allergic rhinitis (Sheikh et al 2006). However, given the sedative effects of first-generation antihistamines they should not be routinely recommended compared to second-generation, non-sedating antihistamines.

Of the second-generation antihistamines, the community pharmacist has a choice between acrivastine, cetirizine, or loratadine. All are equally effective and are considered to be non-sedating, although they are not truly non-sedating and do cause different levels of sedation. Loratadine has been shown to have the lowest affinity for histamine receptors in the brain and a paper published by Mann et al in 2000 reviewing reported sedation with second-generation antihistamines showed loratadine to be least sedating of the non-sedating antihistamines. In comparison, cetirizine was 3.5 times more likely to cause sedation and acrivastine 2.5 times more likely to cause sedation than loratadine. On this basis, loratadine would be the antihistamine of choice.

Topical therapy

A range of topically administered medication is available to combat nasal congestion and ocular symptoms, including antihistamines, corticosteroids, mast cell stabilisers and decongestants. All can be administered intranasally but corticosteroids cannot be administered intraocularly.

Intranasal medication

Corticosteroids Intranasal corticosteroids are the medicine of choice for moderate to severe allergic rhinitis especially where there is nasal congestion. Several studies have shown them to be effective and have superior efficacy compared with oral antihistamines, decongestants and mast cells stabilisers. There is little difference in efficacy between the intranasal corticosteroids in patients with allergic rhinitis and clinical evidence does not support the use of one intranasal corticosteroid over another. They have a slow onset of action and patients should be advised that it will take 2 weeks before maximum clinical efficacy is observed. Patients who regularly suffer from nasal congestion associated with

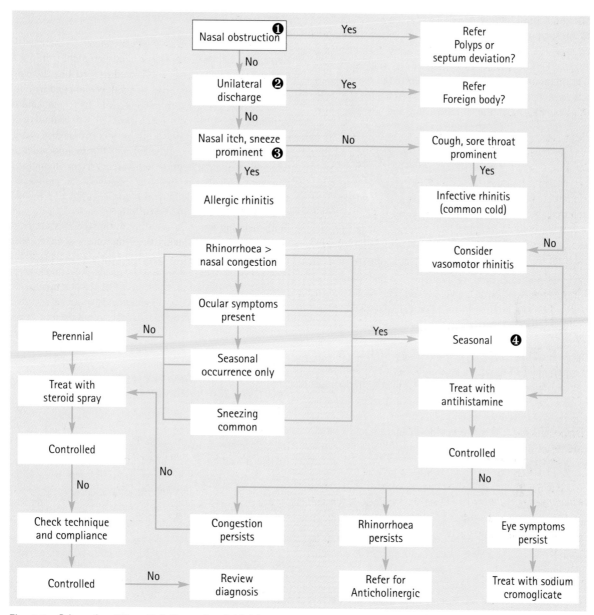

Fig. 1.5 Primer for differential diagnosis of rhinitis

❶ Nasal obstruction
Nasal obstruction differs from nasal congestion in that obstruction refers to a physical blockage of the nasal passage and is normally due to an anatomical fault, whereas congestion refers to the nasal passages being temporarily blocked by nasal secretions that can easily be cleared by nose blowing. Obstruction therefore warrants referral.

❷ Unilateral discharge
Any one-sided nasal discharge must be viewed with suspicion. Accidental lodging of a foreign body by young children is the usual cause.

❸ Nasal itch and sneeze prominent
Nasal itching and sneezing are classically associated with hay fever, although these symptoms are also associated with perennial rhinitis, but to a lesser extent. Sneezing is often said to occur in multiple bouts, which is unlike infective rhinitis. Coughing can occur but is infrequent.

❹ Treatment of vasomotor rhinitis
Because symptoms are similar to hay fever then it is reasonable to assume that first-line therapy for vasomotor rhinitis would be a systemic antihistamine.

allergic rhinitis should be advised to commence therapy before exposure to the allergen to ensure symptom control.

Antihistamines Azelastine is currently the only nasally administered antihistamine that is marketed for OTC sale. Clinical trials have proven its efficacy and a review paper by McNeely (1998) concluded that azelastine was well tolerated and provided an effective alternative to other antihistamine agents as it had a rapid onset of action.

Mast cell stabilisers Like corticosteroids, sodium cromoglicate is a prophylactic agent. However, the effect of sodium cromoglicate is only partial – it is less effective than corticosteroids, although it is not clear why. A further drawback with nasal cromoglicate is the frequency of administration; between four and six times a day. Although no data are available for the compliance with such a regimen it is likely to be poor and result in inadequate symptom control. Mast cell stabilisers' place in allergic rhinitis is therefore limited.

Decongestants Topical decongestants are effective in the treatment of nasal congestion but sympathomimetics are of limited value in treating allergic rhinitis because of their rebound effects. Their place in therapy is probably best reserved for when nasal congestion needs to be treated quickly and can provide symptom relief while corticosteroid therapy is initiated and has time to begin to exert its action.

Intraocular medication

Mast cell stabilisers Sodium cromoglicate has proven efficacy and is significantly better than placebo. It does require four times a day dosing and compliance might be a problem.

Lodoxamide Clinical trials appear to show that lodoxamide is as effective as sodium cromoglicate. It too is given four times a day and therefore compliance is again an issue.

Antihistamines The only ocular antihistamine available OTC is antazoline. It is available in combination with xylometazoline. There appear to be little trial data in the public domain regarding decongestant/antihistamine combinations, although one small trial involving 25 patients concluded that a combination of the two drugs was superior to either alone. At best it should be used in the short term to avoid possible rebound conjunctivitis caused by xylometazoline, which is well documented.

Sympathomimetics OTC ocular sympathomimetics are commonly used to control ocular redness and discomfort. There appear to be no significant differences between ocular decongestants on the basis of their vasoconstrictive effectiveness. They should be restricted to short-term use to avoid rebound effects.

Summary

Loratadine should be recommended as first-line therapy if the patient suffers from general symptoms such as nasal itching, sneezing, rhinorrhoea and associated ocular symptoms. If this fails to control all symptoms then sodium cromoglicate eye drops or a corticosteroid nasal spray should be added to the regimen. If nasal congestion predominates then regular topical nasal corticosteroids are recommended as first-line treatment. A pharmacy protocol recommended by the ARIA guidelines breaks down treatment on the basis of symptom severity and frequency.

Practical prescribing and product selection

Prescribing information relating to the rhinitis medicines reviewed in the section 'Evidence base for over-the-counter medication' is discussed and summarised in Table 1.11 and useful tips relating to patients presenting with rhinitis are given in Hints and Tips Box 1.4.

Systemic antihistamines (acrivastine, cetirizine and loratadine)

Systemic antihistamines selectively inhibit histamine H_1 receptors and suppress many of the vascular effects of histamine. They have rapid onset of action (approximately 30 minutes to 1 hour) and relieve ocular symptoms, rhinorrhoea and nasal irritation, but have little effect on nasal congestion. For maximum effect they are best taken on a regular basis but will have an effect if taken when required. Patient response is variable among the different antihistamines and more than one type may have to be tried to provide symptom control. They possess very few side effects and can be given safely with other prescribed medication. They can also be prescribed to all patient groups, although manufacturers advise against prescribing to the elderly. First-generation, sedating antihistamines are the preferred antihistamines in pregnancy as the risk of foetal toxicity appears low, with chlorphenamine being the medicine of choice. Of the non-sedating antihistamines loratadine is the most widely studied and data available do not indicate an increased risk of teratogenicity, yet manufacturers advise avoidance (presumably on the basis of being outside their product licences). For breast-feeding mothers, non-sedating antihistamines should be avoided as infant drowsiness has been associated with their use. Expert opinion states that cetirizine and loratadine are antihistamines of choice despite manufacturers advising that they should not be used in this patient group.

Acrivastine (Benadryl Allergy Relief)

Acrivastine is recommended for adults and children over 12 years of age. The dose is one capsule (8 mg) as

Table 1.11
Practical prescribing: Summary of rhinitis medicines

Name of medicine	Use in children	Likely side effects	Drug interactions of note	Patients in whom care should be exercised	Pregnancy and breast-feeding
Systemic antihistamines					
Acrivastine	>12 years	Sedation but least likely with loratadine	None	None	Manufacturers advise avoidance, but safety data have shown them to be safe
Cetirizine	>6 years				
Loratadine	>2 years				
Ocular antihistamines					
Antazoline*	>5 years	Local irritation, bitter taste	Avoid concomitant use with MAOIs and moclobemide because of risk of hypertensive crisis	Avoid in glaucoma	Safety not established, but probably OK
Nasal antihistamines					
Azelastine	>5 years	Nasal irritation (5%), bitter taste (3%)	None	None	Safety not established, but probably OK
Nasal corticosteroids					
Beclometasone	>18 years	Nasal irritation, bitter taste, nosebleeds	None	Avoid in glaucoma	Manufacturers advise avoidance, but safety data have shown them to be safe
Fluticasone					
Ocular and nasal mast cell stabilisers					
Lodoxamide	>4 years	Transient burning, stinging and discomfort	None	None	Avoid, insufficient experience
Sodium cromoglicate ocular	>12 years	Local irritation, blurred vision			OK
Sodium cromoglicate nasal	>5 years	Nasal irritation. Rare – wheezing and shortness of breath			OK
Ocular sympathomimetics					
Naphazoline	>12 years	Local irritation	Avoid concomitant use with MAOIs and moclobemide because of risk of hypertensive crisis	None	Not adequately studied but not yet shown to be a risk – probably OK

*Only available in combination with naphazoline.

HINTS AND TIPS BOX 1.4: RHINITIS

Breakthrough symptoms with one-a-day antihistamines

Patients who suffer breakthrough symptoms using a once daily preparation (loratadine, cetirizine) may benefit from changing to acrivastine as three times a day dosing may confer better symptom control necessary, up to three times a day. Acrivastine can also be purchased as a combination product (Benadryl Plus), which contains a sympathomimetic (pseudoephedrine). However, if nasal congestion is a problem, corticosteroids should be used in preference to the addition of a decongestant.

Cetirizine (e.g. Zirtek 7, Benadryl One-a-Day)

Cetirizine is available as either tablets or solution. The dose for adults and children 6 years and over is one tablet (10 mg) daily. The dose for the oral solution can either be 10 mL (10 mg) once daily, or 5 mL (5 mg) twice daily.

Loratadine (e.g. Clarityn Allergy)

Loratadine is available as either a tablet or syrup. The dose for people aged over 6 years is one tablet (10 mg) each day. The syrup (1 mg/mL) can be given to children aged between 2 and 5 years old at a dose of 5 mL (5 mg) each day.

Nasal corticosteroids (beclometasone, fluticasone)

Currently, only beclometasone and fluticasone are available for sale to the public. In addition, flunisolide, budesonide and triamcinolone possess pharmacy status but manufacturers have not produced an OTC product. They can be used in most patient groups, although avoidance is recommended in glaucoma. In addition, manufacturers recommend that they are not used during pregnancy and breast-feeding due to insufficient evidence to establish safety. However, exposure data do suggest that they are safe. Both products can cause unpleasant taste and smell as well as nasal and throat irritation (incidence > 1%). Beclometasone is also reported to cause rashes and urticaria and fluticasone headaches.

Beclometasone (Beconase)

This is licensed for adults and children over 18 years old, although it can be given to children over the age of 6 years on prescription. The recommended dose is two sprays into each nostril twice daily (400 µg/day). Once symptoms have improved it might be possible to decrease the dose to one spray twice daily. However, should symptoms recur, patients should revert to the standard dosage.

Fluticasone (Flixonase)

In common with beclometasone, fluticasone is licensed for adults and children over 18 years old. The dose is two sprays into each nostril once daily (200 µg/day). If symptoms are not controlled, the dose can be increased to twice daily.

Nasal antihistamines

Intranasal antihistamines are useful in treating mild or intermittent nasal symptoms and work more quickly than systemic antihistamines (15 minutes). They appear to have no drug interactions and there is no evidence to show they are unsafe in pregnancy, although manufacturers advise caution. There is a lack of data for use in breast-feeding but it is assumed that if oral antihistamines can be used then intranasal antihistamines, which result in lower blood concentrations, would be safe to use.

Azelastine (Rhinolast Hayfever Nasal Spray)

Azelastine can be given to adults and children over 5 years of age. The dose is one application (0.14 mL) in each nostril twice daily (0.56 mg of azelastine hydrochloride). It should not be recommended to elderly patients.

Mast cell stabilisers (sodium cromoglicate and lodoxamide)

Sodium cromoglicate eye drops and nasal spray are poorly absorbed at therapeutic doses and the amount reaching the systemic circulation is very low. It has no drug interactions and can be given to all patient groups. Clinical experience has shown it to be safe in pregnancy and expert opinion considers sodium cromoglicate to be safe in breast-feeding. Lodoxamide, like sodium cromoglicate, has no drug interactions but manufacturers advise against use in pregnant and breast-feeding women due to lack of data. Both are prophylactic agents and have to be given continuously while exposed to the allergen.

Ocular cromoglicate (e.g. Opticrom Allergy, Optrex Allergy)

One or two drops should be administered in each eye four times a day. Instillation of the drops can cause a transient blurring of vision.

Nasal cromoglicate (Rynacrom 4% Nasal Spray)

The dose for adults and children is one spray into each nostril two to four times daily. Nasal irritation is possible, especially during the first few days of use.

Lodoxamide (Alomide allergy)

Lodoxamide can be given from 4 years of age upwards. The dose is one to two drops into each nostril four times a day. Instillation of the drops can cause a transient burning, stinging and discomfort. Other side effects reported include ocular pruritus, blurred vision and tearing.

Sympathomimetics

For general information about sympathomimetics and product information on nasally administered products see page 14.

Ocular sympathomimetics

Ocular products either contain a combination of sympathomimetic and antihistamine (antazoline/xylometazoline, Otrivine Antistin) or sympathomimetic alone (e.g.

Naphazoline 0.01%). They are useful in reducing redness in the eye but will not treat the underlying pathology that is causing the eye to be red. They should be limited to short-term use to avoid rebound effects. Like all sympathomimetics they can interact with MAOIs and should not be used by patients receiving such treatment or within 14 days of ceasing therapy.

Otrivine Antistin Adults and children over 5 years old should administer Otrivine Antistin two or three times a day. Patients with glaucoma should avoid this product due to the potential of the antihistamine component to increase intraocular pressure. Local transient irritation and a bitter taste after application have been reported.

Naphazoline (e.g. Murine, Optrex Red Eyes Eye Drops)
The use of products containing naphazoline is restricted to adults and children over the age of 12 years. One to two drops should be administered into the eye four times a day.

Complementary therapies

Butterbur is promoted as having anti-allergic properties. Two clinical trials have reported favourable outcomes of butterbur in controlling symptoms. Both trials found butterbur to be as effective as its comparator drug (cetirizine and fexofenadine, respectively) although another trial found it to be no better than placebo. Until further larger studies are conducted to assess butterbur's effect it should not be routinely recommended.

Further reading

Anon. Common questions about hay fever. MeReC Bulletin 2004;14(5):17–20.
Anon. How should seasonal allergic rhinitis be treated during pregnancy? Available at: http://www.druginfozone.nhs.uk/Record%20Viewing/viewRecord.aspx?id=543627

ARIA in the pharmacy. Available at: http://www.blackwell-synergy.com/doi/pdf/10.1111/j.1398-9995.2003.00468.x?cookieSet=1 (accessed 13 Oct 2007).
de Groot H, Brand PLP, Fokkens WF, Berger MY. Allergic rhinoconjunctivitis in children. BMJ 2007;335:985–8.
Jones N. Management of allergic rhinitis in primary care. Prescriber 2001;12:81–96.
Jones NS, Carney AS, Davis A. The prevalence of allergic rhinosinusitis: a review. J Laryngol Otol 1998;112:1019–30.
McNeely W, Wiseman LR. Intranasal azelastine. A review of its efficacy in the management of allergic rhinitis. Drugs 1998;56:91–114.
Mann RD, Pearce GL, Dunn N, et al. Sedation with 'non-sedating' antihistamines: four prescription-event monitoring studies in general practice. BMJ 2000;320:1184–6.
Passalacqua G, Bousquet PJ, Kai-Hakon C, et al. ARIA Update: 1 – Systematic review of complimentary and aternative medicine for rhinitis and asthma. J Allergy Clin Immunol 2006;117:1054–62.
Price D, Bond C, Bouchard J, et al. International Primary Care Respiratory Group (IPCRG) Guidelines: Management of Allergic Rhinitis. Prim Care Resp J 2006;15:58–70.
Saleh HA, Durham SR. Perennial rhinitis. BMJ 2007;335:502–7.
Sheikh A, Panesar SS, Dhami S. Seasonal allergic rhinitis. Br Med J Clin Evidence 2006. Available at http://www.clinicalevidence.com
Sheikh A, Hurwitz B. House dust mite avoidance measures for perennial allergic rhinitis. Cochrane Database of Systematic Reviews 2001, issue 4.
Skoner DP. Allergic rhinitis: definition, epidemiology, pathophysiology, detection, and diagnosis. J Allergy Clin Immunol 2001;108 (Suppl 1):2–8.
Slater JW, Zechnich AD, Haxby DG. Second-generation antihistamines: a comparative review. Drugs 1999;57:31–47.

Web sites
Allergy UK: http://www.allergyuk.org/

Self-assessment questions

The following questions are intended to supplement the text. Two levels of questions are provided: multiple choice questions and case studies. The multiple choice questions are designed to test factual recall and the case studies allow knowledge to be applied to a practice setting.

Multiple choice questions

1.1 Which respiratory condition is characterised by shortness of breath and bronchoconstriction?

    a. Acute bronchitis
    b. Heart failure
    c. Asthma
    d. Chronic bronchitis
    e. Pneumonia

1.2 What course of action would be most appropriate if a baby was suffering with croup-like symptoms?

    a. Take the infant to casualty
    b. Put the infant into a steamy room
    c. Give the infant paracetamol
    d. Give the infant a cough suppressant
    e. Give the infant an antihistamine

1.3 Which patient group is most at risk of pneumothorax?

    a. Elderly women
    b. Young men
    c. Young women
    d. Elderly men
    e. None of the above

1.4 Which one of the following medicines can cause rebound congestion with overuse?

    a. Pseudoephedrine tablets
    b. Guaifenesin cough mixture
    c. Oxymetazoline nasal spray
    d. Chlorphenamine tablets
    e. Codeine linctus

1.5 Which medicine is drug of choice for nasal congestion caused by allergic rhinitis?

    a. Loratadine
    b. Nasal sodium cromoglicate — *most drowsing*
    c. Azelastine
    d. Nasal beclometasone — *who recommends*
    e. Chlorphenamine

1.6 Which patient group is most likely to suffer from infectious mononucleosis?

    a. Infants
    b. Children
    c. Adolescents
    d. Adults
    e. The elderly

1.7 What symptoms are commonly associated with acute sinusitis? *ask tell where the pain is*

    a. Dull, localised unilateral pain that is often worse on bending down
    b. Dull, localised unilateral pain that often eases on bending down
    c. Dull, diffuse bilateral pain that is often worse on bending down
    d. Dull, diffuse bilateral pain that often eases on bending down
    e. Sharp, localised bilateral pain that often eases on bending down

1.8 The most likely cause of acute cough in children is:

    a. Bacterial infection
    b. Viral infection
    c. Postnasal drip
    d. Croup
    e. Asthma

Questions 9 to 11 concern the following conditions:

A.   Tuberculosis
B.   Left ventricular failure
C.   Chronic bronchitis
D.   Pneumonia
E.   Acute bronchitis

Select in which of the above conditions (A to E):

1.9 Is shortness of breath often the main presenting symptom *B*

1.10 Is cigarette smoking the main cause of the condition *C*

1.11 A higher prevalence is seen in ethnic groups *A*

Questions 12 to 14 concern the following medicines:

A.   Codeine
B.   Phenylpropanolamine
C.   Pholcodine
D.   Beclometasone
E.   Benzydamine

Select, from A to E, which of the above medicines:

1.12 Should be avoided by patients taking beta-blockers

1.13 Can be abused by patients

1.14 Has been linked to causing stroke

Questions 1.15 to 1.17: for each of these questions *one or more* of the responses is (are) correct. Decide which of the responses is (are) correct. Then choose:

A.   If a, b and c are correct
B.   If a and b only are correct
C.   If b and c only are correct
D.   If a only is correct
E.   If c only is correct

Directions summarised

A	B	C	D	E
a, b and c	a and b only	b and c only	a only	c only

1.15 Which of the following symptoms are associated with sinusitis:

a. Localised pain
b. Pain is worsened on bending over
c. Pain is described as throbbing

1.16 A pharmacist should refer patients when the following symptoms are associated with the common cold:

a. Duration of more than 5–7 days
b. If fever is present
c. If middle ear involvement is suspected

1.17 Which of the following precautions should a patient take if he or she suffers from perennial rhinitis:

a. Avoid contact with animals, especially household pets

b. Reduce house dust mite by regular cleaning of carpets
c. Close the windows when in the house

Questions 1.18 to 1.20: these questions consist of a statement in the left-hand column followed by a statement in the right-hand column. You need to:

●   decide whether the first statement is true or false
●   decide whether the second statement is true or false

Then choose:

A.   If both statements are true and the second statement is a correct explanation of the first statement
B.   If both statements are true but the second statement is NOT a correct explanation of the first statement
C.   If the first statement is true but the second statement is false
D.   If the first statement is false but the second statement is true
E.   If both statements are false

Directions summarised

	1st statement	2nd statement	
A	True	True	2nd statement is a correct explanation of the first
B	True	True	2nd statement is not a correct explanation of the first
C	True	False	
D	False	True	
E	False	False	

	First statement	*Second statement*
1.18	Carbimazole can cause a sore throat	Carbimazole is used to treat hypothyroidism
1.19	Conjunctivitis is a common symptom in hay fever sufferers	The redness is concentrated in fornices of the eyes
1.20	Pholcodine is an antitussive	It blocks nerve conduction to the medulla

Case study

Mr RT has asked to speak to the pharmacist as he has a troublesome cough.

a. Discuss the appropriately worded questions you will need to ask Mr RT to determine the seriousness of the cough and to establish whether he can be treated or must be referred. Explain your rationale for each question.

Questions should fall broadly into two groups:

- *Those that relate to the presenting complaint, for example, nature, duration, onset, periodicity, sputum colour (if applicable), associated symptoms, aggravating/alleviating symptoms.*
- *Those that look at the medical, family and social history of the patient: current medication regimen (recent changes to medication or dosage adjustment), self-medication, general well-being of the patient, smoking status.*

Discussion with Mr RT indicates he has a productive cough that appeared a few days ago and the sputum is white. His nose is 'a bit blocked'. He has a headache and he does not have any chest pain. Before you can make a recommendation for the symptoms you identify that he is taking the following medication:

- Manerix 150 mg bd – he has taken this for over 6 months.
- Trusopt tds – he has used this for 2 years.
- Paracetamol 2 qds prn – for lower back pain.

b. Compare and contrast the different products available to treat Mr RT's symptoms and indicate which you consider would be the most beneficial to him and those that are contraindicated.

Information related to products to treat a productive cough with nasal congestion should be sought. This involves expectorant medication and sympathomimetics. Mr RT's current drug regimen will have to be taken into consideration and checks for interactions and suitability made. For example, Mr RT is taking Manerix, therefore sympathomimetics should be avoided.

A few weeks later Mr RT returns to the pharmacy complaining that he is still having trouble clearing his blocked nose. A friend at work recommended Otrivine Nasal Spray.

c. The use of local decongestants is associated with the phenomenon known as rhinitis medicamentosa. Explain what this is and what advice you would give to Mr RT?

Rhinitis medicamentosa relates to the problem of overly long use of topical sympathomimetics. Prolonged use (normally more than 7 days continuous use) results in vascular engorgement of the nose on withdrawal of the medication. Patients often believe mistakenly that symptoms have returned and begin to use the medication again and thus perpetuate the problem. This cycle of overuse has to be broken and explained to patients so that they understand why they have continued nasal congestion. Strategies to relieve the problem are, if appropriate, a switch to systemically administered decongestants or, if this is not appropriate, then on withdrawal of the medication the patient is counselled that the symptoms will initially worsen but then gradually resolve. In Mr RT's case he should be advised not to take the nasal spray because of the risk of a drug interaction between the spray and Manerix.

CASE STUDY 1.2

Ms NR, a female patient (about 30 years old), presents to the pharmacist complaining of a bothersome sore throat. The following information is gained from the patient.

Information Gathering	Data Generated
Presenting complaint (possible questions)	
What symptoms have you got?	Pain when trying to swallow
How long have you had the symptoms?	Had for the last 2 days
Do you have any other symptoms?	Headache
Additional questions asked	
Do you have a temperature?	Not sure
Do you have true difficulty swallowing?	No
Previous history of presenting complaint?	Had cough and cold a few months ago
Past medical history?	Eczema
Drugs (OTC, Rx, and compliance)?	Nothing currently
Allergies?	None known
Social history	
Smoking	
Alcohol	
Drugs	
Employment	
Relationships	No questions asked in relation to social history
Family history	N/A
Examination	Throat appears normal. No ulceration or pus obviously visible using pen torch. Glands do not feel swollen. Running low fever (38°C)

Probability	Cause
Most likely	Viral infection
Likely	Streptococcal infection
Unlikely	Thrush, glandular fever, trauma
Very unlikely	Carcinoma, medicines

Using the information gained from questioning and linking this with known epidemiology on sore throat it should be possible to make a differential diagnosis.

Epidemiology of sore throat suggests that viral sore throat is the most likely cause of sore throat in primary care for all ages. However, other conditions are possible and are noted below:

Continued

CASE STUDY 1.2

Diagnostic Pointers with respect to symptom presentation

Below summarises the expected findings for questions when related to the different conditions that can be seen by community pharmacists.

	Age	Tonsillar/ pharyngeal exudate	Duration	Cervical glands	Cough present	Other symptoms
Viral Infection	Any age	Possible but generally limited	3-7 days	Normal	Common	Low grade fever, headache
Bacterial Infection	School children	Often present and can be substantial	3-7 days	Swollen	Rare	High grade fever, possible rash
Thrush	Young and old	No	5-14 days?	Normal	No	No
Glandular fever	Adolescents	Unlikely	>14 days	Swollen	No	Lethargy
Trauma	Any age	Unlikely	Varies depending on cause	Normal	No	None
Carcinoma	Older people	None	>14 days	Normal?	No?	Dysphagia, ear pain
Medicines	Adults	None	depends	Normal	No	

When this information is applied to the information gained from our patient we see that her symptoms most closely match viral infection or trauma. As epidemiology states viral infection is the most prevalent cause of sore throat it seems likely that this is the cause of her symptoms. Trauma appears less likely due to having no systemic symptoms – a supplementary question about precipitating factors should exclude trauma as a cause.

CASE STUDY 1.2

	Age	Tonsillar/ pharyngeal exudate	Duration	Cervical glands swollen	Cough present	Absence of dysphagia	Systemic upset present
Viral Infection	✓	✓?	✓	✓	✗	✓	✓
Bacterial Infection	✗	✗	✓	✗	✗?	✓	✓?
Thrush	✗	✓	✗?	✓	✓	✓	✗
Glandular fever	✗	✓	✗	✗	✓	✓	✗
Trauma	✓	✓	✓?	✓	✓	✓	✗
Carcinoma	✗	✓	✗	✓	✓	✗	✗
Medicines	N/A	N/A	N/A	N/A	N/A	N/A	N/A

Danger Symptoms/signs (Trigger Points for referral)

As a final double check it might be worth making sure the person has none of the 'referral signs or symptoms. This is the case with this patient.

Adverse drug reaction	✗
Associated skin rash	✗
Duration of more than 2 weeks	✗
Dysphagia	✗
Marked tonsillar exudate accompanied with a high temperature and swollen glands	✗

CASE STUDY 1.3

Mr JL, a man in his early sixties (slightly overweight), wants something for his persistent cough. He has tried some stuff from the supermarket but it did not work. The following information is gained from the patient.

Information gathering	Data generated
Presenting complaint (possible questions)	
Describe symptoms	Cough with a little bit of phlegm
How long have you had the symptoms?	Weeks. Just been there in the background. Not really bothered by it but just doesn't seem to want to go. Saw the GP about 6 weeks ago and was given antibiotics. Seemed to help but the cough came back again
Nature of sputum	Not a lot there really. Seems green/brown
Onset/timing	Not noticed it being better or worse at any time
Other symptoms/provokes	Generally feels off colour and has done for a while
Additional questions	No blood in sputum noticed; no weight loss
Previous history of presenting complaint	Gets coughs and colds from time-to-time but not constantly
Past medical history	GORD, hypothyroidism
Drugs (OTC, Rx and compliance)	Pantoprazole 1 od Thyroxine 100 µg 1 od
Allergies	No allergies known

Information gathering	Data generated
Social history	
Smoking	Drinks most nights down
Alcohol	the club plus smokes 20–40
Drugs	a day.
Employment	Unemployed currently
Relationships	
Family history	Lives on own
On examination	N/A

GORD, gastro-oesophageal reflux disease

Epidemiology of cough suggests that viral sore throat is the most likely cause of cough in primary care for all ages. However, other conditions are possible and are noted below:

Probability	Cause
Most likely	Viral infection
Likely	Postnasal drip, allergies, acute bronchitis
Unlikely	Croup, chronic bronchitis, asthma pneumonia, ACE inhibitor
Very unlikely	Heart failure, bronchiectasis, tuberculosis, cancer, pnuemothorax, lung abscess, nocardiasis, GORD

ACE, angiotensin converting enzyme; GORD, gastro-oesophageal reflux disease.

Using the information gained from questioning and linking this with known epidemiology on cough it should be possible to make a differential diagnosis.

CASE STUDY 1.3

Diagnostic pointers with respect to symptom presentation

Below summarises the expected findings for questions when related to the different conditions that can be seen by community pharmacists.

	Acute or chronic	Sputum	Sputum colour	Age	Systemic symptoms	Worse at any particular time of day?
Viral	Acute	Sometimes	White to green or yellowy	Any	Yes	pm
Postnasal drip	Acute	No	N/A	Adults	No	None
Allergy	Either	No	N/A	Any	No	pm
Acute bronchitis	Acute	Sometimes	White to green or yellowy	Adults	Yes	None
Croup	Acute	No	N/A	Young children	No	pm
Chronic bronchitis	Chronic	Yes	Mucopurulent	> 40	No	am
Asthma	Chronic	Sometimes	Yellow	Any	No	pm
Pneumonia	Acute	Yes	Rust tinged	> 50	Yes	pm
Medication	Either	No	N/A	Adults	No	None
Heart failure	Chronic	Yes	Pink tinged	Elderly	No	pm
Bronchiectasis	Chronic	Yes	Mucopurulent	Adults	No	am & pm
Tuberculosis	Chronic	Yes	Blood present	Any	Yes	None
Carcinoma	Chronic	Yes	Dark red	> 50	No	None
Pneumothorax	Acute	No	N/A	Young adults	No	None
Lung abscess	Chronic	No	N/A	Elderly	Yes	None
Nocardiasis	Chronic	Yes	Mucopurulent	Adults	Yes	None

When this information is applied to the information gained from our patient (opposite table) we see that the conditions that most closely fit with the man's symptoms are chronic bronchitis, tuberculosis or nocardiasis. Based on epidemiology, nocardiasis seems highly unlikely so is it chronic bronchitis or tuberculosis? The man does smoke heavily and this fits with chronic bronchitis but he says that he does not have a repeated history of cough. The patient has felt unwell for 'a while' and this suggests systemic involvement. Although rare, tuberculosis appears to be a possibility and it would seem sensible to refer him to his GP because of the long-standing nature of the symptoms coupled with his general malaise.

Continued

CASE STUDY 1.3

	Acute or chronic	Sputum	Sputum colour (productive only)	Age	Systemic symptoms	Worse at any particular time of day (non-specific answer ?)
Viral	✗	✓?	✗?	✓	✓	?
Postnasal drip	✗	✗	N/A	✓	✗	?
Allergy	✗?	✗	N/A	✓	✗	?
Acute bronchitis	✗	✓	✗?	✓	✓	?
Croup	✗	✗	N/A	✗	✗	?
Chronic bronchitis	✓	✓	✓	✓	✗	?
Asthma	✓	✓?	✓?	✓	✗	?
Pneumonia	✗	✓	✓?	✓	✓	?
Medication	✗?	✗	N/A	N/A	N/A	?
Heart failure	✓	✓	✗	✗	✗	?
Bronchiectasis	✓	✓	✓?	✓	✗	?
Tuberculosis	✓	✓	✓?	✓	✓	?
Carcinoma	✓	✓	✓?	✓	✗	?
Pneumothorax	✗	✗	N/A	✗	✗	?
Lung abscess	✓	✗	N/A	✓	✓	?
Nocardiasis	✓	✓	✓?	✓	✓	?

Answers to multiple choice questions

1 = c,　　2 = b,　　3 = b,　　4 = c,　　5 = d,　　6 = c,　　7 = a,　　8 = b,　　9 = b,　　10 = c,
11 = a,　　12 = b,　　13 = a,　　14 = b,　　15 = b,　　16 = e,　　17 = b,　　18 = c,　　19 = b,　　20 = a.

Ophthalmology

In this chapter

Background

The eye is one of the most important and complex organs of the body. Vision is taken for granted and only when our sight is threatened do we truly appreciate what we have. Because of its complicated and intricate anatomy, many things can and do go wrong with the eye, and these manifest as ocular symptoms to the patient.

It is the pharmacist's role to differentiate between minor self-limiting and serious sight-threatening conditions. For pharmacists to undertake this role they need to be familiar with the gross anatomy of the eye, be able to take an eye history and perform a simple eye examination.

In addition, pharmacists can play a major role in health promotion towards eye care. Patients who present with repeat medication for degenerative conditions, such as glaucoma, could have regular contact with the pharmacist, who could check patient concordance, ability to administer eye drops and ointments correctly and, potentially, discover any deterioration of the patient's condition.

General overview of eye anatomy

A basic understanding of the main eye structures is useful to help pharmacists assess the nature and severity of the presenting complaint. Figure 2.1 highlights the principal eye structures.

The eyelids

The eyelids consist mainly of voluntary muscle with a border of thick connective tissue, known as the tarsal plate. This plate is felt as a ridge when everting the eyelid to remove a foreign body. Covering the inner aspect of the eyelids is the conjunctiva, which continues over the surface of the eye.

The sclera and cornea

The sclera encircles the eye, apart from a small 'window' at the very front of the eye where the cornea is located. The sclera is often referred to as the 'white of the eye'. The transparent cornea allows light to enter the eye and helps to converge light onto the retina.

The iris, pupil and ciliary body

The iris is the coloured part of the eye. It is an incomplete circle, with a hole in the middle, which forms the pupil. The iris attaches to the ciliary body, which serves to hold the lens in place. The ciliary body produces the aqueous, a watery solution that bathes the lens. This is manufactured behind the iris, travels through the posterior chamber and the pupil before draining at the anterior chamber angle (where the iris meets the cornea). If this exit becomes blocked then the intraocular pressure of the eye becomes elevated.

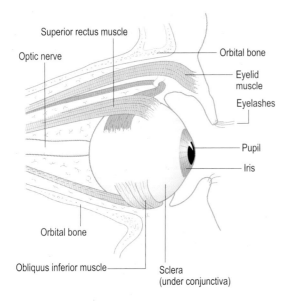

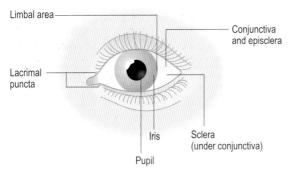

Fig. 2.1　Anatomy of the eye. Above: side view; below: front view

The lens

The lens is responsible for 'fine focusing' light onto the retina. It possesses the ability to vary its focusing power. However, this variable focus power is lost with increasing age as the lens grows harder and less elastic. This is the reason many people require reading glasses as they get older.

The retina

The retina is the light-sensitive layer of the eye; it is the reason for the presence of all the other eye structures. The functioning of the retina can be compromised by many factors, such as underlying disease states, and foreign bodies causing retinal damage and detachment.

History taking and the eye exam

A detailed history should be sought from the patient when attempting to decide on the presenting complaint.

Pay attention to vision, the severity and nature of discomfort and the presence of discharge. Do not forget to ask about any family history of eye disease (e.g. glaucoma) and the person's previous eye and medication history. Answers to these various questions should enable the pharmacist to build up a picture of the problem and arrive at a tentative differential diagnosis.

The history gained should then be supplemented by performing an eye exam. A great deal of information can be learned from a close inspection of the eye. For example, you can check the size of the pupils, their comparative size and reaction to light, the colour of the sclera, the nature of any discharge and if there is any eyelid involvement. It is impossible to agree with a patient's self-diagnosis or for you to differentially diagnose any form of conjunctivitis from behind a counter, however intently you peer at the patient's eye. Pharmacists owe it to their patients to perform a simple eye exam.

The eye can only be examined in good light. This might mean asking the patient to move to an area within the pharmacy where this can be performed. Before performing an eye examination seek the patient's consent and ensure you explain fully what you are about to do.

- First, wash your hands.
- Next, ask the patient to look straight ahead. This allows you to view the pupil, cornea and sclera.
- Then, gently pull down the lower lid and ask the patient to look upwards and to both the left and the right. This enables you to examine the conjunctiva.
- Now ask the patient to look directly into a near light and then to look back at you. This is best performed using a pen-torch. This enables you to examine the reaction of the pupils to light. Any abnormal pupil reaction in the presence of ocular symptoms should always be treated seriously.

You should assess the visual acuity of the patient. Snellen charts (standard charts used to assess visual acuity) will not be available in a community pharmacy; however, you can ask a patient to read small print with the affected eye.

Red eye

Background

Conjunctivitis simply means inflammation of the conjunctva and is characterised by varying degrees of ocular redness, irritation, itching and discharge. Redness of the eye and inflammation of the conjunctiva has been reported as being the most common ophthalmic problem encountered in the Western world. As conjunctivitis (bacterial, viral and allergic forms) is the most common ocular condition encountered by community pharmacists, this section concentrates on recognising the different types of conjunctivitis and differentially diagnosing these from more serious ocular disorders.

Prevalence and epidemiology

The exact prevalence of conjunctivitis is not known, although statistics for GPs show that eye problems account for 2 to 5% of their workload and one small UK community pharmacy-based study found that on average pharmacies saw two cases of red eye per week. Infective (bacterial and viral) red eye accounts for a third of cases seen by GPs with the remainder being allergic in origin; this is not too surprising given that the prevalence of seasonal allergic conjunctivitis (hay fever) in the UK is increasing. Conjunctivitis seems to affect sexes equally and may present in any age of patient although it is more common in children and the elderly. All three types of conjunctivitis are essentially self-limiting, although viral conjunctivitis can be recurrent and persist for many weeks.

Aetiology

The various pathogens that cause bacterial conjunctivitis vary between adults and children. In adults *Staphylococcus* species are most common (over 50% of cases), followed by *Streptococcus pneumoniae* (20%), *Moraxella* species (5%) and *Haemophilus influenzae* (5%). In children, *Streptococcus, Moraxella* and *Haemophilus* are most common. The adenovirus is most commonly implicated in viral conjunctivitis and pollen usually causes seasonal allergic conjunctivitis.

Arriving at a differential diagnosis

Red eye is a presenting complaint of both serious and non-serious causes of eye pathology. Community pharmacists must be able to differentiate between those conditions that can be managed and those that need referral.

Redness of the eye can occur alone or present with accompanying symptoms of pain, discomfort, discharge and loss of visual acuity. Along with an examination of the eye a number of eye-specific questions should always be asked of the patient to aid in diagnosis (Table 2.1).

Clinical features of conjunctivitis

The overwhelming majority of patients presenting to the pharmacy with red eye will have some form of conjunctivitis. Each of the three common types of conjunctivitis has similar but varying symptoms. Each present with the three main symptoms of redness, discharge and discomfort. Table 2.2 and Figures 2.2, 2.3 and 2.4 highlight the similarities and differences in the classical presentations of the three conditions.

Table 2.1
Specific questions to ask the patient: Red eye

Question	Relevance
Discharge present	Most commonly seen in conjunctivitis. Can vary from watery through to mucopurulent, dependent on the form. Mucopurulent discharge is more suggestive of bacterial conjunctivitis especially if the eyes are glued together by discharge in the absence of itching
Visual changes	Any loss of vision or haloes around objects should be viewed with extreme caution, especially if scleral redness is also present
Pain/discomfort/itch	True pain is generally associated with conditions requiring referral, e.g. scleritis, keratitis and acute glaucoma. Pain associated with conjunctivitis is often described as a gritty/foreign body-type pain
Location of redness	Redness concentrated near or around the coloured part of the eye can indicate sinister pathology, for example, uveitis. Generalised redness and redness towards the fornices (corner of the eyes) is more indicative of conjunctivitis. Localised scleral redness can indicate scleritis or episcleritis
Duration	Minor eye problems are usually self-limiting and resolve within a few days. Any ocular redness, apart from subconjunctival haemorrhage, and allergic conjunctivitis that lasts more than 1 week requires referral
Other symptoms	Signs and symptoms of an upper respiratory tract infection point toward a viral cause of conjunctivitis. Vomiting suggests glaucoma

Table 2.2
Symptoms that help to distinguish between the different types of conjunctivitis

	Bacterial *Infection*	Viral	Allergic
Eyes affected	Both, but one eye often affected first by 24–48 hours	Both	Both
Discharge	Purulent	Watery	Watery
Pain	Gritty feeling	Gritty feeling	Itching
Distribution of redness	Generalised and diffuse	Generalised	Generalised but greatest in fornices
Associated symptoms	None commonly	Cough and cold symptoms	Rhinitis (may also have family history of atopy)

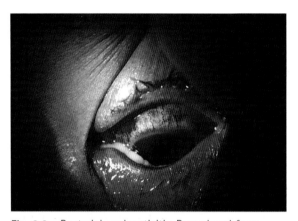

Fig. 2.2 Bacterial conjunctivitis. Reproduced from *Handbook of Ocular Disease Management* by Joseph W Sowka OD, Andrew S Gurwood OD and Alan Kabat OD, Jobson Publishing, with permission

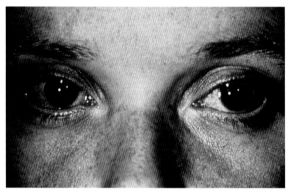

Fig. 2.4 Allergic conjunctivitis. Reproduced from *Handbook of Ocular Disease Management* by Joseph W Sowka OD, Andrew S Gurwood OD and Alan Kabat OD, Jobson Publishing, with permission

Conditions to eliminate

Episcleritis

The episclera lies just beneath the conjunctiva and adjacent to the sclera. If this becomes inflamed the eye appears red, which is segmental affecting only part of the eye (Fig. 2.5). The condition affects only one eye in the majority of cases and is usually painless or a dull ache might be present. It is most commonly seen in young women and is usually self-limiting, but it could take 6 to 8 weeks before symptoms resolve.

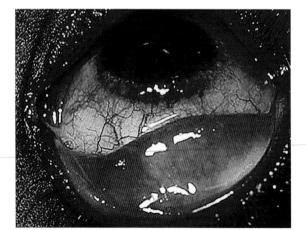

Fig. 2.3 Viral conjunctivitis. Reproduced from *Handbook of Ocular Disease Management* by Joseph W Sowka OD, Andrew S Gurwood OD and Alan Kabat OD, Jobson Publishing, with permission

Scleritis

Inflammation of the sclera is much less common than episcleritis. It is often associated with autoimmune diseases, for example, in 20% of cases the patient has rheumatoid arthritis. It presents similarly to episcleritis but pain is a predominant feature and vision can be affected. Discharge is rare or absent in both episcleritis and scleritis.

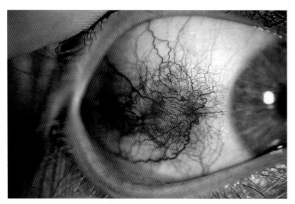

Fig. 2.5 Episcleritis. Reproduced from *Clinical Ophthalmology* by Jack K Kanski, 2007, Butterworth Heinemann, with permission

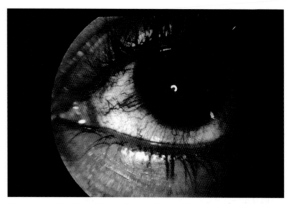

Fig. 2.6 Uveitis. Reproduced from *Handbook of Ocular Disease Management* by Joseph W Sowka OD, Andrew S Gurwood OD and Alan Kabat OD, Jobson Publishing, with permission

Keratitis (corneal ulcer)

Inflammation of the cornea often results from recent trauma (e.g. eye abrasion) or administration of long-term steroid drops. Over wear of soft contact lenses has also been implicated in causing keratitis. Pain, which can be very severe, is a prominent feature. The patient usually complains of photophobia and loss of visual acuity accompanied by a watery discharge. Redness of the eye tends to be worse around the iris. Immediate referral to a medical practitioner is needed as loss of sight is possible if left untreated.

Uveitis (iritis)

Uveitis describes inflammation involving the uveal tract (iris, ciliary body and choroids). The likely cause is an antigen–antibody reaction, which can occur as part of a systemic disease such as rheumatoid arthritis or ulcerative colitis. Photophobia and pain are prominent features along with redness and watering of the eye. Usually, only one eye is affected and the redness is often localised to the limbal area (known as the ciliary flush). On examination, the pupil will appear irregular shaped, constricted or fixed (Fig. 2.6). The patient might also complain of impaired reading vision. Immediate referral to a medical practitioner is needed.

Subconjunctival haemorrhage

The rupture of a blood vessel under the conjunctiva causes subconjunctival haemorrhage. A segment of, or even the whole eye, will appear bright red (Fig. 2.7). It occurs spontaneously but can be precipitated by coughing, straining or lifting. The suddenness of symptoms and the brightness of the blood invariably means patients present very soon after they have noticed the problem. There is no pain and the patient should be reassured that symptoms will resolve in 10 to 14 days without treatment. However, a patient with a history of trauma should be referred to exclude ocular injury.

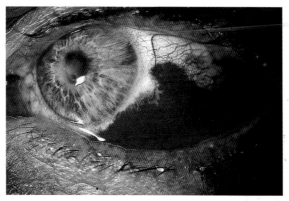

Fig. 2.7 Subconjunctival haemorrhage. Reproduced from *Clinical Ophthalmology*, 2007 by Jack K Kanski, Butterworth Heinemann, with permission

Acute closed-angle glaucoma

There are two main types of glaucoma:

- simple chronic open-angle glaucoma, which does not cause pain
- acute closed-angle glaucoma, which can present with a painful red eye

The latter requires immediate referral to the GP or even casualty. It is due to inadequate drainage of aqueous fluid from the anterior chamber of the eye, which results in an increase in intraocular pressure. The onset can be very quick and characteristically occurs in the evening. The eye appears red and may be cloudy (Fig. 2.8). Vision is blurred and the patient might also notice haloes around lights. Vomiting is often experienced due to the rapid rise in intraocular pressure. As it is such a painful condition, patients are unlikely to present to the community pharmacist.

Figure 2.9 can be used to help differentiate between serious and non-serious red eye conditions.

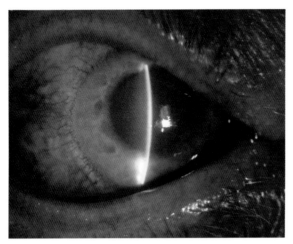

Fig. 2.8 Acute closed-angle glaucoma. Reproduced from *Clinical Ophthalmology*, by Jack K Kanski, 2007, Butterworth Heinemann, with permission

 TRIGGER POINTS indicative of referral: Red eye

- Associated vomiting
- Clouding of the cornea
- Distortion of vision
- Irregular-shaped pupil or abnormal pupil reaction to light
- Photophobia
- Redness caused by a foreign body
- Redness localised around the pupil
- True eye pain

Evidence base for over-the-counter medication

Bacterial conjunctivitis

Bacterial conjunctivitis is regarded as self-limiting – 65% of people will have clinical cure in 2 to 5 days with no treatment – yet antibiotics are routinely given by medical practitioners as they are considered clinically desirable to speed recovery and reduce relapse.

Up until 2005, over-the-counter (OTC) ocular antibiotics consisted of dibromopropamidine isethionate and propamidine. Both compounds are active against a wide range of organisms, including those responsible for bacterial conjunctivitis. However, clinical trials are lacking to substantiate their effectiveness and a further possible limitation is that their licensed dosage regimen (four times a day for drops) has been reported to be too infrequent to achieve sufficient concentrations to kill or stop the growth of the infecting pathogen.

In 2005, chloramphenicol eye drops and in 2007 chloramphenicol ointment were deregulated. Deregulation was probably hindered by case reports linking topical use to cases of aplastic anaemia. However, fears of an association between topical use of chloramphenicol and aplastic anaemia have proven so far to be unfounded. Chloramphenicol has proven efficacy and is currently recommended as first-line treatment in the UK (Prodigy Guidance). However, Rose et al (2005) questioned whether antibiotics were needed in children as no significant difference was seen in the cure rate after 7 days; 86% of the children were clinically cured in the antibiotic group compared with 83% in the placebo group. Even in those children who only had bacterial infection, there was still no significant difference in cure rates. The authors concluded that antibiotics were not needed in children.

Despite the findings from Rose et al the most recent Cochrane review (2006) still concluded that antibiotics are associated with significantly improved clinical rates of remission.

Viral conjunctivitis

Currently, there are no specific OTC preparations available to treat viral conjunctivitis. Chloramphenicol is reported to have some antiviral properties and manufacturer literature advocates its use for any superficial infective conjunctivitis including viral causes, although this is not supported by clinical evidence. As differentiation between bacterial and viral causes of conjunctivitis can be difficult, the use of an antibacterial preparation might be of benefit if uncertainty exists as to the cause of the problem. Viral causes are highly contagious and the pharmacist should instruct the patient to follow strict hygiene measures (e.g. not sharing towels and washing hands), which will help to control the spread of the virus. Current guidance also suggests that if viral conjunctivitis is confirmed, because of its contagious nature, the person should stay off work or school for 2 weeks.

Allergic conjunctivitis

Avoidance of the allergen will, in theory, result in control of symptoms. However, total avoidance is almost impossible and the use of prophylactic medication is usually advocated. The evidence base for mast cell stabilisers, antihistamines and sympathomimetics is discussed in Chapter 1 (page 24).

Practical prescribing and product selection

Prescribing information relating to medication for red eye reviewed in the section 'Evidence base for over-the-counter medication' is discussed and summarised in Table 2.3 and useful tips relating to treatment are given in Hints and Tips Box 2.1.

Products for bacterial conjunctivitis

Chloramphenicol (Optrex Infected Eyes, Brochlor)

Chloramphenicol drops and ointment are licensed for use in children over the age of 2 years. The recommended

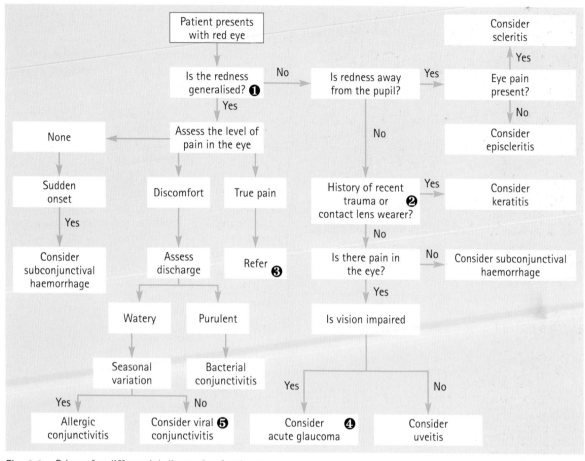

Fig. 2.9   Primer for differential diagnosis of red eye

❶ Generalised redness
Most episodes of conjunctivitis will show generalised redness, although the intensity of redness tends to be worse towards the corners of the eye or away from the pupil. Occasionally, severe conjunctivitis can have marked redness throughout the eye; these cases are best referred.

❷ Contact lens wearers
Contact lens wearers are more predisposed to keratitis because the space between the contact lens and cornea can act as an incubator for bacteria and enhance mechanical abrasion. This is especially true if patients sleep with their lenses in, because contact time for abrasion to occur is prolonged.

❸ True pain
It is important to distinguish true pain from ocular irritation. Red eye caused by conjunctivitis causes discomfort, often described as

gritty or a 'foreign body' sensation. It does not normally cause true eye pain. True pain would indicate more serious ocular pathology, such as scleritis, uveitis or keratitis. It is important to encourage the patient to describe the sensation carefully to enable an accurate assessment of the type of pain experienced.

❹ Glaucoma
This is more common in people aged over 50 years and longsighted people. Dim light can precipitate an attack. It is a medical emergency and immediate referral is needed.

❺ Viral conjunctivitis
Associated symptoms of an upper respiratory tract infection might be present (e.g. cough and cold). Viral conjunctivitis often occurs in epidemics and it is not unusual to see a number of cases in a very short space of time.

dosage for the drops is one drop every 2 hours for the first 48 hours then reducing to four times a day for a maximum of 5 days' treatment. The ointment, if used in conjunction with the drops, should be only applied at night – approximately 1 cm of ointment should be applied to the inside of the eyelid, after which blinking several times will spread the ointment. If used alone, then the ointment should be used three or four times a day. They can be used in most patient groups, although they

should be avoided in pregnancy and breast-feeding, and patients with a family history of blood dyscrasias and glaucoma.

Propamidine isethionate 0.1% (Brolene and Golden Eye drops) and Dibromopropamidine isethionate 0.15% (Brolene and Golden Eye ointment)
Propamidine and dibromopropamidine isethionate are licensed only for adults and children over the age of

Table 2.3
Practical prescribing: Summary of medicines for red eye

Name of medicine	Use in children	Likely side effects	Drug interactions of note	Patients in whom care should be exercised	Pregnancy and breast-feeding
Allergic conjunctivitis Mast cell stabilisers sodium cromoglicate	>12 years	Local irritation, blurred vision	None	None	OK
Antihistamines antazoline	>5 years	Local irritation, bitter taste		Avoid in glaucoma	
Sympathomimetics naphazoline	>12 years	Local irritation	Avoid concomitant use with MAOIs and moclobemide due to risk of hypertensive crisis	None	Not adequately studied but not yet shown to be a risk – probably OK
Bacterial conjunctivitis Chloramphenicol	>2 years	Local burning and stinging	None	Avoid if family history of blood and bone marrow problems	Avoid
Propamidine and dibromopropamidine isethionate	>12 years	Blurred vision	None	None	OK

MAOI, monamine oxidase inhibitor.

HINTS AND TIPS BOX 2.1: EYE DROPS

Contact lens wearers	Patients who wear soft contact lenses should be advised to stop wearing them while treatment continues and for 48 hours afterwards. This is because preservatives in the eye drops can damage the lenses
Brolene and Golden Eye drops	If the patient is instructed to use the drops every 2 hours rather than four times a day then the drops will probably be more efficacious. This is, however, outside their product licences
Choramphenicol drops	These must be stored in the fridge. If they are put into the eye cold it will be uncomfortable so patients should be told to remove them from the fridge prior to use to allow them to warm up to room temperature
Administration of eye drops	1. Wash your hands 2. Tilt your head backwards, until you can see the ceiling 3. Pull down the lower eyelid by pinching outwards to form a small pocket, and look upwards 4. Holding the dropper in the other hand, hold it as near as possible to the eyelid without touching it 5. Place one drop inside the lower eyelid then close your eye 6. Wipe away any excess drops from the eyelid and lashes with the clean tissue 7. Repeat steps 2 to 6 if more than one drop needs to be administered
Administration of eye ointment	1. Repeat eye drop steps 1 and 2 2. Pull down the lower eyelid 3. Place a thin line of ointment along the inside of the lower eyelid 4. Close your eye and move the eyeball from side to side 5. Wipe away any excess ointment from the eyelids and lashes using the clean tissue 6. After using ointment, your vision may be blurred but will soon be cleared by blinking

2

12 years. The dose for eye drops is one or two drops up to four times daily, whereas the ointment should be applied once or twice daily. If there has been no significant improvement after 2 days the person should be referred to a GP. Blurring of vision on instillation may occur but is transient. The manufacturers state that use in pregnancy has not been established but there appear to be no reports of teratogenic effects and therefore these products could be used in pregnancy if deemed appropriate. They are free from drug interactions and can be given to all patient groups.

Products for allergic conjunctivitis

Mast cell stabilisers (sodium cromoglicate)

Intraocular sodium cromoglicate (e.g. Opticrom Allergy, Optrex Allergy) is a prophylactic agent and therefore has to be given continuously when the person is exposed to the allergen. One or two drops should be administered in each eye four times a day. Clinical experience has shown it to be safe in pregnancy and expert opinion considers sodium cromoglicate to be safe in breast-feeding. It has no drug interactions and can be given to all patient groups. Instillation of the drops may cause a transient blurring of vision.

Sympathomimetics

These agents can be used to reduce redness of the eye. Products either contain a combination of sympathomimetic and antihistamine (Otrivine Antistin) or sympathomimetic alone (e.g. Naphazoline 0.01%, Murine, Optrex Red Eyes Eye Drops). They should be limited to short term use (5 days) as prolonged use leads to rebound effects. Like all sympathomimetics they can interact with monoamine oxidase inhibitors and should not be used by patients receiving such treatment or within 14 days of ceasing therapy.

Otrivine Antistin

Adults and children over 5 years old should administer Otrivine Antistin twice or three times a day; one drop for children 5 to 12 years old and one or two drops for adults. Patients with glaucoma should avoid this product due to the potential of the antihistamine component to increase intraocular pressure. Local transient irritation and a bitter taste after application have been reported.

Naphazoline

The use of products containing naphazoline is restricted to adults and children over the age of 12 years. One to two drops should be administered into the eye four times a day.

Further reading

Elton M. Conjunctivitis and chloramphenicol. Pharm J 2005;274:725–8.

Everitt HA, Little PS, Smith PW. A randomised controlled trial of management strategies for acute infective conjunctivitis in general practice. BMJ 2006;333:321.

Kanski JJ, Bolton A. Illustrated tutorials in clinical ophthalmology. Oxford: Butterworth-Heinemann; 2001.

Khaw PT, Elkington AR. ABC of eyes. London: BMJ Publishing Group; 1999.

Rose PW, Harnden A, Brueggemann AB, et al. Chloramphenicol treatment for acute infective conjunctivitis in children in primary care: a randomised double blind placebo controlled trial. Lancet 2005;366:37–43.

Sheikh A, Hurwitz B. Antibiotics versus placebo for acute bacterial conjunctivitis. Cochrane Database of Systematic Reviews 2006, issue 2.

Titcomb L. Over-the counter ophthalmic preparations. Pharm J 2000;264:212–8.

Web sites

Prodigy Guidance: http://www.cks.library.nhs.uk/conjunctivitis_infective

International Glaucoma Association: http://www.iga.org.uk

Uveitis Information Group: http://www.uveitis.net/

Eyelid disorders

Background

A number of disorders can afflict the eyelids, ranging from mild dermatitis to malignant tumours. In the context of community pharmacy consultations, the most common presenting conditions will be blepharitis, hordeola (styes) and chalazion.

Prevalence and epidemiology

Data on the incidence or prevalence of eyelid disorders are limited yet clinical practice suggests that all three conditions are frequently encountered. For example, blepharitis has been reported to account for 5% of primary care ophthalmic consultations and to affect both sexes equally.

Aetiology

Blepharitis is classified into three categories that reflect the aetiology of the condition: staphylococcal, seborrhoeic and meibomian gland dysfunction. Further classification of blepharitis is sometimes used based on anatomical location. For example, anterior blepharitis refers to staphylococcal and seborrhoeic causes as they primarily affect the bases of the eyelashes. Posterior blepharitis refers to meibomian gland dysfunction as these are situated on the posterior lid. However, patients with blepharitis do show overlapping signs and symptoms that suggest mixed aetiology. Furthermore, it appears that many blepharitis sufferers also have dry eye syndrome but the exact relationship between the two conditions is unclear.

Styes are caused by bacterial infection (staphylococcal in 90 to 95% of cases) and can either be internal or external. External styes occur on the outside surface of the eyelid and are due to an infected gland, either the Zeis gland (a type of sebaceous gland) or the gland of Moll (a type of sweat gland), both of which are located near the base of the eyelashes. An internal hordeolum is a secondary infection of the meibomian gland in the tarsal plate. Occasionally, internal styes can evolve into a chalazion, a granulomatous inflammation that develops into a painless lump.

Arriving at a differential diagnosis

Blepharitis and hordeola should be relatively straightforward to recognise, so long as a careful history, eye exam and appropriate questioning are undertaken (Table 2.4).

Clinical features of blepharitis

Typically, blepharitis is bilateral with symptoms ranging from irritation to itching and burning of the lid margins. Lid margins may appear red and raw accompanied by excessive tearing and crusty debris or skin flakes around the eyelashes. Symptoms also tend to be worse in the mornings and patients might complain of eyelids being stuck together (Fig. 2.10). In chronic cases, madarosis (missing lashes) and trichiasis (inturned lash) can occur. This latter symptom can lead to further local irritation and result in conjunctivitis. Seborrhoeic aetiology is likely if greasy crusting of the lashes and oily scale predominates compared to eyelash loss or misdirection, which suggests staphylococcal cause.

Clinical features of styes

Patients with external styes present with a swollen upper or lower lid, which will be painful and sensitive to touch. Over time the swelling develops into a pus-filled lesion. The lesion will then either spontaneously shrink and resolve or burst over the next few days (Fig. 2.11). The primary symptoms of an internal stye are as for external styes (pain, redness and swelling), although pain is often more severe and pus-filled lesions are not obvious due to inward growth.

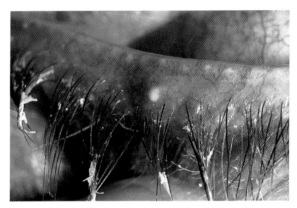

Fig. 2.10 Blepharitis. Reproduced from *Clinical Ophthalmology* by Jack K Kanski, 2007, Butterworth Heinemann, with permission

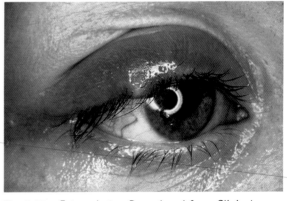

Fig. 2.11 External stye. Reproduced from *Clinical Ophthalmology*, by Jack K Kanski, 2007, Butterworth Heinemann, with permission

Table 2.4
Specific questions to ask the patient: The eyelid

Question	Relevance
Duration	A long-standing history of sore eyes is indicative of blepharitis, a chronic, persistent condition, although it can be intermittent with periods of remission
Lid involvement	If the majority of the lid margin is inflamed and red then this suggests blepharitis. Hordeola tend to show localised lid involvement
Eye involvement	Conjunctivitis is a common complication in blepharitis
Other coexisting conditions	Patients who suffer from blepharitis often have a coexisting skin condition such as seborrhoeic dermatitis or rosacea

Conditions to eliminate for blepharitis and styes

Contact or irritant dermatitis

Many products – especially cosmetics – can be sensitising and result in itching and flaking skin that mimics blepharitis. The patient should be questioned about recent use of such products to allow dermatitis to be eliminated. For further information on dermatitis see Chapter 7, page 226.

Blepharitis unresponsive to therapy

If the patient fails to respond to OTC treatment, or the condition recurs, then it is possible that other causes such as rosacea might be responsible for the symptoms. If OTC treatment has failed then GP referral is needed.

Orbital cellulitis

Inflammation of the skin surrounding the orbit of the eye is usually a complication from a sinus infection, although in extreme cases of stye the infection can spread to involve the entire lid and even the periorbital tissues. The patient will present with unilateral swollen eyelids, be unwell and might show restricted eye movements. This has to be referred immediately because blindness is a potential complication.

Chalazion

A chalazion forms when the meibomian gland becomes blocked, and could be confused with a stye. Styes often have a 'head' of pus at the lid margin and will be tender and sore, whereas a chalazion presents as a painless lump. This should be clearly visible if the eyelid is everted. A chalazion is self-limiting, although it might take a few weeks to resolve completely. No treatment is needed unless the patient complains that it is particularly bothersome and is affecting vision. In these circumstances referral is needed for surgical removal.

Entropion

Entropion is defined as inversion of the eyelid margin. It can occur unilaterally or bilaterally, and the lower eyelid is more frequently affected. The in-turning of the eyelid causes the eyelashes to be pushed against the cornea, resulting in ocular irritation and conjunctival redness (Fig. 2.12). Referral is needed for surgical repair to correct the problem. Taping down the lower lid to draw the eyelid margin away from the eye is sometimes employed as a temporary solution.

Ectropion

Ectropion is the converse to entropion. The eyelid turns outwards exposing the conjunctiva and cornea to the atmosphere (Fig. 2.13). Patients will often present

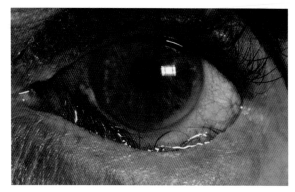

Fig. 2.12 Entropion. Reproduced from *Clinical Ophthalmology* by Jack K Kanski, 2007, Butterworth Heinemann, with permission

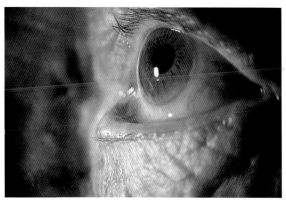

Fig. 2.13 Ectropion. Reproduced from *Clinical Ophthalmology*, by Jack K Kanski, 2007, Butterworth Heinemann, with permission

complaining of a continually watering eye. Paradoxically, this can lead to dryness of the eye, as the eye is not receiving adequate lubrication.

Basal cell carcinoma

This is the commonest form of eyelid malignancy and accounts for over 90% of cases. The lesion is usually nodular with a reddish hue (due to permanent capillary dilation) and most frequently affects the lower lid margin. No pain or discomfort is present. Long-term exposure to the sun is the main cause and for further information on sun-induced skin damage see Chapter 7, page 232.

 TRIGGER POINTS indicative of referral: Blepharitis and styes

- Chalazion that becomes bothersome to the patient
- Inward or outward turning lower eyelid
- Middle aged/elderly patient with painless nodular lesion on or near eyelid
- Patient with swollen eyelids and associated feelings of being unwell

Evidence base for over-the-counter medication

OTC medication is generally not required for blepharitis or styes. No specific products are available and both can respond well to conservative treatment, such as warm compresses.

Practical prescribing and product selection

Blepharitis

The mainstay of treatment for blepharitis is improved lid hygiene. A mild shampoo, such as baby shampoo, is advocated. First the eyelids should be cleaned using a warm compress for 10 minutes. A diluted mixture of baby shampoo should then be applied to the eyelids using a cotton bud. This should be done twice a day initially and can be reduced to once a day if symptoms improve. Failure to respond to hygiene measures requires GP referral for topical antibiotics such as fusidic acid gel applied twice a day or even systemic treatment with oxytetracycline, especially if blepharitis is associated with rosacea.

Styes

Although styes are caused by bacterial pathogens the use of antibiotic therapy is not usually needed. Topical application of ocular antibiotics does not result in speedier symptom resolution but it might prevent a subsequent staphylococcal infection from a lash lower down. A warm compress applied three or four times a day might bring to a head an external stye and, once burst, the pain will subside and the symptoms resolve. The use of dibromopropamidine has been advocated in the treatment of styes but is of unproven benefit.

Further reading
Miller KV, Odufuwa TOB, Liew G, Anderson KL. Interventions for blepharitis. (Protocol) Cochrane Database of Systematic Reviews 2005, issue 4.
Shields SR. Managing eye disease in primary care. Postgrad Med 2000;108:83–6, 91–6.

Web sites
Handbook of Ocular Disease Management: http://www.revoptom.com/handbook/hbhome.htm

Dry eye (keratoconjunctivitis sicca)

Background

Dry eye is a frequent cause of eye irritation causing varying degrees of discomfort, which leads patients to seek medical care. The condition is chronic with no cure.

Prevalence and epidemiology

The exact prevalence of dry eye is unclear due to a lack of consistency in its definition coupled with few population-based studies that used differing criteria for diagnosis. What is clear though is that dry eye syndrome is common. Almost 3% of older adults will develop dry eye each year; it is more common in women than men and is more often associated with people in poor health.

Aetiology

Essentially, a reduction in tear volume or alteration in tear composition causes dry eyes. Underproduction of tears can be the result of increased evaporation from the eye, increased tear drainage and a decrease in tear production by the lacrimal gland. Tear composition is complex; the tear film is made up from three distinct layers:

- innermost mucin layer, which allows tears to adhere to the conjunctival surface
- middle aqueous layer, containing 90% of the tear thickness
- outermost, lipid layer, which helps to slow aqueous layer evaporation

A reduction in any of these layers can lead to dryness but, frequently, the mucin layer is affected due to a reduction in the mucin-producing globlet cells.

Arriving at a differential diagnosis

There are a number of conditions that can cause dry eye; however, keratoconjunctivitis sicca accounts for the vast majority of dry eye cases. From a community pharmacist's perspective many patients will want to buy artificial tears, and good practice would dictate that the pharmacist enquires whether the patient has been instructed from their GP or optician to buy these products or whether this is a self-diagnosis. If it is a self-diagnosis the pharmacist should eliminate underlying pathology and ask a number of eye-specific questions to determine if the self-diagnosis is correct (Table 2.5).

Clinical features of dry eye

Usually affecting both eyes, symptoms reported are eyes that burn, feel tired, itchy, irritated or gritty. The conjunctiva is not red unless irritated (e.g. eye rubbing or allergy). Decreased tear production results in irritation and burning.

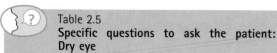

Table 2.5
Specific questions to ask the patient: Dry eye

Question	Relevance
Clarifying questions	• Have you had daily, persistent, troublesome dry eyes for more than 3 months? • Do you have a recurrent sensation of sand or gravel in the eyes? A positive response to at least one of these questions would indicate dry eye syndrome
Aggravating factors	Dry eye is worsened by dry air, wind, dust and smoke
Associated symptoms	Normally no other symptoms are present in dry eye. If the patient complains of a dry mouth, check for medication that can cause dry mouth. If medication is not implicated then symptoms could be due to an autoimmune disease
Amount of tears produced	If the patient complains of watery eyes but states that the eyes are dry and sore, check for ectropion

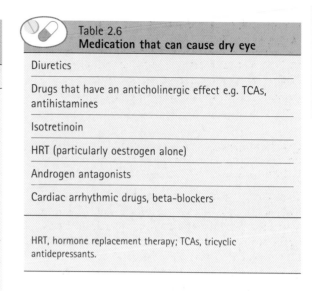

Table 2.6
Medication that can cause dry eye

Diuretics

Drugs that have an anticholinergic effect e.g. TCAs, antihistamines

Isotretinoin

HRT (particularly oestrogen alone)

Androgen antagonists

Cardiac arrhythmic drugs, beta-blockers

HRT, hormone replacement therapy; TCAs, tricyclic antidepressants.

Conditions to eliminate

Blepharitis

Chronic disease of eyelashes, eyelids or margins of eyelids can lead to irritation of the conjunctiva. See page 48 for more information on blepharitis.

Sjögren's syndrome

This syndrome has unknown aetiology but is associated with rheumatic conditions. It occurs in the same patient population as keratoconjunctivitis sicca: elderly patients and more commonly in women. The patient does not have a history of chronic dry eyes but experiences periods of exacerbation and remission. It is also associated with dryness of other mucous membranes such as the mouth. Criteria for diagnosing and classifying Sjögren's syndrome have been proposed (Viteli 2002).

Medicine-induced dry eye

A number of medicines can exacerbate or produce side effects of dry eyes as a result of decreased tear production (Table 2.6). If medication could be causing dry eyes then the pharmacist should contact the GP to discuss possible alternative therapies to alleviate the problem.

Ectropion

Sometimes the lower eyelid turns outward. This overexposes the conjunctiva to the atmosphere leading to eye dryness. For further information see page 49.

Roasacea

Rosacea is a disease of the skin and eye characterised by facial skin findings including erythema, telangiectasia, papules and pustules that mimic acne vulgaris, although many patients also suffer from marginal blepharitis and keratoconjunctivitis sicca. Those patients with rosacea should be questioned about eye involvement to maximise treatment.

Bell's palsy

Bell's palsy is characterised by unilateral facial paralysis, often with sudden onset. A complication of Bell's palsy is that the patient might be unable to close one eye or blink, leading to a decreased tear film and dry eye.

TRIGGER POINTS indicative of referral: Dry eye

- Associated dryness of mouth and other mucous membranes
- Outward turning lower eyelid

Evidence base for over-the-counter medication

Dry eyes are managed by the instillation of artificial tears and lubricating ointments. Products in the UK consist of hypromellose (0.3 to 1.0%), polyvinyl alcohol, carmellose, carbomer 980 and wool fats.

Despite a lack of published trial data, hypromellose products have been in use for over half a century. They possess film-forming and emollient properties but unfortunately do not have ideal wetting characteristics, which results in up to hourly administration to provide adequate relief.

This disadvantage of frequent installation has led to the development of other products. Polyvinyl alcohol in a concentration of 1.4% acts as a viscosity enhancer. At this concentration the products have the same surface tension as normal tears, lending them optimal wetting characteristics and hence less frequent dosing, typically four times a day. Similarly to hypromellose there is a lack of published data confirming their efficacy.

More recently, a synthetic high molecular weight polymer, known as carbomer, has been introduced. Carbomer has been shown to be more efficacious than placebo and as safe as, but better tolerated, than polyvinyl alcohol. In a comparison study between two proprietary brands, Viscotears and GelTears, both were found to be equally effective although neither was significantly better than the other.

Summary

Despite hypromellose lacking trial evidence, its place in the management of dry eye is well established. In addition, it is very cheap and should therefore be recommended as a first-line treatment. However, other newer products, which possess better wetting characteristics, provide useful alternatives to hypromellose because they can be administered less frequently; these products are more expensive.

Practical prescribing and product selection

Prescribing information relating to medication for dry eye that is reviewed in the section 'Evidence base for over-the-counter medication' is discussed and summarised in Table 2.7 and useful tips on medication are given in Hints and Tips Box 2.2.

The dosage of all products marketed for dry eye is largely dependent on the patient's need for lubrication, and is therefore given on a when required basis. None of these products is known to interact with any medicine, they cause minimal and transient side effects and are suitable for all patient groups.

Hypromellose

Hypromellose is widely available as a non-proprietary medicine in a strength of 0.3%; it is also available at 0.5% (Isopto Plain) and 1% (Isopto Alkaline). It might require hourly or even half-hourly dosing initially, which should reduce as symptoms improve. Hypromellose is pharmacologically inert and all patient groups should be

Table 2.7
Practical prescribing: Summary of medicines for dry eye

Name of medicine	Use in children	Likely side effects	Drug interactions of note	Patients in whom care should be exercised	Pregnancy and breast-feeding
Hypromellose Carbomer 940	Can be given but dry eye in children rare. Patients should be referred	Transient stinging and/or burning reported. Blurred vision after instillation of carbomer and polyvinyl alcohol	None	None	OK
Polyvinyl alcohol Wool fats		None	None	None	OK

HINTS AND TIPS BOX 2.2: DRY EYE

Preservatives in eye drops	Many eye drops contain benzalkonium chloride, which itself can cause eye irritation. If symptoms persist or are worsened by the eye drops it may be worth trying a preservative-free formulation
	Prodigy guidance recommends that if more than six applications per day are necessary a preservative-free formulation should be used to overcome ocular irritation

able to use it safely, including pregnant and breast-feeding women. However, because of a lack of data, some manufacturers err on the side of caution and recommend that it should be avoided.

Polyvinyl alcohol

Two proprietary products are available; Liquifilm Tears and Sno Tears. The standard dose is four times a day. Liquifilm is also available as a preservative-free formulation. It can be given to all patient groups.

Carbomer (e.g. GelTears, Liposic, Liquivisc, Viscotears)

Manufacturers recommend that adults and the elderly use one drop three or four times a day or as required, depending upon patient need. Owing to the product's viscosity, carbomer should be used last if other eye drops need to be instilled. Data are limited for use in pregnancy and lactation and so manufacturers advise avoidance.

Lubricants (wool fats e.g. Lacri-Lube, Lubri-Tears and Simple Eye Ointment)

These products contain a mixture of white soft paraffin, liquid paraffin and wool fat. They are useful at bedtime when prolonged lubrication is needed but because they blur vision are unsuitable during the day. They are pharmacologically inert and can be used in pregnancy and breast-feeding.

Further reading

Brodwall J, Alme G, Gedde-Dahl S, et al. A comparative study of polyacrylic acid [Viscotears] liquid gel versus polyvinylalcohol in the treatment of dry eyes. Acta Ophthalmol Scand 1997;75:457-61.

Bron AJ, Daubas P, Siou-Mermet R, et al. Comparison of the efficacy and safety of two eye gels in the treatment of dry eyes: Lacrinorm and Viscotears. Eye 1998;12:839-47.

Moss SE, Klein R, Klein BEK. Incidence of dry eye in an older population. Arch Ophthalmol 2004;122:369-73.

Sullivan LJ, McCurrach F, Lee S, et al. Efficacy and safety of 0.3% carbomer gel compared to placebo in patients with moderate to severe dry eye syndrome. Ophthalmology 1997;104:1402-8.

Viteli C, Bombardieri S, Jonsson R, et al. Classification criteria for Sjogren's syndrome: a revised version of the European criteria proposed by the American-European Consensus Group. Ann Rheum Dis 2002;61:554-8.

Web sites

Prodigy Guidance: http://www.prodigy.nhs.uk/dry_eye_syndrome/view_whole_guidance

Article on dry eye syndrome from emedicine.com: http://www.emedicine.com/oph/topic597.htm

Report on dry eye syndrome from the American Academy of Ophthalmologists: http://www.aao.org/education/library/ppp/dryeye_new.cfm

2

Self-assessment questions

The following questions are intended to supplement the text. Two levels of questions are provided: multiple choice questions and case studies. The multiple choice questions are designed to test factual recall and the case studies allow knowledge to be applied to a practice setting.

Multiple choice questions

2.1 Which of the following would be the *most* appropriate course of action for a patient with a chalazion?

    a. Instillation of Brolene eye drops four times a day
    b. Bathing with salt water three times a day
    c. Application of Golden Eye ointment twice a day
    d. No treatment
    e. Referral to the GP

2.2 Basal cell carcinoma usually affects?

    a. The upper eyelid
    b. The lower lid margin
    c. Upper and lower eyelids equally
    d. The lower lid margin and eye itself
    e. The eye only

2.3 How can visual acuity be assessed in the community pharmacy?

    a. By checking the reaction of the pupils to light
    b. Getting the patient to walk in a straight line
    c. Getting the patient to read print from a book
    d. Getting the patient to read distant print
    e. None of the above

2.4 Which one of the following medicines can cause dry eyes?

    a. Pseudoephedrine
    b. Atenolol
    c. Codeine
    d. Isotretinoin
    e. Pantoprazole

2.5 Symptoms of blurred vision and eye pain that is associated with onset in the evening suggests:

    a. Episcleritis
    b. Keratitis
    c. Uveitis
    d. Glaucoma
    e. Viral conjunctivitis

2.6 In which of the following conditions is severe eye pain experienced?

    a. Subconjunctival haemorrhage
    b. Episcleritis
    c. Keratitis
    d. Ectropion
    e. Viral conjunctivitis

2.7 What viral pathogen is responsible for the majority of viral conjunctivitis cases?

    a. The rhinovirus
    b. The Epstein-Barr virus
    c. The adenovirus
    d. The Norwalk-like virus
    e. The rotavirus

2.8 Subconjunctival haemorrhage is associated with?

    a. A segment or whole eye appearing bright red and no pain
    b. A segment or whole eye appearing bright red and with pain
    c. A segment of the eye only that appears pale red and no pain
    d. A segment of the eye only that appears bright red and with pain
    e. Ciliary flush

Questions 2.9 to 2.11 concern the following conditions:

A. A clear, watery discharge
B. Haloes seen around bright lights
C. Soreness of the surface of the eye
D. A small, hard lump under the skin of the upper lid
E. Grittiness and burning of the eyes in an elderly patient

Select from A to E which of the above statements relate to the following conditions:

2.9 Acute closed-angle glaucoma

2.10 Chalazion

2.11 Allergic conjunctivitis

Questions 2.12 to 2.14 concern the following OTC medications:

A. Hypromellose
B. Naphalazine
C. Carbomer 940
D. Dibromopropamide isethionate
E. Lodoxamide

Select, from A to E, which of the above medicines:

2.12 Is used to treat allergic conjunctivitis

2.13 Can cause rebound conjunctivitis

2.14 May require hourly administration

Questions 2.15 to 2.17: for each of these questions *one or more* of the responses is (are) correct. Decide which of the responses is (are) correct. Then choose:

A. If a, b and c are correct
B. If a and b only are correct
C. If b and c only are correct
D. If a only is correct
E. If c only is correct

Directions summarised

A	B	C	D	E
a, b and c	a and b only	b and c only	a only	c only

2.15 Which condition(s) are associated with autoimmune disease?

   a. Scleritis
   b. Keratitis
   c. Glaucoma

2.16 Subconjunctival haemorrhage is characterised by:

   a. An eye that is red and bloodshot
   b. No pain
   c. Sudden onset

2.17 Patients with dry eye syndrome usually present with:

   a. Itchy/sore eyes
   b. Associated red eye
   c. A long-standing history of dry eye

Questions 2.18 to 2.20: these questions consist of a statement in the left-hand column followed by a statement in the right-hand column. You need to:

● decide whether the first statement is true or false
● decide whether the second statement is true or false

Then choose:

A. If both statements are true and the second statement is a correct explanation of the first statement
B. If both statements are true but the second statement is NOT a correct explanation of the first statement
C. If the first statement is true but the second statement is false
D. If the first statement is false but the second statement is true
E. If both statements are false

Directions summarised

	1st statement	2nd statement	
A	True	True	2nd statement is a correct explanation of the first
B	True	True	2nd statement is not a correct explanation of the first
C	True	False	
D	False	True	
E	False	False	

	First statement	*Second statement*
2.18	Conjunctivitis is caused by infection only	Inflammation of the conjunctiva tends to be away from the pupil
2.19	Ectropion should be referred	It requires surgical intervention
2.20	Blepharitis can cause red eye	Skin flaking results in direct conjunctival irritation

Case study

CASE STUDY 2.1

Mrs JR, a 32-year-old women, asks you for something to treat her 'sore eyes'. She doesn't wear contact lenses.

a. What questions you would ask Mrs JR and what observations would you make of her eyes to help you to diagnose her eye condition?

Questions should fall broadly into two groups:

- *General questions: duration, onset, medication, family history*
- *More specific questions: degree of discomfort, whether there is any discharge, if there have been any changes to vision, if the patient has experienced previous episodes*

You perform a physical examination.

b. What signs or symptoms would cause you to refer Mrs JR, rather than recommend OTC treatment?

- *True eye pain*
- *Sudden distortion of vision*
- *Photophobia*
- *Associated vomiting*
- *Clouding of the cornea*
- *Irregular-shaped pupil*
- *Redness localised around the pupil*
- *Redness caused by a foreign body*
- *Patient with swollen eyelids and associated feelings of being unwell*
- *Inward or outward turning lower eyelid*

You decide that Mrs JR appears to be suffering from allergic conjunctivitis.

c. What OTC preparations are available to treat allergic conjunctivitis?

- *First line: topical mast cell stabilisers*
- *Second line: systemic antihistamines*

CASE STUDY 2.2

Mr DP, a man in his early fifties, presents at lunchtime to the pharmacy with a bright red eye. He wants to ease the redness. The following questions are asked, and responses received.

Information gathering	Data generated
Presenting complaint (possible questions)	
Describe symptoms	Left eye in the lower half of the sclera. Bright red and no blood vessels visible
How long have you had the symptoms	Since mid-morning
Type/severity of pain	None
Other symptoms/ provokes	None
Discharge	None
Additional questions	Done nothing different at work (builder) than he would usually do
Previous history of presenting complaint	No
Past medical history	Takes blood pressure medicines but cannot remember their name
Drugs (OTC, Rx and compliance)	Rennies for indigestion now and then
Allergies	None known
Social history Smoking Alcohol Drugs Employment Relationships	Smokes (10–15 cigarettes a day) and has a pint or two on most days

Information gathering	Data generated
Family history	No history of eye problems in the family (mum and dad)
On examination	Acuity OK. Pupil reaction normal

Epidemiology of red eye suggests that bacterial or allergic conjunctivitis are the most likely causes in primary care. However, other conditions are possible and are noted below:

Probability	Cause
Most likely	Bacterial or allergic conjunctivitis
Likely	Viral conjunctivitis, subconjunctival haemorrhage
Unlikely	Episcleritis, scleritis, keratitis, uveitis
Very unlikely	Acute closed-angle glaucoma

Using the information gained from questioning and linking this with known epidemiology on red eye it should be possible to make a differential diagnosis.

Diagnostic pointers with regard to symptom presentation

The following page summarises the expected findings for questions when related to the different conditions that can be seen by community pharmacists.

Continued

CASE STUDY 2.2

	Discharge	Pain	Visual disturbance	Pupil reflex	Eyes affected	Redness
Conjunctivitis – bacterial	Yes, often mucopurulent	Sore, gritty	No	OK	1 or both	Generalised redness
Conjunctivitis – viral	Yes, sometimes watery	Sore, gritty	No	OK	1 or both	Generalised redness
Conjunctivitis – allergic	Yes, watery	Very itchy	No	OK	Both	Worse in fornices
Subconjunctival haemorrhage	No	No	No	OK	Either	Segmental
Episcleritis	No	Little or none	No	OK	1	Segmental
Scleritis	No	Yes	No	OK	1	Segmental
Keratitis	Watery	Yes, severe	Photophobia	Abnormal	1	Around iris
Uveitis	No	Painful	Photophobia	Abnormal	1	Around iris
Glaucoma	No	Yes, severe	Blurred	Abnormal	1	Haloes (vomiting)

When this information is applied to that gained from our patient (below) we see that his symptoms most closely match subconjunctival haemorrhage or episcleritis. Looking at the presenting history and considering the patient's sex then subconjunctival haemorrhage is most likely (episcleritis is more common in women and is not seen as an 'injection' of bright red blood in the eye). Subconjunctival haemorrhage also has a very sudden onset and fits with the patient's symptoms.

	Discharge	Absence of true pain	Visual disturbance	Pupil reflex	Eyes affected	Redness
Conjunctivitis – bacterial	✗	✓	✓	✓	✓	✓
Conjunctivitis – viral	✗	✓	✓	✓	✓	✓
Conjunctivitis – allergic	✗	✓	✓	✓	✓	✓
Subconjunctival haemorrhage	✓	✓	✓	✓	✓	✓
Episcleritis	✓	✓	✓	✓	✓	✓
Scleritis	✓	✗	✓	✓	✓	✓
Keratitis	✗	✗	✗	✗	✓	✗
Uveitis	✓	✗	✗	✗	✓	✗
Glaucoma	✓	✗	✗	✗	✓	✗

CASE STUDY 2.2

Danger symptoms/signs (trigger points for referral)

As a final double check it might be worth making sure the person has none of the 'referral signs or symptoms', which is the case with this patient.

Associated vomiting	✗
Clouding of the cornea	✗
Distortion of vision	✗
Irregular-shaped pupil or abnormal pupil reaction to light	✗
Photophobia	✗
Redness caused by a foreign body	✗
Redness localised around the pupil	✗
True eye pain	✗

CASE STUDY 2.3

Mrs MS asks for your advice for her 14-year-old daughter. Emma has a sore and red eye.

Questioning reveals that:

- Emma has had the symptoms for 2 to 3 days.
- The redness is located away from the coloured part of the eye.
- There is a slight discharge, although Emma has not noticed much colour in the discharge.
- Her eye feels slightly gritty.
- Her other eye is a little red but not as red as the problem eye.
- She is complaining of slight headaches around her eyes.
- She has taken nothing for the problem and only takes erythromycin for acne from the GP.

- She has not had these types of symptoms before.

Using the information in case study 2.2, what do you think is wrong with her?

Differential diagnosis of bacterial or viral conjunctivitis.

What action are you going to take?

Instigate antibacterial eye drops (e.g. chloramphenicol) and give advice about hygiene measures. If eye drops fail to resolve symptoms after 48 hours then refer for further evaluation. In this instance the patient has been appropriately treated for bacterial conjunctivitis and hygiene measures will hopefully help if it were viral conjunctivitis.

Answers to multiple choice questions									
1 = d	2 = b	3 = c	4 = d	5 = d	6 = c	7 = c	8 = a	9 = b	10 = d
11 = a	12 = e	13 = b	14 = a	15 = d	16 = a	17 = a	18 = d	19 = a	20 = a.

Ear conditions

Background

Currently, community pharmacists can only offer help to patients with conditions that affect the external ear and this chapter therefore concentrates on external ear problems. However, with appropriate training and further POM to P deregulation of medicines, it is not unrealistic to extend the community pharmacists' role to include middle ear problems.

General overview of ear anatomy

The external ear consists of the pinna (Fig. 3.1) and the external auditory meatus (ear canal). Their function is to collect and transmit sound to the tympanic membrane (eardrum).

The pinna consists chiefly of cartilage and has a firm elastic consistency. The external auditory meatus (EAM) opens behind the tragus and curves inward for approximately 3 cm; the inner two-thirds is bony and the outer third cartilaginous. The skin lining the cartilaginous outer portion has a well-developed subcutaneous layer that contains hair follicles and ceruminous and sebaceous glands.

The two portions of the meatus have slightly different directions; the outer cartilaginous portion is upward and backward whereas the inner bony portion is forward and downward. This is important to know when examining the ear.

History taking and physical exam

The pharmacist is dependent on the patient's ability to accurately describe their symptoms as only a limited examination of the ear is possible in a community pharmacy. This necessitates that a thorough and accurate history is taken from the patient. Certain symptoms can help decide what structure of the ear the problem originates from (Table 3.1).

After taking a history of the presenting complaint, the ear should be examined. Initially, inspect the external ear for redness, swelling and discharge. Then apply pressure to the mastoid area (directly behind the pinna). If the area is tender this suggests mastoiditis, a rare complication of otitis media. Also move the pinna up and down and manipulate the tragus. If either is tender on movement then this suggests external ear involvement. Finally, examine the EAM. This is best performed using an otoscope; however, currently most pharmacists have not had appropriate training in their use. Because of the shape of the EAM, when performing an examination the pinna needs to be manipulated to obtain the best view of the ear canal (Fig. 3.2). This should provide some clues as to the origin of the problem (Table 3.2).

Ear wax impaction

Background

Ear wax is produced in the outer third of the cartilaginous portion of the ear canal by the ceruminous glands. Ear wax performs a number of important functions, including mechanical protection of the tympanic membrane, trapping dirt, repelling water and contributing to a slightly acidic medium that has been reported to exert protection against bactericidal and fungicidal infection. Cerumen varies in its composition among individuals but can be broadly divided into two types: a 'wet or sticky'

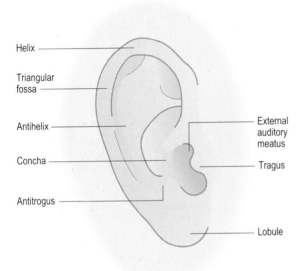

Fig. 3.1 The pinna

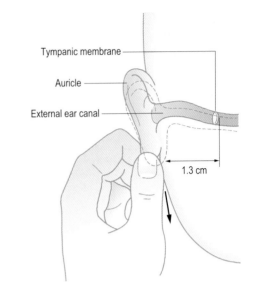

Table 3.1 Ear symptoms and the affected ear structures			
Symptom	**External ear**	**Middle ear**	**Inner ear**
Itch	✓		
Pain	✓	✓	
Discharge	✓	✓	
Deafness	✓	✓	✓
Dizziness		✓	
Tinnitus			✓

Source: Acomb, C, Pharmaceutical Journal, Aug 1991. Adapted with permission

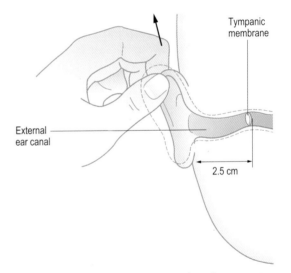

Fig. 3.2 Inspection of the external auditory meatus. Above: in children; below: in adults

type of wax, which is common in Caucasians and African-Americans, or 'dry' wax, which is common in Asian populations.

Prevalence and epidemiology

Ear wax is by far the commonest external ear problem that pharmacists encounter and is the most common ear problem in the general population. Exact prevalence rates of ear wax impaction are not clear but studies have shown that 2 to 6% of the general population suffer from impacted wax and one Scottish survey of GPs reported an average of nine patients per month (range 5 to 50 patients) requesting ear wax removal. However, many more patients self-diagnose and medicate without seeking GP assistance; therefore, pharmacists have an important role in ensuring that treatment is appropriate. The high number of presentations may be due to patient misconception that ear wax needs to be removed.

Additionally, a number of patient groups appear to be more prone to ear wax impaction than the general population, for example, patients with congenital anomalies (narrowed ear canal), patients with learning difficulties and those fitted with a hearing aid. The elderly are more susceptible to impaction due to the decrease in cerumen-producing glands resulting in drier and harder ear wax.

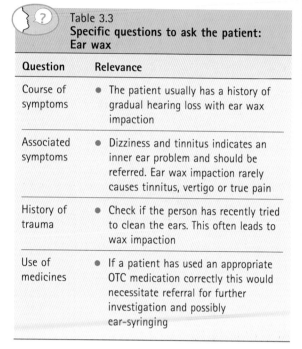

Table 3.2
Examination of the pinna and external auditory meatus: possible causes of presenting complaint

Patient presents with	Possible causes
Redness and swelling	Perichondritis, haematoma
Discharge	Otitis externa or media. If discharge mucinous, originates from middle ear as EAM has no mucous glands
Pain in mastoid area	Otitis media, mastoiditis
Pain when pressing tragus or moving pinna	Otitis externa

Table 3.3
Specific questions to ask the patient: Ear wax

Question	Relevance
Course of symptoms	• The patient usually has a history of gradual hearing loss with ear wax impaction
Associated symptoms	• Dizziness and tinnitus indicates an inner ear problem and should be referred. Ear wax impaction rarely causes tinnitus, vertigo or true pain
History of trauma	• Check if the person has recently tried to clean the ears. This often leads to wax impaction
Use of medicines	• If a patient has used an appropriate OTC medication correctly this would necessitate referral for further investigation and possibly ear-syringing

Aetiology

The skin of the tympanic membrane is unusual. It is not simply shed as skin is from the rest of the body but is migratory. This is because the auditory canal is the body's only 'dead end' and abrasion of the stratum corneum cannot occur. Skin therefore moves outwards away from the ear drum and out along the ear canal. This means that the ears are largely self-cleaning as the ear canal naturally sheds wax from the ear. However, this normal function can be interrupted, usually by misguided attempts to clean ears. Wax therefore becomes trapped, hampering its outward migration.

Arriving at a differential diagnosis

Careful questioning along with inspection of the EAM should mean that wax impaction is readily distinguished from other conditions (Table 3.3).

Clinical features of ear wax impaction

The key features of ear wax impaction are a history of gradual hearing loss, ear discomfort (to variable degrees) and recent attempts to clean ears. Itching, tinnitus and dizziness occur infrequently. Otoscopical examination should reveal excessive wax.

Conditions to eliminate

Trauma of the ear canal

It is common practice for people to use all manner of implements to try and clean the ear canal of wax (e.g. cotton buds, hairgrips and pens). Inspection of the ear canal might reveal laceration of the ear canal and the patient could be experiencing greater conductive deafness because of the wax becoming further impacted. Trauma might also lead to discharge from the ear canal. These cases are probably best referred.

Foreign bodies

Symptoms can mimic ear wax impaction but, over time, discharge and pain is observed. Children are the most likely age group to present with a foreign body in the ear canal and suspected cases need to be referred to a GP.

 TRIGGER POINTS indicative of referral: Ear wax

- Associated trauma-related conductive deafness
- Dizziness or tinnitus
- Fever and general malaise in children
- Foreign body in the EAM
- OTC medication failure
- Pain originating from the middle ear

Evidence base for over-the-counter medication

Cerumenolytics have been used for many years to help soften, dislodge and remove impacted ear wax. Two systematic reviews have been published (Burton & Doree 2003; Hand & Harvey 2004) to determine if pharmacological intervention is effective in wax removal. Each had slightly different inclusion criteria resulting in some trials being included in both and other trials being included in only one of the reviews. All trials reviewed had aspects of poor methodological quality (e.g. lack of clear randomisation and blinding and potential for publication bias as some were company sponsored trials) and were of relatively small size. The findings from these reviews support the use of oil-based softeners, sodium bicarbonate and sterile water over no treatment at all, but no active treatment proved superior over any other. Further trials on oil-based products and saline found oil-based products to be significantly better than saline but no oil-based product was superior to any other oil-based product.

Summary

The evidence from limited trial data suggests simple remedies such as water appear to be equally effective as marketed ear wax products. Additionally, trial data do not clearly point to one particular cerumenolytic having superior efficacy. In the UK, Prodigy guidelines recommend the use of tap water, sodium chloride 0.9%, sodium bicarbonate ear drops or olive and almond oil.

Practical prescribing and product selection

Prescribing information relating to ear wax medicines reviewed in the section 'Evidence base for over-the-counter medication' is discussed and summarised in Table 3.4 and useful tips relating to patients presenting with ear wax are given in Hints and Tips Box 3.1.

Cerumunolytics

Although agents used to soften ear wax have limited evidence of efficacy, they are very safe. They can be given to all patient groups, do not interact with any medicines and can be used in children. They have very few side effects, which appear to be limited to local irritation when first administered. They might, for a short while, increase deafness and the patient should be warned about this possibility.

Table 3.4
Practical prescribing: Summary of medicines for ear wax

Name of medicine	Use in children	Likely side effects	Drug interactions of note	Patients in whom care should be exercised	Pregnancy and breast-feeding
Cerumol/Earex	No lower age limit stated	None	None	None	OK
Exterol/Otex		Irritation			
Waxsol/Molcer		Irritation			
Sodium bicarbonate		None			

HINTS AND TIPS BOX 3.1: EAR WAX

Peanut allergy	Peanut allergy affects approximately 1 in 200 people and patients should be warned about preparations that contain arachis or almond oil
Hypersensitivity reactions to ear drops	Local reactions to the active ingredient or constituents have been reported that may cause severe irritation and pain. If a person has had a previous reaction using ear drops then care must be exercised
Administration of ear drops	1. Hold the bottle in your hands for a few minutes prior to administration to warm the solution. This makes insertion more comfortable
	2. Lie on a bed with the affected ear pointing towards the ceiling or alternatively tilt your head to one side with the affected ear pointing towards the ceiling
	3. With one hand straighten the ear canal. Adults pull the pinna up and back and in children, pull down and back
	4. Holding the dropper in the other hand, hold it as near as possible to the ear canal without touching it and place the correct number of drops into the ear canal
	5. The head should be kept in the same position for several minutes
	6. Once the head is returned to the normal position, any excess solution should be wiped away with a clean tissue

Oil-based products

Cerumol (peanut oil 57.3%)

The standard dose for adults and children is five drops into the affected ear two or three times a day repeated for up to 3 days. In between administrations a plug of cotton wool moistened with Cerumol or smeared with petroleum jelly should then be applied to retain the liquid.

Earex (Arachis – peanut oil – 33.3% and camphor oil 33.33%)

For adults and children, four drops should be instilled twice a day for up to 4 days. Like Cerumol, a cotton wool plug should be gently placed in the ear to retain the liquid.

Peroxide-based products (Exterol and Otex; urea hydrogen peroxide 5%)

For adults and children, five drops should be instilled once or twice daily for at least 3 to 4 days. Unlike Cerumol, the patient should be advised not to plug the ear but retain the drops in ear for several minutes by keeping the head tilted and then wipe away any surplus. Patients might experience mild, temporary effervescence in the ear as the urea hydrogen peroxide complex liberates oxygen.

Water-based products (e.g. sodium bicarbonate)

This is only available as a non-proprietary product and should be instilled two to three times a day for up to 3 days.

Docusate (Waxsol, Molcer)

The manufacturers of Waxsol recommend that adults and children use enough ear drops to fill the affected ear on not more than two consecutive nights.

Further reading

Burton MJ, Doree CJ. Ear drops for the removal of ear wax. Cochrane Database of Systematic Reviews 2003, issue 3.
Corbridge RJ. Essential ENT practice. London: Arnold; 1998.
Hand C, Harvey I. The effectiveness of topical preparations for the treatment of earwax: a systematic review. Br J Gen Pract 2004;54:862–7.
Rodgers R. Hearing loss and wax occlusion in older people. Pract Nurs 2004;15:290–4

Web sites

Prodigy guidance: http://www.cks.library.nhs.uk/earwax
British Tinnitus Association: http://www.tinnitus.org.uk
The ear care centre: http://www.earcarecentre.com/
ENT Nursing: http://www.entnursing.com/

Otitis externa

Background

Otitis externa refers to generalised inflammation throughout the ear canal (EAM) and is often associated with infection. It usually occurs as an acute episode but may become chronic (greater than 3 months) in children.

Prevalence and epidemiology

The lifetime prevalence of acute otitis externa is 10% and a GP will see approximately 16 new cases per year. It is more common in hot and humid climates, and in Western society the number of episodes increases in the summer months. People who swim are five times more likely than non-swimmers to contract it and it is commoner in adults and reported to be slightly more common in women than men.

Aetiology

Primary infection, contact sensitivity or a combination of both causes otitis externa. Pathogens implicated in acute otitis externa include *Pseudomonas aeruginosa*, *Staphylococcus* species and *Streptococcus pyogenes*. Fungal overgrowth with *Aspergillus niger* is also seen especially after prolonged antibiotic treatment.

Certain local or general factors can precipitate otitis externa. Local causes include trauma or discharge from the middle ear and general causes include seborrhoeic dermatitis, psoriasis and skin infections.

Arriving at a differential diagnosis

In common with ear wax impaction, otitis externa is easily recognised providing a careful history and ear examination has been conducted. However, other otological conditions can present with similar symptoms of pain and discharge. It is therefore important to differentiate between otitis externa and conditions that require referral. Table 3.5 highlights some of the questions that should be asked of the patient.

Clinical features of otitis externa

Otitis externa is characterised by itching and irritation, which, depending on the severity, can become intense. This provokes the patient to scratch the skin of the EAM, resulting in trauma and pain. Patients might not present until pain becomes a prominent feature. However, there should be a period when irritation is the only symptom apparent. Chewing and manipulation of the tragus and pinna can exacerbate pain. Otorrhoea (ear discharge) follows and the skin of the EAM can become oedematous,

3

Table 3.5
Specific questions to ask the patient: Otitis externa

Question	Relevance
Symptom presentation	• Principal symptom of acute otitis externa is itch/irritation, which can progress to pain and discharge
Discharge	• Otitis media is the commonest cause of ear discharge, which is usually mucopurulent. If discharge is present with otitis externa, then it is not mucopurulent
Systemic symptoms	• Otitis externa should not present with any systemic symptoms. Fever and cold symptoms usually present in otitis media. In all forms of dermatitis, systemic symptoms should not be present

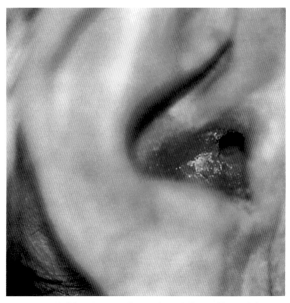

Fig. 3.3 Otitis externa. Reproduced from *Shared Care for ENT* by C Milford and A Rowlands, 1999, Isis Medical Media Ltd, Martin Dunitz Publishers, with permission of Taylor and Francis Books UK

leading to conductive hearing loss. On examination, the ear canal or external ear, or both, appear red, swollen or eczematous (Fig. 3.3).

Conditions to eliminate

Otalgia (earache)

Earache is normally due to a rapidly accumulating effusion in the middle ear (acute otitis media) and is most common in children aged 3 to 6 years old. Ear pain tends to be throbbing and signs of infection are often present (e.g. cough, cold or fever). In young children this is often manifested as irritability or crying with characteristic ear tugging. Systemic symptoms can also be present such as fever and loss of appetite. An examination of the ear should reveal a red and bulging tympanic membrane. Pain resolves on rupture of the tympanic membrane, which releases a mucopurulent discharge. Over three-quarters of episodes resolve within 3 days without treatment and current UK guidelines do not advocate the routine use of antibiotics. Children may develop recurrent otitis media and this is known as 'glue ear'. The condition is symptomless apart from impaired hearing.

Dermatitis

Allergic, contact, seborrhoeic and atopic forms of dermatitis can occur on the external ear. Itch is a prominent symptom and could be mistaken for otitis externa; however, there should be no ear pain or discharge associated with dermatitis. In addition, in seborrhoeic and atopic forms skin involvement elsewhere should be obvious.

Perichondritis

In severe cases of otitis externa the inflammation can spread from the outer ear canal to the pinna, resulting in perichondritis (Fig. 3.4). Referral is needed, as systemic antibiotics are required.

Trauma

Recent trauma (e.g. blow to the head) can cause an auricular haematoma. This is best known as a cauliflower ear and requires non-urgent referral.

Malignant tumours

Basal and squamous cell carcinomas can develop on the pinna of the ear. Typically they are slow growing and associated with increasing age. Any elderly patient presenting with an ulcerative or crusting lesion needs referral.

 TRIGGER POINTS indicative of referral: Otitis externa

- Ear pain in children under 6 years of age (within 24 hours)
- Generalised inflammation of the pinna
- If symptoms persist for 7 days or longer after initiation of treatment
- Impaired hearing in children
- Mucopurulent discharge
- Pain on palpation of the mastoid area
- Slow-growing growths on the pinna in elderly people

Evidence base for over-the-counter medication

Unfortunately, OTC treatment of otitis externa is very limited. Inflammation of the EAM would respond to corticosteroids; however, currently all ear drops/sprays that contain steroids are POM. This limits OTC options to either oral antihistamines – to try and combat itching and irritation – or analgesia to control pain. Choline salicylate is found in two proprietary products (Earex Plus, Audax). Two small trials comparing the analgesic effect of choline salicylate against aspirin and paracetamol have been conducted. Both trials concluded that choline salicylate reduced pain more quickly than oral analgesia.

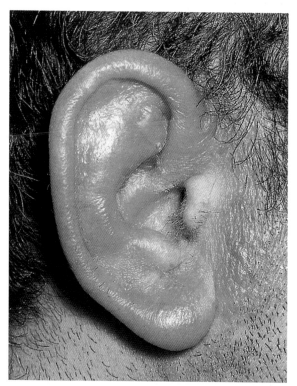

Fig. 3.4 Perichondritis. From *Essential ENT Practice* by R Corbridge, 1998, reproduced by permission of Edward Arnold (Publishers) Ltd

In addition, acetic acid is available OTC (Earcalm Spray, 2% acetic acid) and is indicated for the treatment of superficial infections of the EAM. The *British National Formulary 54* states that it may be useful to treat mild otitis externa but more severe cases should be referred for anti-inflammatory preparations with or without an anti-infective. This advice appears to be taken from a 2003 BMJ article (van Balen et al) who found acetic acid to be far less effective than acetic acid combined with a steroid or a steroid/anti-infective combination. A further review article (Hajioff 2006) found insufficient evidence to demonstrate the effectiveness of acetic acid in treating otitis externa. However, current Prodigy guidance states that acetic acid alone can be used first-line to treat bacterial and/or fungal disease.

Practical prescribing and product selection

Prescribing information relating to otitis externa medicines reviewed in the section 'Evidence base for over-the-counter medication' is discussed below and summarised in Table 3.6. Pain associated with otitis media can be managed with simple analgesics such as paracetamol and ibuprofen.

Choline salicylate (Earex Plus and Audax)

Choline salicylate can be given to adults and children over the age of 1 year. The EAM should be completely filled with drops then plugged with cotton wool soaked with the ear drops. This should be repeated every 3 to 4 hours.

Acetic acid (Earcalm Spray)

This can be given to adults and children aged 12 years and over. The dose is one spray (60 mg) into the affected ear at least three times a day. The maximum dosage frequency is one spray every 2 to 3 hours. Treatment should be continued until 2 days after symptoms have disappeared but if symptoms do not improve or worsen within 48 hours the patient should be referred to a medical practitioner. The spray should not be used for more than 7 days.

Table 3.6
Practical prescribing: Summary of medicines for otitis externa

Name of medicine	Use in children	Likely side effects	Drug interactions of note	Patients in whom care should be exercised	Pregnancy and breast-feeding
Choline salicylate	>1 year	None reported	None	None	OK
Acetic acid	>12 years	Transient stinging or burning sensation			

Further reading

Hajioff D. Otitis media. British Medical Journal Clinical Evidence 2006. Available online at http://www.clinicalevidence.com

Hewitt HR. Clinical evaluation of choline salicylate ear drops. The Practitioner. 1970;204:438–40.

Milford C, Rowlands A. Shared care for ENT. Oxford: Isis Medical Media Ltd; 1999.

Lawrence N. A comparison of analgesic therapies for the relief of acute otalgia. Br J Clin Pract 1970;24:478–9.

Rosenfeld RM, Brown L, Cannon CR, et al. Clinical practice guideline: acute otitis externa. Otolaryngol Head Neck Surg 2006 Apr; 134(4 Suppl):S4–S23.

SIGN (2003) Diagnosis and management of childhood otitis media in primary care. Report No. 66. Scottish Intercollegiate Guidelines Network. Available online at http://www.sign.ac.uk (accessed 14 Nov 2006).

van Balen FA, Smit WM, Zuithoff NP, Verheij TJM. Clinical efficacy of three common treatments in acute otitis externa in primary care: randomised controlled trial. BMJ 2003;327:1201–5.

Web sites

Prodigy guidance: http://www.cks.library.nhs.uk/otitis_externa

Outer and middle ear problems: http://www.pjonline.com/pdf/cpd/pj_20060121_ear01.pdf

Self-assessment questions

The following questions are intended to supplement the text. Two levels of questions are provided; multiple choice questions and case studies. The multiple choice questions are designed to test factual recall and the case studies allow knowledge to be applied to a practice setting.

Multiple choice questions

3.1 Which of the following OTC treatments would you recommend for otitis media?

 a. Hydrocortisone
 b. An astringent
 c. Local analgesia
 d. Emollient
 e. None of the above

3.2 Otitis media is more prevalent in which age group?

 a. 0 to 3 years
 b. 3 to 6 years
 c. 6 to 9 years
 d. 9 to 12 years
 e. Over 12 years

3.3 If a patient complains of tinnitus and deafness, what is the most likely part of the ear that is affected?

 a. Outer ear
 b. Middle ear
 c. Inner ear
 d. Either middle or outer ear
 e. Either inner or middle

3.4 Which patient group is predisposed to otitis externa?

 a. Patients with seborrhoeic dermatitis
 b. Patients with acne vulgaris
 c. Patients with tinea corporis
 d. Patients with discoid eczema
 e. Patients with lichen planus

3.5 Symptoms suggestive of a middle ear problem are?

 a. Itch, pain and discharge
 b. Pain, discharge and deafness
 c. Deafness, dizziness and tinnitus
 d. Pain only
 e. Itch only

3.6 The best way to view the EAM of an adult is to?

 a. Pull the pinna up and back to straighten the EAM
 b. Pull the pinna down and back to straighten the EAM
 c. Pull the pinna up and forward to straighten the EAM

 d. Pull the pinna down and forward to straighten the EAM
 e. Pull the pinna back to straighten the EAM

3.7 Elderly people are more prone to ear wax because?

 a. Of an increase in cerumen production
 b. The skin migrates at a slower rate
 c. Decreased oestrogen concentrations cause less wax to be produced
 d. The number of cerumen glands decreases with age
 e. Greater immobility

3.8 Which of the following contains peanut oil?

 a. Otex
 b. Earcalm
 c. Earex
 d. Molcer
 e. Exterol

Questions 3.9 to 3.11 concern the following conditions:

A. Mastoid area
B. The pinna
C. Tympanic membrane
D. External auditory maetus
E. Helix

Select from A to E, which of the above statements relate to the following conditions:

3.9 When painful on manipulation suggests external ear involvement

3.10 Serves to collect sound

3.11 Appears to bulge if an infection is present

Questions 3.12 to 3.14 concern the following OTC medications:

A. Hydrogen peroxide ear drops
B. Almond oil
C. Hydrocortisone 1% cream
D. Choline salicylate ear drops
E. Sodium bicarbonate ear drops

Select, from A to E, which of the above medicines:

3.12 Should not be given to children

3.13 Can reduce pain

3.14 Should be avoided in peanut allergy

Questions 3.15 to 3.17: for each of these questions *one or more* of the responses is (are) correct. Decide which of the responses is (are) correct. Then choose:

A. If a, b and c are correct
B. If a and b only are correct
C. If b and c only are correct
D. If a only is correct
E. If c only is correct

Directions summarised

A	B	C	D	E
a, b and c	a and b only	b and c only	a only	c only

3.15 Which statements are associated with the EAM:

   a. The outer third consists mainly of cartilage
   b. To inspect the EAM of a child the pinna should be pulled down and back
   c. To inspect the EAM of an adult the pinna should be pulled down and back

3.16 Conductive deafness can be caused by:

   a. Insertion of a foreign body into the EAM
   b. Blockage of the eustachin tube
   c. Poor ear-cleaning technique

3.17 The principal symptom associated with otitis externa is?

   a. Intense ear pain
   b. Mucopurulent discharge
   c. Itch

Questions 3.18 to 3.20: these questions consist of a statement in the left-hand column followed by a statement in the right-hand column. You need to:

- decide whether the first statement is true or false
- decide whether the second statement is true or false

Then choose:

A. If both statements are true and the second statement is a correct explanation of the first statement
B. If both statements are true but the second statement is NOT a correct explanation of the first statement
C. If the first statement is true but the second statement is false
D. If the first statement is false but the second statement is true
E. If both statements are false

Directions summarised

	1st statement	2nd statement	
A	True	True	2nd statement is a correct explanation of the first
B	True	True	2nd statement is not a correct explanation of the first
C	True	False	
D	False	True	
E	False	False	

	First statement	*Second statement*
3.18	Swimmers often get otitis externa	Prolonged exposure to water predisposes people to EAM infections
3.19	Perichondritis is a precursor to otitis externa	Topical antibiotics are ineffective
3.20	All children with ear pain must be referred	Systemic antibiotics are needed

Case study

CASE STUDY 3.1

Mr SW has asked to speak to the pharmacist as his ear is bothering him.

a. Discuss the appropriately worded questions you will need to ask Mr SW to determine the diagnosis of his complaint.

Questions to ask include: duration; medication tried; whether the symptoms are getting better, worse or staying about the same; degree of discomfort; whether there is any discharge. You should also check the order in which the symptoms presented, any precipitating factors and if there is a previous history of symptoms.

b. How would a physical examination help to confirm or refute your diagnosis?

A physical examination will allow, along with questions, differentiation between middle and outer ear involvement.

You decide that Mr SW has impacted wax.

c. Compare and contrast the different products available to treat Mr SW's symptoms?

Cerumunolytics remain the mainstay of treatment in the UK. However, the evidence base for efficacy is poor. The British National Formulary advocates the use of simple agents such as olive and almond oil and Prodigy also recommends tap water, sodium chloride 0.9% and sodium bicarbonate ear drops. Dosing for all products is similar and therefore treatment choice will be driven by patient acceptability.

CASE STUDY 3.2

Mrs PR asks to speak to the pharmacist about her 4-year-old son Luke. She wants some Calpol to treat his earache.

a. How do you respond?

The pharmacist needs to establish the severity of the earache and try to determine the cause of the pain.

b. What questions will you need to ask?

- When was the onset of the earache?
- Describe the pain
- Is any discharge present?
- Are there any associated symptoms (e.g. cough and cold)?
- How is Luke's general condition compared to normal?
- Is this the first episode or is it a recurrent problem?
- Is there any loss of hearing?
- Is the earache associated with any trauma?

You find out that the earache has been present for a day or so and Luke is more irritable than normal. Mrs PR says he has a temperature but she hasn't actually taken it. Apart from this Luke has no other symptoms. However, he had this problem about a year ago and was given Calpol then and it seemed to help.

c. What course of action are you going to take?

It appears Luke has a middle ear infection. Examination of the tympanic membrane would confirm this and if possible should be carried out in the pharmacy. Instigation of Calpol seems reasonable and Mrs PR could buy some for Luke. If symptoms did not subside in the next 24 hours then referral to the GP would be appropriate.

Answers to multiple choice questions

1 = e	2 = b	3 = c	4 = a	5 = b	6 = a	7 = d	8 = c	9 = b	10 = b
11 = c	12 = c	13 = d	14 = b	15 = b	16 = d	17 = e	18 = a	19 = d	20 = e.

The central nervous system

Background

The number of patient requests for advice and or products to treat headache and insomnia make up a smaller proportion of a pharmacist's workload than other conditions such as coughs and colds yet sales for analgesics and hypnotics are extremely high. The vast majority of patients will present with benign and non-serious conditions and only in very few cases will sinister pathology be responsible.

General overview of CNS anatomy

The central nervous system (CNS) comprises the brain and spinal cord. Its major function is to process and integrate information arriving from sensory pathways and communicate an appropriate response back via afferent pathways. CNS anatomy is complex and outside the scope of this book. The reader is referred to any good anatomical text for a comprehensive description of CNS anatomy.

History taking

A differential diagnosis for all CNS conditions will be made solely from questions asked of the patient. It is especially important that a social and work-related history is sought alongside questions asking about the patient's presenting symptoms because pressure and stress are implicated in the cause of CNS conditions.

Headache

Background

Headache is not a disease state or condition but rather a symptom, of which there are many causes. Headache can be the major presenting complaint, for example, in migraine, tension and cluster headache, or one of many symptoms, for example, in an upper respiratory tract infection.

Headache classification

If the pharmacist is to advise on appropriate treatment and referral then it is essential to make an accurate diagnosis. However, with so many disorders having headache as a symptom pharmacists should endeavour to follow an agreed classification system. The 2nd edition of the International Headache Society (IHS) classification is now almost universally accepted (Table 4.1). The system first distinguishes between primary and secondary headache disorders. This is useful to the community pharmacist, as any secondary headache disorder is symptomatic of an underlying cause and would normally require referral. In the IHS system, primary headaches are classified on symptom profiles, relying on careful questioning coupled with epidemiological data on the distribution a particular headache disorder has within the population.

Prevalence and epidemiology

The exact prevalence of headache is not precisely known. However, virtually everyone will have suffered from a

Table 4.1
The International Headache Society classification of headache

Primary headaches	1. Migraine, *including:* 　1.1　Migraine without aura 　1.2　Migraine with aura 2. Tension-type headache, *including:* 　2.1　Infrequent episodic tension-type 　　　 headache 　2.2　Frequent episodic tension-type 　　　 headache 　2.3　Chronic tension-type headache	3. Cluster headache and other trigeminal 　　autonomic cephalalgias, *including:* 　3.1　　Cluster headache 4. Other primary headaches
Secondary headaches	5. Headache attributed to head and/or neck 　 trauma, *including:* 　5.2　Chronic post-traumatic headache 6. Headache attributed to cranial or cervical 　 vascular disorder, *including:* 　6.2.2 Headache attributed to subarachnoid 　　　 haemorrhage 　6.4.1 Headache attributed to giant cell 　　　 arteritis 7. Headache attributed to non-vascular 　 intracranial disorder, *including:* 　7.1.1 Headache attributed to idiopathic 　　　 intracranial hypertension 　7.4　 Headache attributed to intracranial 　　　 neoplasm 8. Headache attributed to a substance or its 　 withdrawal, *including:* 　8.1.3 Carbon monoxide-induced headache 　8.1.4 Alcohol-induced headache	8.2 Medication-overuse headache 　8.2.1　Ergotamine-overuse headache 　8.2.2　Triptan-overuse headache 　8.2.3　Analgesic-overuse headache 9. Headache attributed to infection, *including:* 　9.1　　Headache attributed to intracranial 　　　　infection 10. Headache attributed to disorder of 　　homoeostasis 11. Headache or facial pain, atributed to 　　disorder of cranium, neck, eyes, ears, nose, 　　sinuses, teeth, mouth or other facial or 　　cranial structures *including:* 　11.2.1 Cervicogenic headache 　11.3.1 Headache attributed to acute 　　　　 glaucoma 12. Headache attributed to psychiatric disorder
Neuralgias and other headaches	13. Cranial neuralgias, central and primary 　　facial pain and other headaches *including:* 　13.1　Trigeminal neuralgia	14. Other headache, cranial neuralgia, central 　　or primary facial pain

Source: adapted by the British Association of Headache (BASH) from the International Headache Society Classification Subcommittee,
The International Classification of Headache Disorders, 2nd ed. Cephalalgia 2004, Blackwell Publishing, with permission

headache at some time; it is probably the most common pain syndrome experienced by man. It has been estimated that up to 80 to 90% of the population will experience one or more headaches per year.

Tension-type headache has been reported to affect between 40 and 90% of people in Western countries. Migraine affects approximately 15 to 20% of women and is approximately three times more common than in men. Prevalence peaks between 30 to 40 years of age. Conversely, cluster headache, which is also most prevalent in the 30- to 40-year-old age group is five to six times more common in men.

Aetiology

Considering headache affects almost everyone, the mechanisms that bring about headache are still poorly under-

stood. Pain control systems modulate headaches of all types, independent of the cause. However, the exact aetiology of tension-type headache and migraine are still to be fully elucidated. Tension-type headache is commonly referred to as muscle contraction headache as electromyography has shown pericranial muscle contraction, which is often exacerbated by stress. However, similar muscle contraction is noted in migraine sufferers and this theory has now fallen out of favour. Consequently, no current theory for tension-type headache is unanimously endorsed but recent studies suggest a neurobiological basis.

Traditionally, migraine was thought to be a result of abnormal dilation of cerebral blood vessels but this vascular theory cannot explain all migraine symptoms. The use of 5 HT_1 agonists to reduce and stop migraine attacks suggests some neurochemical pathophysiology.

Migraine is therefore probably a combination of vascular and neurochemical changes – the neurovascular hypothesis. Migraine also appears to have a genetic component with about 70% of patients having a first-degree relative with a history of migraine.

Arriving at a differential diagnosis

Given that headache is extremely common, and most patients will self-medicate, any patient requesting advice should ideally be questioned by the pharmacist, as it is likely that the headache has either not responded to OTC medication or is troublesome enough for the patient to seek advice. Arrival at an accurate diagnosis will rely exclusively on questioning, therefore a number of headache-specific questions should be asked (Table 4.2). In addition to these symptom-specific questions, the pharmacist should also enquire about the person's social history because social factors – mainly stress – play a

significant role in headache. Ask about the person's work and family status to determine if the person is suffering from greater levels of stress than normal.

Clinical features of headache

In a community pharmacy the overwhelming majority of patients (80 to 90%) will present with tension-type headache. A further 10% will have migraine. Very few will have other primary headache disorders and fewer still will have a secondary headache disorder. This text therefore concentrates on migraine, tension-type headache and cluster headache.

Tension-type headache

Tension-type headaches can be classed as either episodic or chronic. Episodic tension-type headache can be further subdivided into infrequent and frequent forms. Most

---

Table 4.2
Specific questions to ask the patient: Headache

Question	Relevance
Onset of headache	In early childhood or as young adult, primary headache is most likely. After 50 years of age the likelihood of a secondary cause is much greater Headache and fever at same time imply an infectious cause Headache that follows head trauma might indicate post-concussive headache or intracranial pathology
Frequency and timing	Headache associated with the menstrual cycle or certain times, e.g. weekend or holidays, suggests migraine Headaches that occur in clusters at the same time of day/night suggest cluster headache Headaches that occur on most days with the same pattern suggest tension-type headache
Location of pain (see Fig. 4.1)	Cluster headache is nearly always unilateral in frontal, ocular or temporal areas Migraine headache is unilateral in 70% of patients but can change from side to side from attack to attack Tension-type headache is often bilateral, either in frontal or occipital areas, and described as a tight band Very localised pain suggests an organic cause
Severity of pain	Pain is a subjective personal experience and there are therefore no objective measures. Using a numeric pain intensity scale should allow you to assess the level of pain the person is experiencing: 0 represents no pain and 10 the worst pain possible Dull and band-like suggests tension-type headache Severe to intense ache or throbbing suggests haemorrhage or aneurysm Piercing, boring, searing eye pain suggests cluster headache Moderate to severe throbbing pain that often starts as dull ache suggests migraine
Triggers	Pain that worsens on exertion, coughing and bending suggests a tumour Food (in 10% of sufferers), menstruation and relaxation after stress are indicative of migraine Lying down makes cluster headache worse
Attack duration	Typically migraine attacks last between a few hours and 3 days Tension-type headaches last between a few hours and several days, e.g. a week or more Cluster headache will only normally last 2 to 3 hours

patients will present to the pharmacist with the infrequent episodic form. Headaches last from 30 minutes to up to 7 days in duration and often the patient will have a history of recent headaches. They might have tried OTC medication without complete symptom resolution or say that the headaches are becoming more frequent. Pain is bifrontal or bioccipital, generalised and non-throbbing (Fig. 4.1). The patient might describe the pain as tightness or a weight pressing down on their head. The pain is gradual in onset and tends to worsen progressively through the day. Pain is normally mild to moderate and not aggravated by movement, although it is often worse under pressure or stress. Nausea and vomiting are not associated with tension-type headache and it rarely causes photo- or phonophobia. Overall, the headache has only a limited impact on the individual.

Patients who have frequent episodic tension-type headaches suffer more frequent headaches that last longer and over time these can develop into chronic tension-type headache. These headaches occur for more than 15 days per month, and might occur daily and last for at least 3 months. These types of headaches can severely affect the patient's quality of life and should not be managed by the community pharmacist.

Migraine

There are an estimated 5 million migraine sufferers in the UK, half of whom have not been diagnosed by their GP. The peak onset for a person to have their first attack is in adolescence or as a young adult. Migraines are rare over the age of 50 and anyone in this age group presenting for the first time with migraine-like symptoms should be referred to the GP to eliminate secondary causes of headache. If this is not their first attack they will normally have a history of recurrent and episodic attacks of headache. Attacks last for anything between a few hours and up to 3 days. The average length of an attack is 24 hours. The IHS classification recognises several subtypes of migraine but the two major subtypes are migraine with aura (classical migraine) and migraine without aura (common migraine). A migraine attack can be divided into three phases:

- Phase one: premonitory phase (prodrome phase), which can occur hours or possibly days before the headache. The patient might complain of a change in mood or notice a change in behaviour. Feelings of well-being, yawning, poor concentration and food cravings have been reported. These prodromal features are highly individual but are relatively consistent to each patient. Identification of 'triggers' is sometimes possible (Table 4.3).

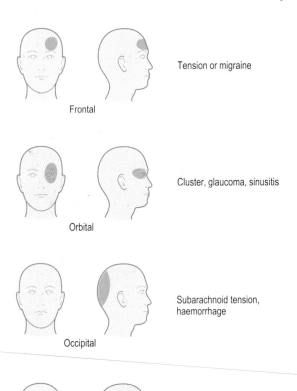

Frontal — Tension or migraine

Orbital — Cluster, glaucoma, sinusitis

Occipital — Subarachnoid tension, haemorrhage

Temporal — Migraine, temporal arteritis

Fig. 4.1 Location of pain in headache

Table 4.3 **Triggers and strategies to reduce migraine attacks**	
Trigger	**Strategy**
Stress	• Maintain regular sleep pattern • Take regular exercise • Modify work environment • Relaxation techniques, e.g. yoga
Diet – any food can be a potential trigger but foods implicated include: 　cheese 　citrus fruit 　chocolate	• Maintain a food diary. If an attack occurs within 6 hours of food ingestion and is reproducible it is likely that it is a trigger for migraine • Eat regularly and do not skip meals

Note: detecting triggers is complicated because they appear to be cumulative, jointly contributing to a 'threshold' above which attacks are initiated

- Phase two: headache with or without aura.
- Phase three: as the headache subsides the patient can feel lethargic, tired and drained before recovery, which might take several hours and is termed the resolution phase.

Headache with aura (classic migraine)

This accounts for less than 25% of migraine cases. The aura, which are fully reversible, develop over 5 to 20 minutes and can last for up to 1 hour. They can either be visual or neurological. Visual auras can take many guises, such as scotomas (blind spots), fortification spectra (zig-zag lines) or flashing and flickering lights. Neurological auras (pins and needles) typically start in the hand, migrating up the arm before jumping to the face and lips. Within 60 minutes of the aura ending the headache usually occurs. Pain is unilateral, throbbing and moderate to severe. Sometimes the pain becomes more generalised and diffuse. Physical activity and movement tends to intensify the pain. Nausea affects almost all patients but less than a third will vomit. Photophobia and phonophobia often mean patients will seek out a dark quiet room to relieve their symptoms. The patient might also suffer from fatigue, find concentrating difficult and be irritable.

Headache without aura (common migraine)

The remaining 75% of sufferers do not experience an aura but do suffer from all the other symptoms described above.

Cluster headache

Cluster headache is predominantly a condition that affects men over the age of 30 years. Typically the headache occurs at the same time each day with abrupt onset and lasts between 10 min and 3 hours, with 50% of patients experiencing night-time symptoms. Patients are woken 2 to 3 hours after falling asleep with very intense unilateral orbital boring pain. Additionally, conjunctival redness, lacrimation, nasal congestion (which laterally becomes watery) and sweating are observed on the pain side of the head. Patients tend to be restless and irritable and move about to relieve the pain.

The condition is characterised by periods of acute attacks, typically lasting a number of weeks to a few months with sufferers experiencing between one to three attacks per day. This is then followed by periods of remission, which can last months or years. During acute phases, alcohol can trigger an attack. Nausea is usually absent and a family history uncommon.

The key differences between the three conditions is shown in Table 4.4.

Conditions to eliminate

All suspected secondary causes of headache except sinusitis need to be referred. In addition, patients suffering from cluster headache must also be referred as sumatriptan, the drug of choice, does not have an OTC licence for cluster headache.

Table 4.4
Differences in symptom presentation for primary headaches

	Duration	Timing and nature	Location	Severity (pain score from 0 to 10)*	Precipitating factors	Who is affected
Tension-type headache	Can last days	Symptoms worsen as day progresses. Non-throbbing pain	Bilateral & most often at back of head	2–5	Stress due to changes in work or home environment	All age groups and both sexes equally affected
Migraine	Average attack lasts 24 hours	Associated with menstrual cycle and weekends. Throbbing pain & nausea. Dislike of bright lights and loud noise	Usually unilateral	4–7	Food (in 10% of sufferers) & family history	Three times more common in women. Rare in children
Cluster headache	1–3 hours	Attacks occur at same time of day. Intense boring pain	Unilateral	>7	Alcohol	Three to five times more common in men

*These are rough guides set by the author and are not evidence-based

Sinusitis

The pain tends to be relatively localised, usually orbital, unilateral and dull. A course of decongestants could be tried but if treatment failure occurs referral to the GP for possible antibiotic therapy would be needed. For further information on sinusitis see Chapter 1, page 12.

Eye strain

People that perform prolonged close work, for example VDU operators, can suffer from frontal aching headache. In the first instance, patients should be referred to an optician for a routine eye check.

Medication overuse headache

Patients with long-standing symptoms of headache who regular medicate can develop medication overuse headache. Pain receptors (nociceptors) instead of being 'switched off' when analgesics are taken are in fact 'switched on'. The consequence is a cycle where patients take more and more painkillers that are stronger and stronger in order to control the pain. Patients will experience daily or near daily headaches that are described as dull and nagging. Obviously in these cases a medication history is essential and should prompt the pharmacist to refer the patient to the GP. Treatment is to stop all analgesia for a number of weeks and requires careful planning.

Glaucoma

Patients experience a frontal/orbital headache with pain in the eye. Sometimes, but not often, the eye appears red and is painful. Vision is blurred and the cornea can look cloudy. In addition, the patient might notice haloes around the vision. For further information on glaucoma see Chapter 2, page 43.

Meningitis

Severe generalised headache associated with fever, an obviously ill patient, neck stiffness, a positive Kernig's sign (pain behind both knees when extended) and latterly a purpuric rash are classically associated with meningitis. However, meningitis is notoriously difficult to diagnose early and any child that has difficulty in placing their chin on their chest, has a headache and running a temperature above 102°F (38.9°C) should be referred urgently.

Subarachnoid haemorrhage

The patient will experience very intense and severe pain, located in the occipital region. Nausea and vomiting are often present and a decreased lack of consciousness is prominent. Patients often describe the headache as the worst headache they have ever had. It is extremely unlikely that a patient would present in the pharmacy with such symptoms but if one did then immediate referral is needed.

Temporal arteritis

The temporal arteries that run vertically up the side of the head, just in front of the ear, can become inflamed. When this happens, they are tender to touch and might be visibly thickened. Unilateral pain is experienced and the person generally feels unwell with fever, myalgia and general malaise. Scalp tenderness is also possible, especially when combing the hair. It is most commonly seen in the elderly, especially women. Prompt treatment with oral corticosteroids is required as the retinal artery can become compromised, leading to blindness. Urgent referral is needed.

Conditions causing raised intracranial pressure

Space-occupying lesions (brain tumour, haematoma and abscess) can give rise to varied headache symptoms, ranging from severe chronic pain to intermittent moderate pain. Pain can be localised or diffuse and tends to be more severe in the morning with a gradual improvement over the next few hours. Coughing, sneezing, bending and lying down can worsen the pain. Nausea and vomiting are common. After a prolonged period of time neurological symptoms start to become evident, such as drowsiness, confusion, lack of concentration, difficulty with speech and paresthesia.

Any patient with a recent history (last 2 to 3 months) of head trauma, headache of long-standing duration or insidious worsening of symptoms, especially decreased consciousness and vomiting, must be referred for fuller evaluation.

Trigeminal neuralgia

Pain follows the course of either the second (maxillary; supplying the cheeks) or third (mandibular; supplying the chin, lower lip and lower cheek) division of the nerve leading to pain experienced in the cheek, jaws, lips or gums. Pain is short-lived, usually lasting only a couple of minutes, but is severe and lancing and is almost always unilateral. It is three times more common in women than men.

Depression

Depression often presents with tension-type headaches. Check for loss of appetite, weight loss, decreased libido, sleep disturbances and constipation. If the patient exhibits these characteristics then referral to the GP would be necessary to determine if the patient is suffering from depression. Recent changes to the patient's social circumstances, for example loss of job, might also support your differential diagnosis.

Figure 4.2 will help in the differentiation of serious and non-serious causes of headache.

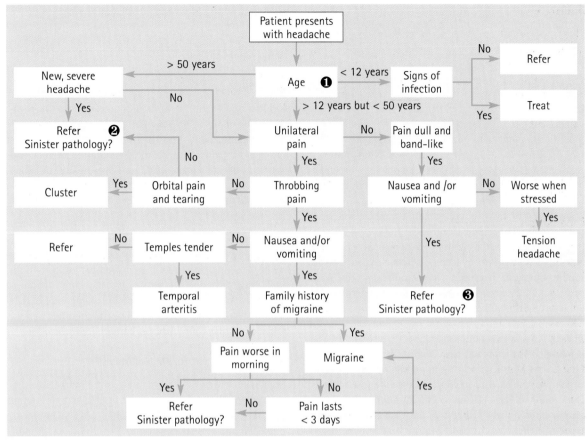

Fig. 4.2 Primer for differential diagnosis of headache

❶ Age
Caution should be exercised in children who present with headache. Although the majority of headaches will not have an organic cause, children under 12 are probably best referred if they show no signs of a systemic infection (e.g. fever, malaise).

❷ Referral for suspected sinister pathology
With increasing age it is more likely that a sinister cause of headache is responsible for the symptoms, especially if the patient has not experienced similar headache symptoms before. Mass lesions (tumours and haematoma) and temporal arteritis should be considered.

❸ Referral for suspected sinister pathology
Nausea and vomiting in the absence of migraine-like symptoms should be treated seriously. Mass lesions and subarachnoid haemorrhage need to be eliminated.

❗ TRIGGER POINTS indicative of referral: Headache

- Headache unresponsive to analgesics
- Headache in children under 12 who have a stiff neck or skin rash
- Headache occurs after recent (1 to 3 months) trauma injury
- Headache that has lasted for more than 2 weeks
- Nausea and/or vomiting in the absence of migraine symptoms
- Neurological symptoms, if migraine excluded, especially change in consciousness
- New or severe headache in patients over 50
- Progressive worsening of headache symptoms over time
- Symptoms indicative of cluster headache
- Very sudden and/or severe onset of headache

Evidence base for over-the-counter medication

Four UK products are specifically marketed to aid relief from pain and nausea associated with migraine: Migraleve, Midrid, Buccastem and Imigran Recovery. The evidence for these products is reviewed. Simple analgesia (paracetamol, aspirin and ibuprofen) has shown clinical benefit in relieving some migraine attacks and should be taken as early as possible. Approximately 60% of patients can expect a reduction in the severity of pain from moderate/severe to mild/none 2 hours after treatment but only a quarter of patients will be pain-free within 2 hours. Because migraine is associated with gastric stasis standard OTC doses might be inadequate to relieve migraine symptoms.

A recent systematic review (Verhagen et al 2006) investigating comparative efficacy of simple analgesics for episodic tension-type headache concluded that all simple analgesics had similar efficacy (measured as >50% pain relief). However, the authors did suggest that ibuprofen might be more effective than paracetamol.

Migraleve

Migraleve is available as either Migraleve Pink tablets, which contain a paracetamol codeine combination (500/8) plus buclizine 6.25 mg, or Migraleve Yellow tablets, which contain only the analgesic combination. A number of trials have investigated Migraleve Pink tablets against placebo, buclizine and ergotamine products in an attempt to establish clinical effectiveness.

A review of two trials in which Migraleve was compared against buclizine (Jorgensen 1974) and placebo (Scopa 1974) showed Migraleve was as effective as buclizine and superior to placebo in reducing severity of migraine attacks. However, patient numbers were small (n = 21 and 20, respectively) and statistical significance was not reported. Migraleve has also been compared to ergotamine-containing products; the standard drug at the time the trial was conducted. Results from a GP research group (1973) concluded that Migraleve was equally as effective as Migril in treating migraine. However, results should be viewed with caution because the trial suffered from poor design, lacked randomisation, placebo or proper blinding. A further trial by Carasso (1984) also reported beneficial effects of Migraleve. The most recent trial (Adam 1987) was well designed, being double-blind, randomised and placebo controlled. The author concluded that, compared with placebo, Migraleve did reduce the severity of attacks significantly but not their total duration.

Midrid

Midrid capsules contain isometheptene mucate 65 mg and paracetamol 325 mg. A number of trials have investigated the effect of Midrid on reducing the severity of migraine attacks. Trials date back to 1948, although it was not until the 1970s that soundly designed trials were performed. Two studies (Diamond 1975, 1976) using similar methodology investigated isometheptene versus placebo and paracetamol. Both were double-blind, placebo controlled and had identical inclusion criteria. The 1975 trial concluded that isometheptene was superior in relieving headache severity compared to placebo, although the dose of isometheptene used was double that found in Midrid. The 1976 trial also concluded that isometheptene was significantly superior to placebo and appeared to be better than paracetamol alone, but this did not reach statistical significance. A further trial (Behan 1978) compared Midrid against placebo and ergotamine. Fifty patients who suffered four or more migraine attacks per month were recruited to the study. Diary cards were completed for six attacks in which patients rated relief from headache on a four-point rating

scale. The author concluded that Midrid was as effective as ergotamine and that both were more beneficial than placebo, although it is unclear whether this was statistically significant.

Summary

Limited trial data for both products suggest that they might be more effective than placebo. They could be recommended but it is not known which product is most efficacious. However, with the deregulation of sumatriptan in 2006 their place in therapy is now questionable.

Prochlorperazine (Buccastem M)

The deregulation of prochlorperazine (UK) in 2001 represented a significant step forward in treatment options for pharmacists to manage migraine. It has been found to be a potent anti-emetic in a number of conditions, including migraine. It works by blocking dopamine receptors found in the chemoreceptor trigger zone. It is administered via the buccal mucosa and therefore patients will need to be counselled on correct administration.

Sumatriptan (Imigran Recovery)

Sumatriptan was the first 'triptan' to be marketed in the UK and subsequently deregulated to OTC status. Triptans are $5HT_1$ agonists and stimulate $5HT1_B$ and $5HT1_D$ receptors. Triptans cause constriction of the cranial blood vessels, stop the release of inflammatory neurotransmitters at the trigeminal nerve synapses and reduce pain signal transmission. As a class of medicines they have been extensively researched. Most trials with sumatriptan (and other triptans) use end point data of 2-hour pain-free response, headache relief and functional disability. In all end points sumatriptan 100 mg was significantly superior to placebo. At the lower 50 mg OTC dose evidence of efficacy is less strong than that for 100 mg but it is still effective (McCrory & Gray 2003). In head-to-head trials, other POM triptans, e.g. rizatriptan 10 mg and eletriptan 80 mg, show better efficacy than sumatriptan 100 mg (Ferrari).

Practical prescribing and product selection

Prescribing information relating to specific products used to treat migraine in the section 'Evidence base for over-the-counter medication' is discussed and summarised in Table 4.5 and useful tips relating to patients presenting with migraine are given in Hints and Tips Box 4.1.

Migraleve

Migraleve is recommended for children aged 10 years and over. The dose for adults and children over 14 years is two Migraleve Pink tablets taken when the attack is imminent or has begun. If further treatment is required, one or two Migraleve Yellow tablets can be taken every

Table 4.5
Practical Prescribing: Summary of medicines for migraine

Name of medicine	Use in children	Likely side effects	Drug interactions of note	Patients in whom care shold be exercised	Pregnancy and breast-feeding
Migraleve	>10 years	Dry mouth, sedation and constipation	Increased sedation with alcohol, opioid analgesics, anxiolytics, hypnotics and antidepressants	Glaucoma, prostate enlargement	Avoid in 3rd trimester
Midrid	>12 years	Dizziness, rash	Avoid concomitant use with MAOIs and moclobemide due to risk of hypertensive crisis. Avoid in patients taking beta-blockers and TCAs	Control of hypertension and diabetes may be affected, but a short treatment course is unlikely to be clinically important	Avoid
Buccastem M	>18 years	Drowsiness	Increased sedation with alcohol, opioid analgesics, anxiolytics, hypnotics and antidepressants	Patients with Parkinson's disease, epilepsy and glaucoma	Manufacturers advise avoidance but it has been used safely in both pregnancy and breast-feeding
Imigran Recovery	>18 years	Dizziness, drowsiness, tingling feeling, warm, flushed or weak, sensation of heaviness in any part of the body, and pressure in the throat, neck, chest and arms or legs	MAOIs, ergotamine	Avoid in people with a previous MI, ischaemic heart disease, transient ischaemic attack, peripheral vascular disease, cardiac arrhythmias, hypertension; history of seizures; hepatic and renal impairment; atypical migraines	Avoid

MAOI, monoamine oxidase inhibitor; MI, myocardial infarction; TCA, tricyclic antidepressants

HINTS AND TIPS BOX 4.1: MIGRAINE

Simple analgesia	Recommend a soluble or orodispersible formulation to maximise the absorption of analgesic before it is inhibited by gastric stasis
Administration of buccal tablets	1. Place the tablet either between the upper lip and gum above the front teeth or between the cheek and upper gum 2. Allow the tablet to dissolve slowly. The tablet will soften and form a gel-like substance after 1 to 2 hours 3. The tablet will take between 3 to 5 hours to completely dissolve. If food or drinks are to be consumed in this time, place the tablet between the upper lip and gum, above the front teeth 4. The tablets should not be chewed, crushed or swallowed 5. Touching the tablet with the tongue, or drinking fluids can cause the tablet to dissolve faster

4

4 hours. The dose for children aged between 10 and 14 years is half that of the adult dose. The maximum adult dose is eight tablets (two Migraleve Pink and six Migraleve Yellow) in 24 hours and for children aged between 10 and 14 years of age, the maximum dose is four tablets (one Migraleve Pink and three Migraleve Yellow) in 24 hours.

The buclizine component of Migraleve Pink tablets can cause drowsiness and antimuscarinic effects, whereas the codeine content might result in patients experiencing constipation. Buclizine and codeine can interact with POM and OTC medication, especially those that cause sedation. The combined effect is to potentiate sedation and it is important to warn the patient of this. It appears that Migraleve is safe in pregnancy but because of the codeine component, it is best avoided in the third trimester.

Midrid

Midrid is licensed for use only in adults. The dose is two capsules at the start of an attack followed by one capsule every hour until relief is obtained. A maximum of five capsules can be taken in a 12-hour period. It is a sympathomimetic agent, therefore, like decongestants, it interacts with MAOIs, which might lead to fatal hypertensive crisis, and it can affect diabetes and hypertension control (see Chapter 1, page 13). Side effects reported with Midrid include transient rashes and other allergic reactions.

Buccastem M

Buccastem M is indicated for previously diagnosed migraine sufferers aged 18 years and over who experience nausea and vomiting. The dose is one or two tablets twice daily. Side effects include drowsiness, dizziness, dry mouth, insomnia, agitation and mild skin reactions. Because it crosses the blood–brain barrier it will potentiate the effect of other CNS depressants and interact with alcohol. Prochlorperazine has been safely used in pregnancy, although the manufacturer advises avoidance unless absolutely necessary during the first trimester of pregnancy.

Imigran Recovery

Patients over the age of 18 years, but younger than 65, should take a single tablet (50 mg) as soon as possible after the onset of the headache. If the headache clears and then recurs a second tablet can be taken, provided there was a response to the first tablet and more than 2 hours have elapsed between the first and second tablet. No more than 100 mg can be taken during any 24-hour period. If there is no response to the first tablet, a second tablet should not be taken for the same attack. Sumatriptan is associated with a well-recognised side effect profile with the commonest adverse events (classified as occurring in 1 to 10% of patients) being dizziness, drowsiness, tingling, feeling warm, flushed or weak and sensation of heaviness in any part of the body, and pressure in the throat, neck, chest and arms or legs. Triptans are associated with rare cases of cardiac disorders and therefore to allow wider availability via OTC sales the warnings associated with prescription use have become contraindications. Therefore, patients ineligible for OTC use are those with:

- a previous myocardial infarction, ischaemic heart disease, peripheral vascular disease, cardiac arrhythmias and history of transient ischaemic attack and stroke
- known hypertension
- a history of seizures
- hepatic and renal impairment
- atypical migraines
- concomitant administration of MAOIs and ergotamine, or other $5-HT_1$ receptor agonists.

To facilitate pharmacists in the diagnosis of migraine and the appropriate supply of sumatriptan the manufacturer has produced a migraine questionnaire (http://www.imigranrecovery.co.uk/questionnaire.aspx). This should prove useful as sumatriptan supply is associated with various product license restrictions, which might be difficult to remember.

Further reading

Adam EI. A treatment for the acute migraine attack. J Int Med Res 1987;15:71–5.

[Anonymous] Reports from the general practitioner clinical research group. Migraine treated with an antihistamine-analgesic combination. Practitioner 1973;211:357–61.

Behan PO. Isometheptene compound in the treatment of vascular headache. Practitioner 1978;221:937–9.

Carasso RL, Yehuda S. The prevention and treatment of migraine with an analgesic combination. Br J Clin Pract 1984;38:25–7.

Coutin IB, Glass SF. Recognizing uncommon headache syndromes. Am Fam Physician 1996;54:2247–52.

Diamond S, Medina JL. Isometheptene – a non-ergot drug in the treatment of migraine. Headache 1975;15:211–3.

Diamond S. Treatment of migraine with isometheptene, acetaminophen, and dichloralphenazone combination: a double blind crossover trial. Headache 1976;15:282–7.

Ferrari MN, Goadsby PJ, Roon KI, et al. Triptans in migraine: detailed results and methods of a meta-analysis of 53 trials. Cephalagia 2002;22:633–58.

Goadsby PJ. Recent advances in the diagnosis and management of migraine. BMJ 2006;332;25–9.

Jorgensen PB, Weightman D, Foster JB. Comparison of migraleve and buclizine in prophylaxis of migraine. Curr Ther Res 1974;16:1276–80.

McCrory DC, Gray RN. Oral sumatriptan for acute migraine. Cochrane Database of Systematic Reviews 2003, issue 3.

Merrington DM. Comments on Migraleve trial reports. Curr Ther Res Clin Exp 1975;18:222–5.

Scopa J, Jorgensen PB, Foster JB. Migraleve in the prophylaxis of migraine. Curr Ther Res 1974;16:1270–5.

Verhagen AP, Damen L, Berger MY, et al. Is any one analgesic superior for episodic tension-type headache? J Fam Pract 2006:55;1064–72.

Web sites

The Migraine Trust: http://migrainetrust.org

Migraine Action Association: http://www.migraine.org.uk/index.aspx

International Headache Society: http://www.i-h-s.org/

International Headache Society Classification Guidelines: http://ihs-classification.org/en/

Migraine in Primary Care Advisors (MIPCA): http://www.mipca.org.uk

British Association for the Study of Headache: http://www.bash.org.uk

World Headache Alliance: http://www.w-h-a.org/wha2/index.asp

Organisation for the Understanding of Cluster Headaches (OUCH-UK): http://www.ouchuk.org

National Headache Foundation: http://www.headaches.org/consumer/index.html

Prodigy guidance: http://www.prodigy.nhs.uk/migraine

Bandolier migraine special issue: http://www.jr2.ox.ac.uk/Bandolier/booth/booths/migraine.html

Triptan guidance: http://www.rpsgb.org/pdfs/otcsumatriptanguid.pdf

Migraine articles: http://www.pharmj.com/pdf/cpd/pj_20020202_migraine1.pdf and http://www.pharmj.com/pdf/cpd/pj_20020209_migraine2.pdf

Insomnia

Background

The length of sleep people need varies but typically people aged between 20 and 45 years require 7 to 8 hours per day, although 10% of people can function on less than 5 hours per night. Sleep requirements also decrease with increasing age and people over 70 commonly have 6 hours sleep per day. Insomnia is classified by its duration: transient (a few days), short-term (up to 3 weeks) or chronic (greater than 3 weeks).

It is likely that everyone at some point will experience insomnia as it can arise from many different causes (Fig. 4.3) but for most people the problem will be of nuisance value, affecting next day alertness. The pharmacist can manage most patients with transient or short-term insomnia; however, cases of chronic insomnia are best referred to the GP, as there is usually an underlying cause.

Prevalence and epidemiology

Approximately 20 to 40% of adults report occasional sleep difficulty and half of them consider it to be significant. It is twice as common in women than men. It is reported that only 5 to 10% of patients go on to develop chronic insomnia, although chronic insomnia is more common in the elderly, affecting approximately 20% of people over 65 years of age.

Aetiology

Sleep is essential to allow the body to repair and restore brain and body tissues. The mechanisms controlling sleep

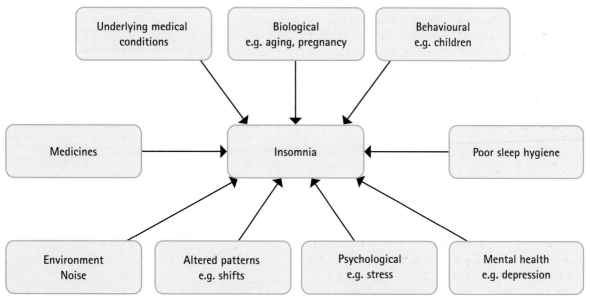

Fig. 4.3 Causes of insomnia

are complex and not yet fully understood but reflect disturbances of arousal and/or sleep-promoting systems in the brain. Their relative activities determine the degree of alertness during wakefulness and depth and quality of sleep. Therefore, insomnia may be caused by any factor that increases activity in arousal systems or decreases activity in sleep systems.

Arriving at a differential diagnosis

The key to arriving at a differential diagnosis is to take a detailed sleep history. Asking symptom-specific questions will help the pharmacist to determine if referral is needed (Table 4.6). Two key features of insomnia need to be determined: the type of insomnia and how it affects the person. Transient insomnia is often caused by a

change of routine, for example, time zone changes or a change to shift patterns, excessive noise, sleeping in a new environment (e.g. hotel) or extremes of temperature. Short-term insomnia is usually related to acute stress such as sitting exams, bereavement, loss of job, forthcoming marriage or house move. Asking the patient to tell you what they are thinking about before they fall asleep and when they awake will give you a clue to the cause of the insomnia. Often it can be difficult to determine a cause of the insomnia and getting the patient to keep a sleep diary (retiring and waking times, time taken to fall asleep, etc.) is sometimes beneficial as it allows an objective measure of the person's habits compared to their subjective perceptions.

Clinical features of insomnia

Insomnia is a subjective complaint of poor sleep in terms of its quality and duration. Patients will complain of difficulty in falling asleep, staying asleep or lack refreshment by sleep. Sometimes patients will experience daytime fatigue but not generally sleepiness. This tiredness can lead to poor performance at work.

Conditions to eliminate

Insomnia in children

Bedwetting is the most common sleep arousal disorder in children. If this is not the cause, then insomnia invariably stems from a behavioural problem such as fear of the dark, insecurity or nightmares. Children should not be given sleep aids but referred to their GP for further evaluation, as the underlying cause needs to be addressed.

Medicine-induced insomnia

Medication can cause all three types of insomnia (Table 4.7). The mild stimulant effects of caffeine, contained in chocolate, tea, coffee and cola drinks, are frequently implicated in causing transient insomnia. It is therefore advisable to instruct patients to avoid products containing caffeine after 6 or 7 pm.

Underlying medical conditions

Many medical conditions may precipitate insomnia. It is therefore necessary to establish a medical history from the patient. A key role for the pharmacist in these situations is to ensure that the condition is being treated optimally and check that the medication regime is appropriate. If improvements to prescribing could be made then the prescriber should be contacted to discuss possible changes to the patient's medication.

Depression

It is well known that between one-third and two-thirds of patients suffering from chronic insomnia will have a

Table 4.6
Specific questions to ask the patient: Insomnia

Question	Relevance
Pattern of sleep	• An emotional disturbance (predominantly anxiety) is commonly associated in patients who find it difficult to fall asleep; patients who fall asleep but wake early and cannot fall asleep again, or who are then restless, are sometimes suffering from depression
Daily routine	• Has there been any change to the work routine – changes to shift patterns, additional workload resulting in longer working hours and greater daytime fatigue • Too much exercise or intellectual arousal prior to going to bed can make sleep more difficult
Underlying medical conditions	• Medical conditions likely to cause insomnia are gastro-oesophageal reflux disease, pregnancy, pruritic skin conditions, asthma, Parkinson's disease, painful conditions (osteoarthritis), hyperthyroidism (night sweats), menopausal symptoms (hot flushes) and depression
Recent travel	• Time zone changes will affect the person's normal sleep pattern and it can take a number of days to re-establish normality
Daytime sleeping	• Elderly people might 'nap' through the day, which results in less sleep needed in the evening, making patients believe they have insomnia

Table 4.7
Medication that can cause insomnia

Stimulants	Caffeine, theophylline, sympathomimetic amines (e.g. pseudoephedrine), MAOIs (especially in early treatment)
Anti-epileptics	Carbamazepine, phenytoin
Alcohol	Low to moderate amounts can promote sleep but when taken in excess or over long periods of time can disturb sleep
Beta-blockers	Can cause nightmares, especially propranolol. Limit by swapping to a beta-blocker that does not readily cross the blood–brain barrier
SSRIs	Especially fluoxetine
Diuretics	Ensure doses are not taken after midday to stop the need to urinate at night
Griseofulvin	

MAOI, monoamine oxidase inhibitor; SSRI, selective serotonin reuptake inhibitors

recognisable psychiatric illness, most commonly depression. Many of these patients do not seek medical help and will self-medicate. The patient will complain of having difficulty in staying asleep and suffer from early morning waking. The pharmacist should look for other symptoms of depression such as fatigue, loss of interest and appetite, feelings of guilt, low self-esteem, difficulty in concentrating and constipation. The National Institute for Clinical Excellence (NICE) recommends using the ICD-10 criteria for diagnosing and assessing the severity of depression and could be applied to those patients the pharmacist suspects might have depression.

Figure 4.4 will help.

> **TRIGGER POINTS indicative of referral: Insomnia**
>
> - Children under 12
> - Duration of more than 3 weeks
> - Insomnia for which no cause can be ascertained
> - Previously undiagnosed medical conditions
> - Symptoms suggestive of anxiety or depression

Evidence base for over-the-counter medication

Many cases of transient and short-term insomnia should be managed initially by non-pharmacological measures.

If these fail to rectify the problem then short-term use of sedating antihistamines may be tried.

Sleep hygiene

Once a diagnosis of insomnia has been reached, underlying causes ruled out and any misconceptions about normal sleep addressed then education about patient behaviour and practice that affects sleep should be tackled (Table 4.8).

Medication

The sedating antihistamines diphenhydramine (DPH) and promethazine are the mainstay of OTC pharmacological treatment.

Diphenhydramine
A substantial body of evidence exists to support the clinical effectiveness of DPH as a sleep aid. At doses of 50 mg DPH has been shown to be consistently superior to placebo in inducing sleep, and as effective as 60 mg of sodium pentobarbital. Doses higher than 50 mg DPH do not produce a statistically superior clinical effect and night-time doses should therefore not exceed this amount. It appears to be most effective at shortening sleep-onset time but is less effective than GABA-A receptor-acting hypnotics (e.g. the 'z' drugs available on prescription).

Promethazine
Promethazine is widely accepted to cause sedation when used for its licensed indications; however, only one trial that investigated its use as a hypnotic could be found. The study by Adam & Oswald (1986) recruited 12 healthy volunteers who took placebo or promethazine 20 or 40 mg in a blinded fashion. The authors concluded that both doses of promethazine increased the length of sleep and sleep disturbances were reduced when compared to

Table 4.8
Key steps to good sleep hygiene

- Maintain a routine, with a regular bedtime and wakening time
- Food snacks, alcoholic and caffeine-containing drinks should be avoided
- Avoid sleeping in very warm rooms
- Daytime and not evening exercise
- No daytime naps
- No sleeping in to catch up on sleep
- No strenuous mental activity at bedtime (e.g. doing a crossword in bed)
- Solve problems before retiring

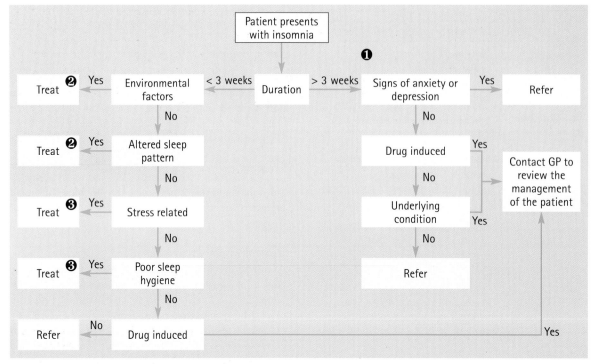

Fig. 4.4 Primer for differential diagnosis of insomnia

❶ No cases of insomnia lasting longer than 3 weeks should be treated with OTC medication. If a previously undiagnosed medical condition is suspected, most often anxiety or depression or if insomnia has been possibly caused by the patient's pre-existing condition/medicines, then the GP should be consulted and treatment options discussed/suggested.

❷ Patients should not take antihistamines for more than 7 to 10 continuous days as tolerance to their effect can develop.

❸ In the first instance, strategies to manage the patient's insomnia should be suggested rather than issuing medication.

placebo. However, it was not clear if this reached statistical significance.

Summary

Of the two sedating antihistamines, DPH has by far the stronger evidence base to substantiate its use as a hypnotic. It therefore seems prudent to use this as the treatment of choice.

Herbal remedies

Herbal remedies containing hops, German chamomile, skullcap, wild lettuce, lavender, passiflora and valerian are available and widely used. In one study of elderly patients, over 11% of respondents had used herbal remedies within the last year. However, there is little evidence to support their use. The majority of information available in the literature relates to hypothesised action of chemical constituents or studies in animals. Valerian appears to be the only product in which more than one trial has been conducted on humans. One systematic review (Stevinson & Ernst 2000) found some evidence of efficacy in long-term studies (14–28 nights of therapy) but inconclusive evidence in the short term (1–4 nights of therapy). In addition, the trials were often of short duration, used volunteers or patients with different criteria, and were usually methodologically poor. A number of branded products containing combinations of herbal ingredients are available OTC (e.g. Kalms sleep tablets, Nytol herbal tablets, Potters Nodoff, Stressless).

Melatonin

Melatonin is advocated for use in sleep disturbance, particularly in association with jet lag. What evidence is available for melatonin is not very convincing and two systematic reviews have concluded that it is not effective in treating insomnia.

Practical prescribing and product selection

Prescribing information relating to medicines for insomnia in the section 'Evidence base for over-the-counter medication' is discussed and summarised in Table 4.9 and useful tips relating to patients presenting with insomnia are given in Hints and Tips Box 4.2.

Both the antihistamines that are used for insomnia are first-generation antihistamines and interact with other sedating medication, resulting in potentiation of sedation. Additionally, they possess antimuscarinic side effects, which commonly lead to dry mouth and possibly

Table 4.9
Practical Prescribing: Summary of medicines for insomnia

Name of medicine	Use in children	Likely side effects	Drug interactions of note	Patients in whom care should be exercised	Pregnancy and breast-feeding
Diphenhydramine	>16 years	Dry mouth, sedation, and grogginess next day	Increased sedation with alcohol, opioid analgesics, anxiolytics, hypnotics and antidepressants	Glaucoma, prostate enlargement	Some manufacturers advise avoidance but safety data show antihistamines to be OK

HINTS AND TIPS BOX 4.2: INSOMNIA

Antihistamines	Tolerance can develop with continuous use
Patients who self-treat for depression	St John's wort (hypericum) is used by many patients to treat depression. There is a growing body of evidence that it is more effective than placebo for mild depression and is comparable in effect to tricyclic antidepressants. However, pharmacists should not recommend it routinely. If depression is suspected then the patient should be referred for further assessment. St John's wort also interacts with other medicines including warfarin, SSRIs, anti-epileptics, digoxin, ciclosporin, theophylline and contraceptives
Melatonin	Despite the poor evidence for melatonin, it is used in other countries, e.g. USA, for jet lag. It is available in the UK through health food shops

to constipation. It is these antimuscarinic properties that mean patients with glaucoma and prostate enlargement should ideally avoid their use as it could lead to increased intraocular pressure and precipitation of urinary retention.

Diphenhydramine (e.g. Nytol, Nightcalm)

Diphenhydramine is made by a number of manufacturers to aid the relief of temporary sleep disturbance. It is licensed only for adults and children over 16 years of age, and should be taken 20 minutes before going to bed.

Promethazine

Proprietary brands of promethazine on sale to the public include Sominex (20 mg) and Phenergan (10 or 25 mg). Adults and children over 16 years of age should take one tablet an hour before bedtime.

Further reading
Adam K, Oswald I. The hypnotic effects of an antihistamine: promethazine. Br J Clin Pharmacol 1986;22:715–7.
Byrne J. Insomnia in older people: current approaches to treatment. The Prescriber 2006;17:54–6.

Buscemi N, Vandermeer B, Hooton N, et al. Efficacy and safety of exogenous melatonin for secondary sleep disorders and sleep disorders accompanying sleep restriction: meta-analysis. BMJ 2006 doi:10.1136/bmj.38731.532766.F6.
Buscemi N, Vandermeer B, Hooton N, et al. The efficacy and safety of exogenous melatonin for primary sleep disorders: A meta-analysis. J Gen Internal Med 2005;20:1151–8.
Gillin JC, Byerley WF. The diagnosis and management of insomnia. NEJM 1990;322:239–48.
Mellinger GD, Balter MB, Uhlenhuth EH. Insomnia and its treatment. Prevalence and correlates. Arch Gen Psychiatry 1985;42:225–32.
Rickels K, Morris RJ, Newman H, et al. Diphenhydramine in insomniac family practice patients: a double-blind study. J Clin Pharmacol 1983;23:234–42.
Sproule BA, Busto UE, Buckle C, et al. The use of non-prescription sleep products in the elderly. Int Geriatr Psychiatry 1999;10:851–7.
Stevinson C, Ernst E. Valerian for insomnia: a systematic review of randomized clinical trials. Sleep Med 2000;1:91–9.

Web sites
National Sleep Foundation: http://www.sleepfoundation.org/
Prodigy Guidance: http://www.prodigy.nhs.uk/insomnia

Nausea and vomiting

Background

Nausea is an unpleasant sensation, which may be a precursor to the forceful expulsion of gastric contents (vomiting). They are common symptoms of many disorders, especially gastrointestinal conditions. However, infection, acute alcohol ingestion, anxiety, severe pain, labyrinth and cardiovascular causes can also produce nausea and vomiting.

Deregulation of domperidone and prochlorperazine has meant that community pharmacists can now more effectively manage nausea and vomiting. Until their deregulation, treatment choices were limited to anticholinergics and first-generation antihistamines, used as prophylactic agents for the prevention of motion sickness (see Chapter 10, page 295).

Prevalence and epidemiology

Nausea and vomiting are symptoms of other conditions and therefore their prevalence and epidemiology within the population are determined by that condition. Needless to say nausea and vomiting are common and most people at some point in time will experience these symptoms.

Aetiology

Nausea occurs because activity in the vomiting centre (located in the medulla oblongata) increases. Information received from the receptor cells in the walls of the gastrointestinal tract and parts of the nervous system reach a 'threshold value' that induces the vomiting reflex. Additionally, further input is received at the vomiting centre from an area known as the chemoreceptor trigger zone. This is highly sensitive to certain circulating chemicals, for example substances released by damaged tissues as a result of bacterial infection.

Arriving at a differential diagnosis

Nausea and/or vomiting rarely occur in isolation. Other symptoms are usually present and should therefore allow a differential diagnosis to be made. Most cases will have a gastrointestinal origin, with gastroenteritis being the commonest acute cause in all age groups. However, questioning the patient about associated symptoms should be made as other causes of nausea and vomiting need to be eliminated (Table 4.10).

Clinical features associated with gastroenteritis

Gastroenteritis is characterised by acute onset, vomiting and/or diarrhoea and systemic illness (e.g. fever). Most cases, regardless of infecting pathogen, resolve in a few days and rarely last more than 10 days. In children under 5 years old, over 60% of cases are viral in origin with the rotavirus and small round structured virus most commonly identified. Vomiting usually precedes diarrhoea by several hours. Bacterial gastroenteritis presents with similar symptoms although fever is usually a more prominent feature.

Conditions to eliminate

Gastritis

Gastritis is often alcohol or medicine induced and can present as acute or chronic nausea and vomiting. Epigastric pain is usually present. For further information on gastritis see Chapter 6, page 136.

Nausea and vomiting associated with headaches

Vomiting, and especially nausea, is a common symptom in patients who suffer from migraines. However, other causes of headache such as raised intracranial pressure

Table 4.10 Specific questions to ask the patient: Nausea and vomiting	
Question	Relevance
Presence of abdominal pain	• Certain abdominal conditions, e.g. appendicitis, cholecystitis and cholelithiasis, can also cause nausea and vomiting. However, for all three conditions abdominal pain would be the presenting symptom and not nausea and vomiting. The severity of the pain alone would trigger referral
Timing of nausea and vomiting	• Early morning vomiting is often associated with pregnancy and excess alcohol intake. If vomiting occurs immediately after food this suggests gastritis and if vomiting begins 1 or more hours after eating food then peptic ulcers are possible
Signs of infection	• Acute cases of gastroenteritis will normally have other associated symptoms such as diarrhoea, fever and abdominal discomfort. If infection is due to food contamination then other people are often affected at the same time

can also cause nausea and vomiting. For further information on nausea and vomiting associated with headaches see pages 75–77.

Nausea and vomiting in neonates (up to 1 month old)

Vomiting in neonates should always be referred because it suggests some form of congenital disorder, for example Hirschsprung's disease.

Nausea and vomiting in infants (1 month to 1 year old)

In the first year of life the most common causes of nausea and vomiting are feeding problems and gastrointestinal and urinary tract infection. Vomiting in infants needs to be differentiated from regurgitation. Regurgitation is an effortless back flow of small amounts of liquid and food between meals or at feed times; vomiting is the forceful expulsion of gastric contents. The infant will usually have a fever and be generally unwell if vomiting is associated with infection. If projectile vomiting occurs in an infant under 3 months of age then pyloric stenosis should be considered. Owing to the higher risk of dehydration in this age group it is prudent to refer to a doctor if symptoms persist for more than 24 hours.

Nausea and vomiting in children (1 year to 12 years old)

Children under 12 years who experience nausea and vomiting will usually have gastroenteritis, fever or otitis media. In most instances the conditions are self-limiting and medication designed to reduce pain and temperature (analgesia) and replace fluid (oral rehydration therapy) will help resolve symptoms.

Pregnancy

Pregnancy should always be considered in women of childbearing age if nausea and vomiting occur in the absence of other symptoms. Sickness tends to be worse in the first trimester and in the early morning.

Excess alcohol consumption

The patient should always be asked about recent alcohol intake, as excess quantities are associated with nausea and early morning vomiting.

Medicine-induced nausea and vomiting

Many medications can cause nausea and vomiting. Frequently implicated medicines are cytotoxics, opiates, iron, antibiotics, NSAIDs, potassium supplements, selective serotonin reuptake inhibitors (SSRIs), nicotine gum (ingestion of nicotine rather than buccal absorption), theophylline and digoxin toxicity. If medication is sus-

pected then the pharmacist should contact the prescriber to discuss alternative treatment options.

Middle ear diseases

Any middle ear disturbance or imbalance may produce nausea and vomiting. Tinnitus, dizziness and vertigo are suggestive of Meniere's disease.

TRIGGER POINTS indicative of referral: Nausea and vomiting

- Children who fail to respond to OTC treatment
- Moderate to severe abdominal pain
- Suspected pregnancy
- Unexplained nausea and vomiting in any age group
- Vomiting in children under 1 year old lasting longer than 24 hours

Evidence base for over-the-counter medication

Currently, there are only two medicines available OTC that have licensed indications for the treatment of nausea and vomiting. For information on fluid replacement by oral rehydration solutions see Chapter 6, page 145.

Domperidone

Domperidone is licensed for pharmacy sale for the relief of post prandial symptoms that include nausea. A number of small studies have suggested that domperidone is more effective than placebo. The studies were of variable design, with differing inclusion criteria and methodology, making judgement on its effectiveness difficult to determine. However, it remains the only medication available to pharmacists to treat nausea associated with overeating and, as such, is a useful treatment option.

Prochlorperazine

Prochlorperazine is licensed for the relief of nausea and vomiting associated with migraine. It has potent antiemetic properties in a number of conditions including migraine.

Practical prescribing and product selection

Prescribing information relating to medicines for nausea and vomiting in the section 'Evidence base for over-the-counter medication' is discussed and summarised in Table 4.11.

Domperidone (Motilium 10)

Motilium 10 is only licensed for use in adults and children aged over 16 years. The dose is one tablet four times

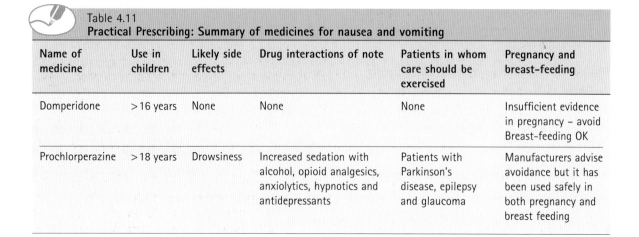

Table 4.11
Practical Prescribing: Summary of medicines for nausea and vomiting

Name of medicine	Use in children	Likely side effects	Drug interactions of note	Patients in whom care should be exercised	Pregnancy and breast-feeding
Domperidone	>16 years	None	None	None	Insufficient evidence in pregnancy – avoid Breast-feeding OK
Prochlorperazine	>18 years	Drowsiness	Increased sedation with alcohol, opioid analgesics, anxiolytics, hypnotics and antidepressants	Patients with Parkinson's disease, epilepsy and glaucoma	Manufacturers advise avoidance but it has been used safely in both pregnancy and breast feeding

a day, preferably after meals. Its safety in pregnant women has not been established, although there appear to be no reports of domperidone being teratogenic. Side effects are rare but galactorrhoea, and less frequently gynaecomastia, breast enlargement or soreness, reduced libido, dystonia and rash have been reported.

Domperidone does not appear to have any important clinical drug interactions; however, as it is a dopamine antagonist it could theoretically alter the peripheral actions of dopamine agonists such as bromocriptine.

Prochlorperazine (Buccastem M)

For dosing and counselling on Buccastem M please refer to page 80.

Further reading

Bekhti A, Rutgeerts L. Domperidone in the treatment of functional dyspepsia in patients with delayed gastric emptying. Postgrad Med J 1979;55:S30–2.

Dollery C. Therapeutic drugs, 2nd edition. Edinburgh: Churchill Livingstone, 1999.

Haarmann K, Lebkuchner F, Widmann A, et al. A double-blind study of domperidone in the symptomatic treatment of chronic post prandial upper gastrointestinal distress. Postgrad Med J 1979;55:S24–7.

Sarin SK, Sharma P, Chawla YK, et al. Clinical trial on the effect of domperidone on non-ulcer dyspepsia. Indian J Med Res 1986;83:623–8.

Self-assessment questions

The following questions are intended to supplement the text. Two levels of questions are provided: multiple choice questions and case studies. The multiple choice questions are designed to test factual recall and the case studies allow knowledge to be applied to a practice setting.

Multiple choice questions

4.1 The most common cause of nausea and vomiting is:

a. Migraine
b. Gastroenteritis
c. Gastritis
d. Medicine induced
e. Excess alcohol consumption

4.2 Which product does not contain an ingredient that can be useful for nausea?

a. Mintec
b. Midrid
c. Motilium 10 √
d. Migraleve
e. Buccastem M

4.3 Cluster headache could be best described as:

a. Bilateral piercing pain that lasts for a matter of only minutes
b. Unilateral piercing pain that lasts for a matter of only minutes
c. Unilateral orbital piercing pain with associated unilateral nasal congestion
d. Bilateral orbital piercing pain with associated nasal congestion
e. Bilateral orbital piercing pain only

4.4 Nausea and vomiting is associated with:

a. Tension headache
b. Trigeminal neuralgia
c. Cluster headache
d. Subarachnoid haemorrhage
e. Sinusitis

4.5 What herbal remedy is used to help treat insomnia?

a. Golden Rod
b. Tolu Balsam
c. Burdock
d. Mugwort
e. Passion Flower

4.6 Which trigger sign or symptom warrants referral?

a. Headache lasting 7 to 10 days
b. Headache described as vice-like
c. Headache associated with the work place environment
d. Headache in under 12 with no sign of infection
e. Headache associated with fever

4.7 The amount of sleep needed with increasing age:

a. Increases
b. Decreases
c. Stays the same

4.8 Which of these statements is true when giving advice on sleep hygiene?

a. Drinking coffee and tea is OK before bedtime
b. Try to vary the time when you go to bed
c. Sleep in a warm room
d. Try not to nap through the day
e. Take light exercise before going to bed

Questions 4.9 to 4.11 concern the following anatomical locations of the brain:

A. Orbital
B. Temporal
C. Occipital
D. Generalised
E. Unilateral and frontal

Select, from A to E, which of the above locations

4.9 Is associated with cluster headache
A

4.10 Is associated with subarachnoid haemorrhage
C

4.11 Is associated with tension-type headache
?

Questions 4.12 to 4.14 concern the following medicines:

A. Motilium 10
B. Midrid
C. Maxolon
D. Marvelon
E. Migraleve

Select, from A to E, which of the above medicines

4.12 Should be avoided by patients taking paracetamol

4.13 Is licensed for nausea associated with gastritis

4.14 Has been linked to causing migraine

Questions 4.15 to 4.17: for each of these questions *one or more* of the responses is (are) correct. Decide which of the responses is (are) correct. Then choose:

A. If a, b and c are correct
B. If a and b only are correct
C. If b and c only are correct
D. If a only is correct
E. If c only is correct

Directions summarised

A	B	C	D	E
a, b and c	a and b only	b and c only	a only	c only

4.15 Tension headache can be described as:

  a. Dull ache, not normally throbbing
  b. Worsens as day progresses
  c. Unilateral

4.16 Symptoms of the aura associated with migraine include:

  a. Scotomas
  b. Flashing lights
  c. Pins and needles

4.17 Which statements relating to headache are true:

  a. Common migraine is more common in women than men
  b. Cluster headache is more common in women than men
  c. Temporal arteritis affects mainly middle-aged men

Questions 4.18 to 4.20: these questions consist of a statement in the left-hand column followed by a statement in the right-hand column. You need to:

- decide whether the first statement is true or false
- decide whether the second statement is true or false

Then choose:

A. If both statements are true and the second statement is a correct explanation of the first statement
B. If both statements are true but the second statement is NOT a correct explanation of the first statement
C. If the first statement is true but the second statement is false
D. If the first statement is false but the second statement is true
E. If both statements are false

Directions summarised

	1st statement	2nd statement	
A	True	True	2nd statement is a correct explanation of the first
B	True	True	2nd statement is not a correct explanation of the first
C	True	False	
D	False	True	
E	False	False	

	First statement	Second statement
4.18	Common migraine is more common in men than women	Trigger factors may precipitate attacks
4.19	Insomnia can be caused by depression	Patients should be advised to try St. John's wort
4.20	Headache in VDU operators is common	Throbbing headache is caused by flickering of VDU screens

Case study

CASE STUDY 4.1

Mr AM, a male patient in his early thirties, presents to the pharmacy at lunch time complaining of headaches. The following questions are asked and responses received.

Information gathering	Data generated
Presenting complaint (possible questions)	
What symptoms/ describe the symptoms	General aching feeling all over the head
How long had the symptoms	Had for the last week
Other symptoms	No problems with lights, etc. No sickness. No recent trauma.
Where exactly	As above
Any time worse/better	Seems to get worse as day goes on.
Severity of pain (1–10)	4
Frequency of pain	Most of the time
Eye test; recent trauma	Eyes OK, no need for glasses; no
Previous history of presenting complaint	None
Past medical history	None
Drugs (OTC, Rx and compliance)	None
Allergies	Penicillin

Information gathering	Data generated
Social history	
Smoking	Non-smoker, drinks red wine (a couple of glasses each night). Works in marketing. Married with two young children. Job OK but busy with new promotion
Alcohol	
Drugs	
Employment	
Relationships	
Family history	Not known
On examination	Not applicable

Epidemiology dictates that tension-type headache is the most likely cause in primary care. However, other conditions are possible and are noted below:

Probability	Cause
Most likely	Tension headache
Likely	Migraine, sinusitis, eye strain
Unlikely	Cluster headache, temporal arteritis, trigeminal neuralgia, depression
Very unlikely	Glaucoma, meningitis, subarachnoid haemorrhage, raised intracranial pressure

Diagnostic pointers with regard to symptom presentation

The expected findings for questions when related to the different conditions that can be seen by community pharmacists are summarised on the following page.

Continued

CASE STUDY 4.1

	Duration	Timing and nature	Location	Severity (pain score from 0 to 10)*	Precipitating factors	Who is affected
Tension-type headache	Can last days	Symptoms worsen as day progresses. Non-throbbing pain	Bilateral & most often at back of head	2–5	Stress due to changes in work or home environment	All age groups and both sexes equally affected
Migraine	Average attack lasts 24 hours	Associated with menstrual cycle and weekends. Throbbing pain & nausea. Dislike of bright lights and loud noise	Usually unilateral	4–7	Food (in 10% of sufferers) & family history	Three times more common in women. Rare in children
Cluster headache	1–3 hours	Attacks occur at same time of day. Intense boring pain	Unilateral	>7	Alcohol	Three to five times more common in men
Sinusitis	Days	Dull ache that starts off being unilateral	Frontal	2–6	Valsava movements	Adults
Eye strain	Days	Aching	Frontal	2–5	Close vision work	All ages
Temporal arteritis	Hours to days	Variable	Unilateral around temples	3–6	None	Elderly
Trigeminal neuralgia	Minutes	Lancing pain at any time	Face	>7	None	Adults
Depression	Days to months	Non-throbbing pain	Generalised	2–5	Social factors	Adults
Glaucoma	Hours	Often in the evening and sudden onset	Unilateral and orbital	>7	Darkness	Older adults
Meningitis	Hours to days	Associated with systemic infection	Generalised	>7	None	Children
Subarachnoid haemorrhage	Minutes to hours	Variable	Occipital	>7	None	Adults
Raised intracranial pressure	Days to months	Worse in the mornings	Variable	>4/5	None	Older adults

*Scores set by the author and are not evidence-based.

When this information is applied to that gained from our patient (below) we see that his symptoms most closely match tension-type headache, which may (or may not) be triggered by extra pressure at work.

Depression is also a possibility, although less likely. It might be worth checking symptoms relating to the ICD-10 classification to eliminate depression.

CASE STUDY 4.1

	Duration	Timing and nature	Location	Severity (pain score from 0 to 10)	Precipitating factors	Who is affected
Tension	✓	✓	✓	✓	✓	✓
Migraine	✗	✗	✗	✓	✗	✓?
Cluster	✗	✗	✗	✗	?	✓
Sinusitis	✓	✓?	✗	✓	✗	✓
Eye strain	✓	✓	✗	✓	✗	✓
Temporal arteritis	✓	✓?	✗	✓	N/A	✗
Trigeminal neuralgia	✗	✗	✗	✗	N/A	✓
Depression	✓	✓?	✓	✓	✓?	✓
Glaucoma	✗	✗	✗	✗	✗	✗
Meningitis	✗	✗	✓	✗	N/A	✗
Subarachnoid haemorrhage	✗	✗	✗	✗	N/A	✓
Raised intracranial pressure	✓	✗	✓	✓	N/A	✗

Danger symptoms/signs (trigger points for referral)

As a final double check it might be worth making sure the person has none of the 'referral signs or symptoms'; this is the case with this patient.

Headache unresponsive to analgesics	Not yet tried
Headache in children under 12 with no signs of systemic infection or who have a stiff neck or skin rash	✗
Headache occurs after recent (1 to 3 months) trauma injury	✗
Headache that has lasted for more than 2 weeks	✗
Nausea and/or vomiting in the absence of migraine symptoms	✗
Neurological symptoms, if migraine excluded, especially change in consciousness	✗
New or severe headache in patients over 50	✗
Progressive worsening of headache symptoms over time	✗
Very sudden and/or severe onset of headache	✗

CASE STUDY 4.2

Mrs PC, a 36-year-old woman, asks you for something to treat her headache. On questioning you find out the following:

- She has had the headache for about 5 days
- The pain is located mainly behind left eye and the front of head but also at back of head
- Mrs PC is experiencing aching, no sickness or visual disturbances
- She has tried paracetamol, which helps for a while but the pain comes back after a few hours
- She has not had this type of headache before
- Work at the moment is busy because of a conference she is organising
- She takes nothing from GP except the mini-pill
- There is no recent history of head trauma
- The pain is about the same during the day

a. Using the information on epidemiology and data on signs and symptoms of each condition from Case Study 4.1, what is the likely differential diagnosis?

Tension-type headache, probably as a result of additional stress at work while organising the conference.

b. From the above responses, which symptoms allowed you to rule out other conditions?

- *Age (36): most likely causes are tension-type and migraine headaches based solely on age.*
- *Sex (female): women experience more migraines than men and less cluster headache. Therefore migraine is a possibility.*
- *Duration (5 days): most migraines do not last beyond 72 hours. Cluster headache duration is even less. More sinister causes of headache tend to last longer than 5 days. Therefore, tension-type headache likely.*
- *Location (behind eye and back of head): the pain seems fairly generalised, which is indicative of tension headache.*

- *Nature of pain (ache): again tension headaches are often described as non-throbbing. Pain does not appear to be severe, which means sinister pathology less likely.*
- *Associated symptoms (none): no nausea or vomiting. This tends to exclude migraine and conditions causing raised intracranial pressure.*
- *Medication (paracetamol): this appears to work but doesn't really help in establishing the cause of the headache.*
- *New headache (yes): the patient has not suffered from this type of headache before, a fact that might be suggestive of a more serious cause of headache. Further questioning is needed to make a judgement on whether referral would be appropriate.*
- *Lifestyle (work is busy): stress is a contributing factor to tension-type headache. It appears the patient is suffering from more stress than normal and could be a cause of the headache.*
- *Medication from GP (mini-pill): unlikely to cause the headache but further questions should be asked of the patient about how long she has been taking the medication. Most ADRs normally coincide with new medication or an alteration to the dosage regimen.*
- *Recent trauma (none): this tends to exclude headache caused by space-occupying lesions. It is worth remembering that symptoms manifest themselves once pressure is exerted on adjacent structures to a haematoma, tumour or abscess. It might therefore take several weeks for the patient to notice symptoms. Therefore, always ask about trauma over the last 6 to 12 weeks.*
- *Periodicity (worse as day goes on): this is suggestive of tension-type headache. It therefore appears that the majority of questions point to tension-type headache as the most likely cause of headache.*

you for a strong
as had the
doesn't seem to be
he man you find

ontal area and is

g
this before
es in the past
of upper

ful lifestyle
or vomiting
but much success

ogy and data on
on from Case
itial diagnosis?

It appears that tension headache and migraine can be ruled out. Cluster headache is a possibility but the type of pain and location is not right. This suggests the headache might be a secondary type of headache requiring referral. Sinusitis is a secondary cause of headache but the patient shows no recent symptoms of URTI. From the remaining secondary causes of headache it appears the symptoms most closely match temporal arteritis.

b. What extra questions could you have asked to support this conclusion?

Enquire about tenderness in the temple region or if the scalp was tender to touch.

CASE STUDY 4.4

Mrs SP, the wife of a 54-year-old man, enters the pharmacy and asks for Imigran Recovery; she has seen it advertised in the paper and her husband seems to have all the symptoms.

Information gathering	Data generated
Presenting complaint (Possible questions)	
Describe symptoms	Very painful headache. Worst towards the back of the head; feels nauseous and vomited twice but vomiting seems to have subsided
How long had you had the symptoms	12–24 hours
Severity of pain	Very painful (7–8 out of 10)
Nature of the pain	Just said it is very painful
Other symptoms/ provokes	Can't do anything. Painful even to do 'normal' things like shower, dress, etc.
Eye test; recent trauma	Not had eye test for a year but eyes OK; no recent trauma
Any symptoms before headache	No
Additional questions	Nothing seems to ease the pain
Previous history of presenting complaint	None
Past medical history	Hypercholesterolaemia

Information gathering	Data generated
Drugs (OTC, Rx and compliance)	Simvastatin 40 mg 1 one at night Ezetrol 10 mg 1 one each day Uses antihistamines OTC during spring/summer
Allergies	No allergies known
Social history	
Smoking	Married
Alcohol	Executive for a marketing firm
Drugs	Smokes 20 a day
Employment	Approx 20 units a week alcohol
Relationships	
Family history	None for presenting complaint
On examination	He generally looks tired and pain is aggravated by light

a. Given the information the lady has given you, is her husband a suitable candidate for Imigran Recovery?

   Imigran Recovery is not indicated in this instance because this is the first presentation of symptoms and he has heart disease.

b. If the patient was suitable for Imigran Recovery, given the symptoms would you sell them to his wife?

   No. Symptoms are not fully consistent with migraine. Severity, location and lack of previous history suggest it is not migraine. Symptoms are suggestive of sinister pathology.

Answers to multiple choice questions

1 = b	2 = a	3 = c	4 = d	5 = e	6 = d	7 = b	8 = d	9 = a	10 = c
11 = d	12 = e	13 = a	14 = d	15 = b	16 = a	17 = d	18 = d	19 = c	20 = c.

Women's health

Background

Women have unique healthcare needs ranging from pregnancy to menstrual disorders. Most of these conditions are outside the remit of the community pharmacist and specialist care is needed. However, a small number of conditions can be adequately treated OTC, providing an accurate diagnosis is made. This chapter explores such conditions and attempts to outline when referral should be made.

History taking

As with all conditions that present in the community pharmacy, it is essential to take an accurate history from the patient. However, for conditions affecting women's health this is especially important. The pharmacist will rely entirely on information gained by thorough questioning. There are no opportunities for any form of physical examination or access to diagnostic tests, unlike the GP. Additionally, the patient might feel uncomfortable or embarrassed about discussing symptoms, especially in a busy pharmacy. Male pharmacists may find that this level of embarrassment is heightened.

Cystitis

Background

Cystitis literally means inflammation of the bladder, although in practice cystitis refers to inflammation of the urethra and bladder. The majority of patients who present in the community pharmacy will have accurately self-diagnosed cystitis but confirmation of the patient diagnosis is essential to eliminate other potential causes. Before moving on to discuss cystitis in women further it is prudent to mention that men can also suffer from cystitis. However, in men cystitis is uncommon because of the longer urethra, which provides a greater barrier to bacteria entering the bladder; fluid from the prostate gland also confers some antibacterial property. This is especially so in men under the age of 50. After 50 years of age urinary tract infections in men become more common due to prostate enlargement.

Prevalence and epidemiology

Urinary tract infections (UTI) are one of most common infections treated in general medical practice and will affect up to 15% of women each year. Patients aged between 15 and 34 account for the majority of cases seen within a primary care setting and it is estimated that up to 50% of all women will experience at least one episode of cystitis in their lifetime; half of whom will have further attacks. Certain factors do increase the risk of a UTI: in young women, frequent or recent sexual activity and previous episodes of cystitis; the use of diaphragms or spermicidal agents; and diabetes (can indicate poor diabetic control). Additionally, cystitis affects 1 to 2% of pregnant women.

Recurrent cystitis (usually defined as three episodes in the past 12 months or two episodes in the past 6 months) is relatively common even though no identifiable risk factors are present.

Aetiology

Infection is caused, in the majority of cases, by the patient's own bowel flora that ascend the urethra from the perineal and perianal areas. Bacteria are thus transferred to the bladder where they proliferate. The most common bacterial organisms implicated in cystitis are *Escherichia coli* (>80% of cases), *Staphylococcus* (up to 10%) and *Proteus*. However, several studies have shown that up to 50% of women do not have positive urine cultures according to traditional criteria (>10^5 bacteria per millilitre of urine), although they do have 'low count bacteriuria' and therefore do have a urinary tract infection.

Arriving at a differential diagnosis

The majority of patients presenting to the community pharmacist will have acute uncomplicated cystitis. Therefore, the pharmacist's aims are to confirm a patient self-diagnosis, rule out upper urinary tract infection (pyelonephritis) and identify patients who are at risk of complications as a result of cystitis. Asking symptom-specific questions will help the pharmacist to determine if referral is needed (Table 5.1).

Table 5.1
Specific questions to ask the patient: Cystitis

Question	Relevance
Duration	Symptoms that have lasted longer than 5 to 7 days should be referred because of the risk that the person might have developed pyelonephritis
Age of the patient	Cystitis is unusual in children and should be viewed with caution. This might be a sign of a structural urinary tract abnormality. Referral is needed Elderly female patients (>70 years) have a higher rate of complications associated with cystitis and are therefore best referred
Presence of fever	Referral is needed if the person presents with fever associated with dysuria, frequency and urgency, as fever is a sensitive indicator of an upper urinary tract infection
Vaginal discharge	If a patient reports vaginal discharge then the likely diagnosis is not cystitis but a vaginal infection
Location of pain	Pain experienced in the loin area suggests an upper urinary tract infection

Clinical features of acute uncomplicated cystitis

Cystitis is characterised by pain when passing urine and causes frequency, urgency, nocturia and haematuria. The diagnostic probability of cystitis is over 90% if patients exhibit dysuria and frequency without vaginal discharge or irritation. In addition, the patient might report only passing small amounts of urine, with pain worsening at the end of voiding urine. Symptoms usually start suddenly. Suprapubic discomfort not associated with passing urine might also be present but is not common. Haematuria, although common, should be viewed with caution because it might indicate stones or a tumour. Such cases are best referred.

Conditions to eliminate

Pyelonephritis

Involvement of the ureter or kidney by the invading pathogen is the most frequent complication and results from the bacteria ascending from the bladder to these higher anatomical structures. The patient will show signs of systemic infection such as fever, chills, flank or loin pain and possibly nausea and vomiting. Referral is needed to confirm the diagnosis, exclude pelvic inflammatory disease and issue appropriate treatment (7-day course of ciprofloxacin – SIGN 2006 guidance).

Vaginitis

Vaginitis exhibits similar symptoms to cystitis in that dysuria, nocturia and frequency are common. However, all patients should be questioned about an associated vaginal discharge. The presence of vaginal discharge is highly suggestive of vaginitis and referral is needed.

Chemical vaginitis

This is a common cause of dysuria in younger women. The patient should be asked about the use of vaginal sprays and toiletries, e.g. bubble baths.

Sexually transmitted diseases

Sexually transmitted diseases can be caused by a number of pathogens, for example *Chlamydia trachomatis* and *Niesseria gonorrhoea*. Symptoms are similar to acute uncomplicated cystitis but they tend to be more gradual in onset and last for a longer period of time. In addition pyuria (pus in the urine) is usually present.

Medicine induced cystitis

Non-steroidal anti-inflammatory agents (especially tiaprofenic acid), allopurinol, danazol and cyclophosphamide have been shown to cause cystitis.

Oestrogen deficiency

Postmenopausal women experience thinning of the endo-metrial lining as a result of a reduction in the levels of circulating oestrogen in the blood. This increases the likelihood of irritation or trauma leading to cystitis symptoms. If the symptoms are caused by intercourse, symptomatic relief can be gained with a lubricating product. Referral for possible topical oestrogen therapy would be appropriate if the symptoms recur.

Figure 5.1 will aid the differentiation of cystitis from other conditions.

> **TRIGGER POINTS indicative of referral: Cystitis**
>
> - Children under 16
> - Diabetics
> - Duration longer than 7 days
> - Immunocompromised
> - Men
> - Patients with associated fever, nausea, vomiting and flank pain
> - Pregnancy
> - Vaginal discharge
> - Women older than 70

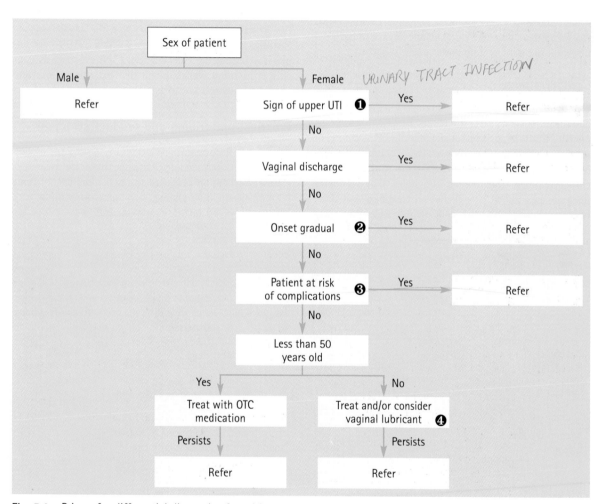

Fig. 5.1 Primer for differential diagnosis of cystitis

❶ Involvement of the higher urinary tract structures
Symptoms such as fever, flank pain, nausea and vomiting suggest conditions such as pyelonephritis.

❷ Gradual onset
STDs should be considered in patients whose symptoms are not sudden.

❸ At-risk patients
Patients at risk of developing upper UTI include those with diabetes, pregnant women, the immunocompromised, the elderly and those patients in whom symptoms have been present for more than 5 to 7 days.

❹ Patients over 50 years old
Oestrogen deficiency might account for the patient's symptoms resulting in local atrophy of the vagina.

Evidence base for over-the-counter medication

Alkalinising agents

Current OTC treatment is limited to products that contain alkalinising agents, namely sodium citrate, sodium bicarbonate and potassium citrate. (However, an application to reclassify trimethoprim in the UK is currently ongoing (December 2007) – see page 311.) Alkalinising agents are used to return the urine pH back to normal thus relieving symptoms of dysuria. However, they have dubious efficacy with little trial data to support their use. Only one trial by Spooner (1984) could be found to support their efficacy. Spooner concluded that, when treated with a 2-day course of Cymalon, 80% of patients with cystitis for whom there was no clear clinical evidence of bacterial infection did gain symptomatic relief.

Cranberry juice

Cranberry juice is a popular alternative remedy to treat and prevent urinary tract infections. However, few robust clinical trials have been conducted to substantiate or refute its clinical effectiveness. Two Cochrane reviews (2000 and updated 2004) have looked into the effects of cranberry juice. The reviews concluded that cranberry juice appears not to be effective in treatment but there is some evidence from two good-quality RCTs that cran-

berry juice might reduce the risk of symptomatic recurrent infection in women. However, the optimal dose and form of administration have not yet been established, although Car (2006) recommends drinking 200 to 750 mL of cranberry juice per day or taking cranberry concentrate tablets. Studies involving cranberry juice were not associated with any serious adverse events but widespread use of cranberry juice has resulted in the identification of possible interaction with warfarin, although evidence is conflicting. In March 2007, the National Patient Safety Agency (http://www.npsa.nhs.uk/) issued guidance on the interaction between cranberry juice and warfarin. They stated that the amount of cranberry juice needed to cause a significant drug interaction was too great to consider it important yet the current edition of the *British National Formulary* and the Medicines and Healthcare Products Regulatory Agency (MHRA) recommend avoiding the combination. Until evidence is conclusive it would seem prudent that patients on warfarin should be advised not to take cranberry products.

Practical prescribing and product selection

Prescribing information relating to cystitis medicines reviewed in the section 'Evidence base for over-the-counter medication' is discussed and summarised in Table 5.2 and useful tips relating to patients presenting with cystitis are given in Hints and Tips Box 5.1.

Table 5.2
Practical prescribing: Summary of medicines for cystitis

Name of medicine	Use in children	Likely side effects	Drug interactions of note	Patients in whom care should be exercised	Pregnancy and breast-feeding
Potassium citrate					
Effercitrate	>1 year	Gastric irritation	None	Patients taking ACE inhibitors, potassium sparing diuretics and ~~spironolactone~~ *Hyperkalemia!*	OK, but best avoided
Cystopurin	>6 years	None			
Sodium citrate					
Cymalon	Not recommended	None reported	None	Patients with heart disease, hypertension or renal impairment *Sodium Retention!*	OK, but best avoided
Cystemme					
Canesten Oasis					

HINTS AND TIPS BOX 5.1: CYSTITIS

Fluid intake	Patients should be advised to drink about 5 L of fluid during every 24-hour period. This will help promote bladder voiding, which is thought to help 'flush' bacteria out of the bladder
Product taste	The taste of potassium citrate mixture is unpleasant. Patients should be advised to dilute the mixture with water to make the taste more acceptable

Alkalinising agents

All marketed products are presented as a 2-day treatment course. The majority are presented as sachets (Effercitrate are dissolvable tablets) and the dose is one sachet to be taken three times a day, although potassium citrate can be bought as a ready made solution (the dose is 10 mL three times a day diluted well with water). They possess very few side effects and can be given safely with other prescribed medication, although in theory products containing potassium should be avoided in patients taking ACE inhibitors, potassium-sparing diuretics and spironolactone. However, in practice, it is highly unlikely that a 2-day course of an alkalinising agent will be of any clinical consequence. They can also be prescribed to most patient groups and can be given in pregnancy; although most manufacturers advise against prescribing in pregnancy, presumably on the basis that pregnant women have a higher incidence of complications resulting from cystitis. The manufacturers of Effercitrate and Cystopurin state they can be used in children but good practice would dictate that children under 16 should be referred to a medical practitioner.

Further reading

Bent S, Nallamothu BK, Simel DL, et al. Does this woman have an acute uncomplicated urinary tract infection? JAMA 2002;287:2701–10.

Car J. Urinary tract infections in women: diagnosis and management in primary care. BMJ 2006;332:94–7.

Jepson RG, Mihaljevic L, Craig J. Cranberries for preventing urinary tract infections. Cochrane Database of Systematic Reviews 2004, issue 2.

Milo G, Katchman EA, Paul M, et al. Duration of antibacterial treatment for uncomplicated urinary tract infection in women. Cochrane Database of Systematic Reviews 2005, issue 2.

Spooner JB. Alkalinisation in the management of cystitis. J Int Med Res 1984;12:30–4.

Web sites

General sites on women's health: http://www.womenshealthlondon.org.uk and http://www.womens-health-concern.org

Cystitis and Overactive Bladder Foundation: http://www.cobfoundation.org

Vaginal discharge

Background

Patients of any age can experience vaginal discharge. The three most common causes of vaginal discharge (in order of incidence) are bacterial vaginosis, vulvovaginal candidiasis (thrush) and trichomoniasis. Because thrush is the only condition that can be treated OTC, the text concentrates on differentiating this from other conditions.

Prevalence and epidemiology

It has been reported that sexually active women have a 75% chance of experiencing at least one episode of thrush during their childbearing years, and half of these will have more than one episode. Most cases are acute attacks but some women will develop recurrent thrush defined as four or more attacks each year. The condition is uncommon in prepubertal girls unless they have been receiving antibiotics. In adolescents it is the second most common cause of vaginal discharge after bacterial vaginosis.

Aetiology

The vagina naturally produces a watery discharge (physiological discharge), the amount and character of which varies depending on many factors, such as ovulation, pregnancy and concurrent medication. At the time of ovulation the discharge is greater in quantity and of higher viscosity. Normal secretions have no odour. The epithelium of the vagina contains glycogen, which is broken down by enzymes and bacteria (most notably lactobacilli) into acids. This maintains the low vaginal pH, creating an environment inhospitable to pathogens. The glycogen concentration is controlled by oestrogen production; therefore any changes in oestrogen levels will result in either increased or decreased glycogen concentrations. If oestrogen levels decrease glycogen concentration also decreases giving rise to an increased vaginal pH and making the vagina more susceptible to opportunistic infection such as *Candida*; 95% of thrush cases are caused by *C. albicans*. The remaining cases are caused by *C. glabrata* although symptoms are indistinguishable.

Arriving at a differential diagnosis

Many patients will self-diagnose their condition. The availability of efficacious OTC products and direct consumer mass marketing by pharmaceutical companies will mean that the pharmacists' role will often be to confirm a self-diagnosis of thrush. This is very important as studies have shown that misdiagnosis by patients is common (Ferris et al 2002) and can have important consequences because other conditions can lead to greater health concerns. For example, bacterial vaginosis has been linked with pelvic inflammatory disease and an increased risk of preterm birth and *C. trachomatis* can cause infertility. Symptoms of pruritus, burning and discharge are possible in all three common causes of vaginal discharge. Therefore, no one symptom can be relied upon with 100% certainty to differentiate between thrush, bacterial vaginosis and trichomoniasis. However, certain

Table 5.3
Specific questions to ask the patient: Vaginal discharge

Question	Relevance
Discharge	Any discharge with a strong odour should be referred. Bacterial vaginosis is associated with a white discharge that has a strong fishy odour and trichomoniasis is malodorous with a green-yellow discharge. By contrast, discharge associated with thrush is often described as 'curd-like' or 'cottage cheese-like' with little or no odour
Age	Thrush can occur in any age group, unlike bacterial vaginosis and trichomoniasis, which are rare in premenarchal girls. In addition, trichomoniasis is rare in women aged over 60
Pruritus	Vaginal itching tends to be most prominent in thrush compared with bacterial vaginosis and trichomoniasis
Onset	In thrush, the onset of symptoms is sudden, whereas bacterial vaginosis and trichomoniasis onset tends to be less sudden

symptom clusters are strongly suggestive of diagnosis. Asking symptom-specific questions will help the pharmacist to determine if referral is needed (Table 5.3).

Clinical features of thrush

The dominant feature of thrush is vaginal itching. This is often accompanied with soreness of the vulval lips and discharge in up to 20% of patients. The discharge has little or no odour and is curd-like. Symptoms are generally acute in onset.

Conditions to eliminate

Bacterial vaginosis

The exact cause of bacterial vaginosis is unknown although *Gardnerella vaginalis* is often implicated. It is the commonest cause of vaginal discharge with approximately 50% of patients experiencing a thin white discharge with a strong fishy odour. Odour might be worse during menses and after sexual intercourse. Itching can be present but is not common. Certain risk factors such as multiple sexual partners, use of an IUD and race (more common in black women) increase the risk of bacterial

vaginosis. Referral for metronidazole (400 mg bd for 5 days) is required.

Trichomoniasis

Trichomoniasis, a protozoan infection, is primarily transmitted through sexual intercourse. It is uncommon compared to bacterial vaginosis and thrush, and up to 50% of patients are asymptomatic. If symptoms are experienced a profuse, frothy, greenish-yellow and malodorous discharge accompanied by vulvar itching is typical. Other symptoms can include vaginal spotting, dysuria and urgency. Referral for metronidazole (400 mg bd for 5 to 7 days) is required.

Cystitis

Dysuria can affect up to one in three women with vaginal infection. However, the patient will often be able to sense that it is an external discomfort, rather than an internal discomfort located in the urethra or bladder that occurs with urinary tract infections.

Recurrent thrush

After treatment a minority of patients will present with recurrent symptoms. This may be due to poor compliance, misdiagnosis, resistant strains of *Candida*, undiagnosed diabetes or the patient having a mixed infection (it has been reported that 14% of women have mixed infections of thrush, bacterial vaginosis or trichomonas). Such cases require referral.

Atrophic vaginitis

Symptoms consistent with thrush in postmenopausal women, especially vaginal itching and burning, may be due to atrophic vaginitis. However, clinically significant atrophic vaginitis is uncommon in postmenopausal women, and should be referred to rule out malignancy.

There are also several factors that predispose women to thrush, which require consideration prior to instigating treatment.

Medicine-induced thrush

Broad-spectrum antibiotics, corticosteroids, immunosuppressants and medication affecting the oestrogen status of the patient (oral contraceptives, HRT, tamoxifen and raloxifene) can predispose women to thrush. It is not unusual to see a patient prescribed an antibiotic and treatment for thrush at the same time.

Diabetes

Patients with poorly controlled diabetes (type 1 or 2) are more likely to suffer from thrush because hyperglycaemia can enhance production of protein surface receptors on *C. albican* organisms. This hinders phagocytosis

hyperglycaemia

by neutrophils, thus making thrush more difficult to eliminate.

Pregnancy

Hormonal changes during pregnancy will alter the vaginal environment and have been reported to make eradication of *Candida* more difficult. Topical agents are safe and effective in pregnancy but OTC licensed indications do not allow sale to pregnant women and therefore these patients must be referred to the GP.

Chemical and mechanical irritants

Ingredients in feminine hygiene products, for example, bubble baths, vaginal sprays and douches can precipitate attacks of thrush by altering vaginal pH. Condoms have also been found to irritate and alter the vaginal pH.

Figure 5.2 will help in the differentiation of vaginal thrush from other conditions in which vaginal discharge is a major presenting complaint.

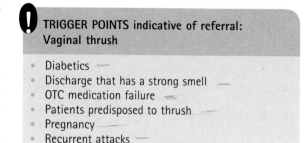

TRIGGER POINTS indicative of referral: Vaginal thrush

- Diabetics
- Discharge that has a strong smell
- OTC medication failure
- Patients predisposed to thrush
- Pregnancy
- Recurrent attacks
- Women under 16 and over 60

Evidence base for over-the-counter medication

Topical imidazoles and one systemic triazole (fluconazole) are available OTC to treat vaginal thrush. They are potent and selective inhibitors of fungal enzymes

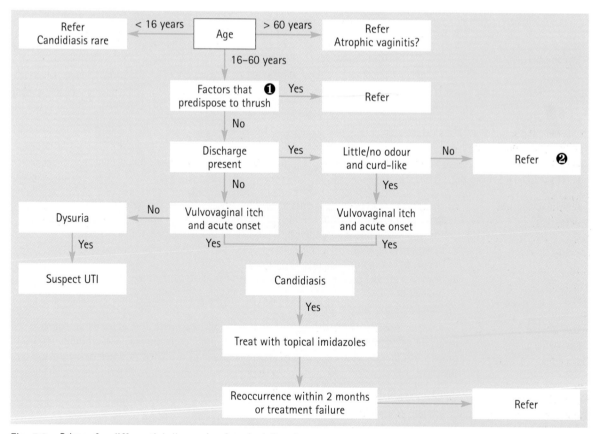

Fig. 5.2 Primer for differential diagnosis of vaginal thrush

❶ If the person is pregnant or has diabetes then referral is the most appropriate option. If the person is suffering from medicine-induced candidiasis the prescriber should be contacted to discuss suitable treatment options and, if appropriate, alternative therapy.

❷ Discharge that has a strong odour and is not white and curd-like should be referred, as trichomoniasis or bacterial vaginosis are more likely causes.

necessary for the synthesis of ergosterol, which is needed to maintain the integrity of cell membranes.

All antifungals used to treat vaginal thrush have proven and comparable efficacy with clinical cure rates between 85 and 90%. Additionally, cure rates between single or multiple dose therapy and multiple day therapy show no differences (Nurbhai et al 2007). Treatment choice will therefore be driven by patient acceptability.

Practical prescribing and product selection

Prescribing information relating to medicines for thrush reviewed in the section 'Evidence base for over-the-counter medication' is discussed below and summarised in Table 5.4; useful tips relating to patients presenting with thrush are given in Hints and Tips Box 5.2.

Topical imidazoles (clotrimazole, econazole, miconazole)

A number of formulations are available for local application including creams, vaginal tablets and pessaries. Pharmacists and the public are probably most familiar with the Canesten range of products. All internal preparations should be administered at night. This gives the medicine time to be absorbed and eliminates the possibility of accidental loss, which is more likely to occur if the person is mobile. Slight irritation on application is infrequently reported (about 5% of users) and has been linked to the vehicle and not the active ingredient. Systemic absorption is minimal and therefore there are no interactions of note, although they may damage latex condoms and diaphragms. Consequently the effectiveness of such

Table 5.4
Practical prescribing: Summary of medicines for thrush

Name of medicine	Use in children	Likely side effects	Drug interactions of note	Patients in whom care should be exercised	Pregnancy and breast-feeding
Canesten	Not applicable	Irritation	None	None	OK but pregnant women should be referred
Fluconazole		GI disturbances	Anticoagulants, ciclosporin, rifampicin, phenytoin, tacrolimus		Avoid

HINTS AND TIPS BOX 5.2: THRUSH

Administration of pessaries	As the dosage is at night, patients should be advised to use the pessary when in bed 1. Remove the pessary from the packaging and place firmly into applicator (the end of the applicator needs to be gently squeezed to allow the pessary to fit) 2. Lying on your back, with knees drawn towards the chest, insert the applicator as deeply as is comfortable into the vagina 3. Slowly press the plunger of the applicator until it stops. Remove and dispose of the applicator 4. Remain in the supine position
Use of yoghurt	Some people recommend live yoghurt as a 'natural' treatment. This is based on sound rationale as lactobacilli contained in the yoghurt produce lactic acid, which inhibits the growth of *Candida*. However, to date, there is a lack of evidence to prove or disprove this theory
General advice to help prevent infection	Avoid tight clothing, e.g. underwear, jeans etc. Use simple non-perfumed soaps when washing
Symptom resolution	The symptoms of thrush (burning, soreness or itching of the vagina) should disappear within 3 days of treatment. If no improvement is seen after 7 days the patient should see their GP
Vaginal douching	This should not be encouraged as there is no evidence of efficacy and it is associated with serious complications such as pelvic inflammatory disease

contraceptives may be reduced. Topical imidazoles do have a number of product licence restrictions that should be observed when recommending these products and these are listed below:

Product licence restriction	Rationale
Is under 16 or over 60 years of age	Thrush less common in these age groups
Has systemic symptoms	Suggests infection from a cause other than thrush
Has symptoms that are not entirely consistent with a previous episode (e.g. discharge is coloured or malodorous, there are ulcers or blisters)	Suspect bacterial vaginitis or trichomoniasis
Has had two episodes in 6 months, and has not consulted her GP about the condition for more than a year	Good practice as repeat infection may be due to misdiagnosis or predisposing risk factors
May be pregnant or is breast-feeding	Safe in both pregnancy and breast-feeding, although thrush is more common during pregnancy and it is also important to rule out gestational diabetes
Has had a previous sexually transmitted infection (or her partner has)	Rule out STD
Has had abnormal menstrual bleeding or lower abdominal pain	Symptoms not suggestive of thrush
Does not experience complete resolution of symptoms after 7 days of treatment	Imidazoles are highly effective and continuing symptoms point to misdiagnosis

Fluconazole (Diflucan One, Canesten oral)

Fluconazole is a single oral dose treatment that can be taken at any time of the day. It is generally well tolerated but it can cause gastrointestinal disturbances, such as nausea, abdominal discomfort, diarrhoea and flatulence in up to 10% of patients. There are a number of established clinically important drug interactions with fluconazole. These include anticoagulants, ciclosporin, rifampicin, phenytoin and tacrolimus. However, these

drug interactions relate to the use of multiple-dose fluconazole and the relevance to single-dose fluconazole has not yet been established. It would be prudent to avoid these combinations until further evidence is available with single-dose fluconazole.

Further reading

Brown D, Binder GL, Gardner HL, et al. Comparison of econazole and clotrimazole in the treatment of vulvovaginal candidiasis. Obstet Gynecol 1980;56:121–3.

Eschenbach DA, Hillier S, Critchlow C, et al. Diagnosis and clinical manifestations of bacterial vaginosis. Am J Obstet Gynecol 1988;158:819–28.

Fidel PL, Sobel JD. Immunopathogenesis of recurrent vulvovaginal candidiasis. Clin Microbiol Rev 1996;9:335–48.

Ferris DG, Dekle C, Litaker MS. Women's use of over-the-counter antifungal medications for gynecologic symptoms. J Fam Pract 1996;42:595–600.

Ferris DG, Nyirjesy P, Sobel JD, et al. Over-the-counter antifungal drug misuse associated with patient-diagnosed vulvovaginal candidiasis. Obstet Gynecol 2002;99:419–25.

Floyd R, Hodgson C. One-day treatment of vulvovaginal candidiasis with a 500-mg clotrimazole vaginal tablet compared with a three-day regimen of two 100-mg vaginal tablets daily. Clin Ther 1986;8:181–6.

Lebherz TB, Goldman L, Wiesmeier E, et al. A comparison of the efficacy of two vaginal creams for vulvovaginal candidiasis, and correlations with the presence of Candida species in the perianal area and oral contraceptive use. Clin Ther 1983;5:409–16.

Nurbhai M, Grimshaw J, Watson M, et al. Oral versus intra-vaginal imidazole and triazole anti-fungal treatment of uncomplicated vulvovaginal candidiasis (thrush). Cochrane Database of Systematic Reviews 2007, issue 4.

Sobel JD, Faro S, Force RW, et al. Vulvovaginal candidiasis: epidemiologic, diagnostic, and therapeutic considerations. Am J Obstet Gynecol 1998;178:203–11.

Spence D, Melville C. Vaginal discharge. BMJ 2007;335:1147–51.

Tobin MJ. Vulvovaginal candidiasis: topical vs. oral therapy. Am Fam Physician 1995;51:1715–20, 1723–4.

Web sites

R U Thinking about it?: http://www.ruthinking.co.uk
Society of Sexual Health Advisers: http://www.ssha.info
Prodigy guidance: http://cks.library.nhs.uk/candida_female_genital

Primary dysmenorrhoea (period pain)

Background

Menstruation spans the years between menarche to menopause. Typically this will last 30 to 40 years, starting around the age of 12 and ceasing around the age of 50.

The menstrual cycle usually lasts 28 days but this varies and it can last anything between 21 and 45 days. Menstruation itself lasts between 3 and 7 days. Individuals can also exhibit differences in menstrual cycle length and blood flow. Dysmenorrhoea is usually categorised as primary or secondary; primary dysmenorrhoea (PD) is defined as menstrual pain without organic pathology whereas in secondary dysmenorrhoea pathologic condition can be identified.

Prevalence and epidemiology

PD is very common in adolescents but exact prevalence rates vary due to differing definitions of dysmenorrhoea used in studies. However, it is likely to affect over 50% of women, and 7 to 15% of these women report symptoms severe enough to cause school and work absence.

Aetiology

Overproduction of uterine prostaglandins E_2 and $F_{2-alpha}$ are major contributory factors in causing painful cramps. Prostaglandin production is controlled by progesterone and before menstruation starts progesterone levels decrease allowing prostaglandin production to increase, and if over produced cramps occur. Ovulation inhibition can also improve symptoms (by using the oral contraceptive pill) as it lessens the endometrial lining of the uterus reducing menstrual fluid volume and reducing prostaglandin production.

Arriving at a differential diagnosis

The main consideration of the community pharmacist is to exclude conditions that have a pathological cause (secondary dysmenorrhoea). It is essential to take a detailed history of the patient's menstrual history as PD is a diagnosis based on exclusion. This should be done in a quiet area of the pharmacy away from other patients because of the potential for embarrassment. The frequency, severity and relationship of symptoms to the menstrual cycle need to be established. Asking symptom-specific questions will help the pharmacist to determine if referral is needed (Table 5.5).

Clinical features of PD

A typical presentation of PD is of lower abdominal cramping pains shortly before (6 hours) and for 2 or possibly 3 days after the onset of bleeding. Associated back pain, nausea and/or vomiting may also occur in up to 50% of patients. It is classically associated with young women who have recently (6–12 months) started having regular periods. However, there may be a gap of months or years between menarche and onset of symptoms. This is due to as many as 50% of women being anovulatory

Table 5.5
Specific questions to ask the patient: Primary dysmenorrhoea

Question	Relevance
Age	PD is most common in adolescents and women in their early twenties. Secondary dysmenorrhoea usually affects women many years after the menarche, typically after the age of 30
Nature of pain	A great deal of overlap exists between PD and secondary dysmenorrhoea but generally PD results in cramping whereas secondary causes are usually described as dull, continuous, diffuse pain
Severity of pain	Pain is rarely severe in PD; the severity decreases with the onset of menses. Any patient presenting with severe lower abdominal pain should be referred
Onset of pain	PD starts very shortly before or within 24 hours of the onset of menses and rarely lasts for more than 3 days. Pain associated with secondary dysmenorrhoea typically starts a few days before the onset of menses

in the first year (and still 10% of women 8 years after the menarche). This is important to know, as anovulatory cycles are usually pain-free.

Conditions to eliminate

Secondary dysmenorrhoea (e.g. endometriosis)

Endometriosis simply means presence of endometrial tissue outside of the uterus. The exact incidence of endometriosis is unclear; however, it is the most common cause of secondary dysmenorrhoea. Reports suggest it may occur in up to 50% of menstruating women but many are asymptomatic. Any person over the age of 30 either presenting for the first time with dysmenorrhoea or has noticed worsening symptoms should be viewed with caution. Patients experience lower abdominal pain (aching rather than cramping) that usually starts 5 to 7 days before menstruation begins and can be constant and severe. The pain often worsens at the onset of menstruation. Referred pain into the back and down the thighs is also possible.

Dysfunctional uterine bleeding

Dysfunctional uterine bleeding is a non-specific medical term defined as abnormal uterine bleeding that is not due to structural or systemic disease and includes conditions such as amenorrhoea (lack of menstruation) and menorrhagia (heavy periods), with the majority of cases attributable to menorrhagia. The pharmacist should ask the patient if their periods are different from usual.

Pelvic inflammatory disease

PID is an important cause of infertility and ectopic pregnancy with many women being asymptomatic and only diagnosed during infertility investigation. It most commonly occurs in sexually active women aged between 15 and 24 years old. Symptomatic cases show variable clinical presentation but it is associated with dull bilateral lower abdominal pain and dysmenorrhoea; however, other symptoms such as fever, malaise, vaginal discharge, irregular menses and dyspareunia are present.

Endometrial carcinoma

This is characterised by inappropriate uterine bleeding, and usually occurs in postmenopausal women. Bleeding starts as slight and intermittent but over time becomes heavy and continuous. Discharge and pain are rare.

TRIGGER POINTS indicative of referral: Primary dysmenorrhoea

- Heavy or unexplained bleeding
- Pain experienced before menses
- Pain that increases at the onset of menses
- Signs of systemic infection (e.g. fever, malaise)
- Vaginal bleeding in postmenopausal women
- Women over the age of 30 with new or worsening symptoms

Evidence base for over-the-counter medication

Non-steroidal anti-inflammatories

The use of non-steroidal anti-inflammatories (NSAIDs) would be a logical choice because raised prostaglandin levels cause PD. In multiple clinical trials these agents, when given orally, have been shown to be effective in 80 to 85% of women and a Cochrane review (Marjoribanks et al 2003) concluded that NSAIDs were significantly more effective in relieving moderate to severe pain associated with PD compared to placebo. However, there was little evidence of superiority of any individual NSAID.

Hyoscine butylbromide (Buscopan)

In one study, Buscopan was given to 17 patients in a double-blind placebo-crossover trial. The study failed to demonstrate a significant effect compared to placebo, or the comparator drug (aspirin), although in the author's opinion Buscopan was a good alternative to NSAIDs. Feminax, a combination analgesic product, has been marketed for many years for period pain. It used to contain hyoscine hydrobromide in low dose but was reformulated in December 2005 at the request of the UK regulatory authority to contain only the analgesic as the dose of hyoscine was subtherapeutic.

Alverine (Spasmonal) is licensed for the treatment of dysmenorrhoea. It is an anticholinergic antispasmodic that relaxes the uterine smooth muscle; however, there is a lack of published evidence regarding its efficacy.

Low dose combined oral contraceptives

Although not available OTC, oral contraceptives have been reported to be effective in treating PD, although a recent Cochrane review stated that trials reviewed were small, poor quality and used higher doses of hormones than those commonly prescribed, and therefore not enough evidence was available to conclude either way if they are useful in treating dysmenorrhoea. Despite this, if standard OTC treatment is not controlling symptoms adequately the patient should be referred as contraceptives might provide an alternative treatment option.

Non-drug treatments

A number of alternative treatments have been tested in PD, most notably transcutaneous electrical nerve stimulation (TENS), acupuncture, exercise and dietary supplements. Of these, high-frequency TENS appears to have the strongest body of evidence to support its use, although acupuncture in one small trial did show significant reduction in pain; the evidence for exercise is conflicting. A wide range of dietary intervention is frequently recommended and includes vitamin B and E, fish oils and magnesium. Most trials were conducted on low patient numbers and have reported limited or no benefit except vitamin B_1 (thiamine – 100 mg), which saw a significant proportion of women with no pain compared with placebo.

Practical prescribing and product selection

Prescribing information relating to the medicines reviewed in the section 'Evidence base for over-the-counter medication' is discussed and summarised in Table 5.6; useful tips relating to patients presenting with PD are given in Hints and Tips Box 5.3.

Table 5.6
Practical prescribing: Summary of medicines for primary dysmenorrhoea

Name of medicine	Use in children	Likely side effects	Drug interactions of note	Patients in whom care should be exercised	Pregnancy and breast-feeding
Ibuprofen	Not recommended	GI discomfort, nausea and diarrhoea	Lithium, anticoagulants, methotrexate	Elderly (increased risk of side effects)	Not applicable in pregnancy as patients do not menstruate when pregnant. Ibuprofen and Feminax OK in breast-feeding but avoid hyoscine if possible
Naproxen					
Buscopan		Dry mouth, sedation and constipation	Increase in side effects with anticholinergic medicines, e.g. TCAs	Glaucoma	
Feminax		Constipation	None	None	

HINTS AND TIPS BOX 5.3: PRIMARY DYSMENORRHOEA

Hot water bottles	The application of warmth to the lower abdomen may confer some relief from the pain

Ibuprofen

Ibuprofen should be used as first-line therapy unless the patient is contraindicated from using an NSAID. A trial of two to three cycles should be long enough to determine if NSAID therapy is successful.

There are a plethora of marketed ibuprofen products (e.g. Nurofen and Cuprofen) all of which have a standard dose for the relief of PD. Adults should take 200 to 400 mg (one or two tablets) three times a day, although most patients will need the higher dose of 400 mg three times a day. Because ibuprofen is only used for a few days each cycle it is generally well tolerated. However, gastric irritation is possible and ibuprofen can cause peptic ulcers and bronchospasm in asthmatics with a history of hypersensitivity to aspirin or any other NSAID. It is therefore contraindicated in these patient groups. Ibuprofen can interact with many medicines although the vast majority are not clinically significant.

Naproxen (Feminax Ultra)

Naproxen became available OTC in the UK in April 2008. It is indicated for primary dysmenorrhoea for women aged between 15 and 50 years old. The dose is two tablets (500 mg) initially, followed 6 to 8 hours later by a second tablet (250 mg) if needed. If further medication is needed then the dose is one tablet (250 mg) every 6 to 8 hours as required. The maximum pack size will be equivalent to 3 days' supply (nine tablets).

Buscopan

The dosage frequency for Buscopan in adults is two tablets four times a day, commencing 2 days before the expected onset of the period and continuing for 3 days after menstruation has begun. It is contraindicated in patients with narrow-angle glaucoma and myasthenia gravis and care should be exercised in patients whose conditions are characterised by tachycardia, for example hyperthyroidism and cardiac problems. Anticholinergic side effects such as dry mouth, visual disturbances and constipation can be experienced but are generally mild and self-limiting. Side effects are potentiated if Buscopan is given with tricyclic antidepressants, antihistamines, butyrophenones, phenothiazines and disopyramide.

Feminax

Adults should be advised to take two tablets every 4 hours, to a maximum of eight in 24 hours. Feminax has very few side effects but the codeine component can cause constipation.

Further reading

Auld B, Sinha P. Dysmenorrhoea: diagnosis and current management. Available at http://www.escriber.com/Prescriber/Features.asp?ID=817&GroupID=6&Action=View

Harlow SD, Ephross SA. Epidemiology of menstruation and its relevance to women's health. Epidemiol Rev 1995;17:265–86.

Kemp JH. "Buscopan" in spasmodic dysmenorrhoea. Curr Med Res Opin 1972;1:19–25.

Marjoribanks J, Proctor ML, Farquhar C. Nonsteroidal anti-inflammatory drugs for primary dysmenorrhoea. Cochrane Database of Systematic Reviews 2003, issue 4.

Proctor ML, Murphy PA. Herbal and dietary therapies for primary and secondary dysmenorrhoea. Cochrane Database of Systematic Reviews 2001, issue 2.

Web sites

Endometriosis UK: http://www.endo.org.uk/
Endometriosis SHE Trust: http://www.shetrust.org.uk/

Premenstrual syndrome

Background

Premenstrual syndrome (PMS) is a broad term that encompasses a wide range of symptoms – both physical and psychological. Symptoms start around the time of ovulation and are apparent during the luteal phase (second half) of the menstrual cycle. Symptoms range from mild to very severe; severe symptoms, especially mood symptoms, affect approximately 5% of patients and can interfere with day-to-day functioning and relationships. In these women a diagnosis of premenstrual dysphoric disorder is given.

Prevalence and epidemiology

The exact prevalence of PMS is hard to determine because of varying definitions attributed to PMS and the number of people that do not seek medical help. Surveys have shown that over 90% of women have experienced PMS symptoms but only a fifth seek medical help, yet 13 to 25% have taken time off work because of PMS symptoms. There appears to be no marked racial or ethnic differences in the prevalence but age appears to be a risk factor – most women tend to be over 30 years old.

Aetiology

The precise pathophysiology of PMS is still unclear. A number of theories have been put forward, for example, excess oestrogen, a lack of progesterone or ovarian function. Most researchers now believe PMS is a complex interaction between ovarian steroids and the neurotransmitters serotonin and GABA.

Arriving at a differential diagnosis

Owing to the varying and wide-ranging symptoms associated with PMS the pharmacist must endeavour to differentiate PMS from other gynaecological and mental health disorders. Careful questioning of when the symptoms occur and what symptoms are experienced will hopefully give rise to a differential diagnosis of PMS, although this might not be easy. It is important not to focus on one cycle's symptoms but ask the patient to describe their symptoms over previous cycles. A diary over three cycles should be maintained to allow a fuller picture of symptoms to be elucidated (diaries can be downloaded from the web site of The National Association for Premenstrual Syndrome). Asking symptom-specific questions will help the pharmacist to determine if referral is needed (Table 5.7).

Clinical features of PMS

Many symptoms have been attributed to PMS, although the most common symptoms are listed in Table 5.8.

Conditions to eliminate

Primary dysmenorrhoea

Abdominal cramps and suprapubic pain might be experienced by PMS sufferers, although these symptoms are uncommon. Key distinguishing features between PMS and primary dysmenorrhoea are the lack of behavioural and mood symptoms in primary dysmenorrhoea and the difference in timing of symptoms in relation to the menstrual cycle.

Table 5.7
Specific questions to ask the patient: Premenstrual syndrome

Question	Relevance
Onset of symptoms	Symptoms that are experienced 7 to 14 days before, and that disappear a few hours after the onset of menses, are suggestive of PMS
Age of patient	PMS is most common in women aged in their thirties and forties
Presenting symptoms	Patients with PMS will normally have symptoms suggestive of mental health disorders such as low mood, insomnia and irritability. This can make excluding mental health disorders such as depression difficult. However, the cyclical nature of the symptoms in conjunction with symptoms such as breast tenderness, bloatedness and fluid retention point to PMS

Table 5.8
Common symptoms of PMS

Physical	Behavioural	Mood
Swelling	Sleep disturbances	Irritability
Breast tenderness	Appetite changes	Mood swings
Aches	Poor concentration	Anxiety/tension
Headache	Decreased interest	Depression
Bloating/weight	Social withdrawal	Feeling out of control

Mental health disorders

Depression and anxiety are common mental health disorders, which often go undiagnosed and can be encountered by community pharmacists. Patients with PMS might experience symptoms similar to such conditions, namely low or sad mood, loss of interest or pleasure and prominent anxiety or worry. Other symptoms may include disturbed sleep and appetite, dry mouth and poor concentration. However, the symptoms are not cyclical and are not associated with other symptoms of PMS such as breast tenderness and bloatedness.

TRIGGER POINTS indicative of referral: Premenstrual syndrome

- Psychological symptoms alone
- Severe or disabling symptoms
- Symptoms that either worsen or stay the same after the onset of menses
- Women under the age of 30

Evidence base for over-the-counter medication

There are many drug and non-drug treatments advocated for the treatment of PMS yet most lack evidence from well-conducted random controlled trials. A lack of evidence or no evidence exists to support the use of reflexology, exercise, chiropractic manipulation, bright light therapy, relaxation, evening primrose oil and magnesium supplements. Only vitamin B_6 and calcium supplements have, to date, been shown to be more effective than placebo.

Trials involving vitamin B_6 have shown that overall symptoms of PMS improve over a period of 2 to 6 months and also help with behavioural/mood symptoms such as depression (Wyatt et al 1999). Vitamin B_6 is therefore worth trying for patients who experience relatively minor symptoms. Those patients who exhibit moderate to severe symptoms are best referred as treatment with selective serotonin reuptake inhibitors has proven to be effective in many cases.

Calcium supplementation at a dose of 1200 mg per day for 3 months has been shown to significantly reduce PMS symptoms overall in the luteal phase compared to placebo (Ward & Holimon 1999).

Practical prescribing and product selection

Prescribing information relating to medicines for PMS reviewed in the section 'Evidence base for over-the-counter medication' is discussed and summarised in Table 5.9; useful tips relating to patients presenting with heavy menstrual bleeding are given in Hints and Tips Box 5.4.

Vitamin B_6 (pyridoxine)

There is no definitive dose of vitamin B_6 required to alleviate symptoms of PMS. However, doses of up to 100 mg daily have been shown to help reduce symptoms. Side effects are extremely rare with doses at this level, although at higher doses it can cause numbness and peripheral neuropathy. A number of drug interactions have been observed in patients taking vitamin B_6, most notably phenytoin, phenobarbitone and levodopa. Only the vitamin B_6/levodopa interaction is significant and should be avoided. Although doses as low as 5 mg vitamin B_6 will reduce the effects of levodopa, the problem

Table 5.9
Practical prescribing: Summary of medicines used in premenstrual syndrome

Name of medicine	Use in children	Likely side effects	Drug interactions of note	Patients in whom care should be exercised	Pregnancy and breast-feeding
Pyridoxine	Not applicable	Very high doses can cause toxicity (>500 mg daily)	Levodopa when administered alone	None	Not applicable in pregnancy as patients do not menstruate when pregnant. OK in breast-feeding
Calcium		Nausea and flatulence	None	Renally impaired patients	

HINTS AND TIPS BOX 5.4: HEAVY MENSTRUAL BLEEDING

Which treatment?	If menorrhagia/heavy menstrual bleeding coexists with dysmenorrhoea, the use of NSAIDs should be preferred to tranexamic acid
Treatment failure (NICE guidance)	If there is no improvement in symptoms within three menstrual cycles then use of NSAIDs and/or tranexamic acid should be stopped

of this interaction in clinical practice is almost always negated as combinations of levodopa/carbidopa (Sinemet) or levodopa/benserazide (Madopar) are unaffected by vitamin B_6.

Calcium

Calcium supplementation should provide at least one 200 mg tablet of elemental calcium per day. It is important to ensure that a product taken by the patient provides the required amount of elemental calcium. For example, a calcium lactate 300 mg tablet provides only 39 mg of elemental calcium; calcium carbonate 1.25 g tablets (e.g. Calcichew) provide 500 mg of elemental calcium. Calcium supplements can cause mild gastrointestinal disturbances such as nausea and flatulence. If the patient is taking tetracycline antibiotics or iron then a 2-hour gap should elapse between doses to avoid decreased absorption of the antibiotic or iron.

Further reading

Gianetto-Berruti A, Feyles V. Premenstrual syndrome. Minerva Ginecol 2002;54:85–95.

Thys-Jacobs S, Starkey P, Bernstein D, Tian J. Calcium carbonate and the premenstrual syndrome: effects on premenstrual and menstrual symptoms. Am J Gynecol 1998;179:444–52.

Ward MW, Holimon TD. Calcium treatment for premenstrual syndrome. Ann Pharmacother 1999;33:1356–8.

Wyatt KM, Dimmock PW, Jones PW, et al. Efficacy of vitamin B-6 in the treatment of premenstrual syndrome: systematic review. BMJ 1999;318:1375–81.

Wyatt KM, Dimmock PW, O'Brien PMS. Selective serotonin reuptake inhibitors for premenstrual syndrome. Cochrane Database of Systematic Reviews 2002, issue 3.

Web sites

National Association for Premenstrual Syndrome: http://www.pms.org.uk/

Heavy menstrual bleeding (menorrhagia)

Background

Tranexamin acid was deregulated from POM to P control in late 2007/early 2008. The product launch was due at the same time that this book went to press (the third quarter of 2008), and is therefore included.

NICE guidance (Jan 2007) defines heavy menstrual bleeding (HMB) as excessive menstrual blood loss that interferes with a woman's physical, social, emotional and/or material quality of life, and which can occur alone or in combination with other symptoms. Other definitions exist and include excessive menses in an otherwise normal menstrual cycle that are associated with clots, the use of towels rather than tampons and dysmenorrhoea. Blood loss can be measured and used in research (menorrhagia defined as 60 to 80 mL of blood loss per cycle) but this is impractical in a clinical setting and does not correlate to subjective assessments. Although heavy blood loss is rarely associated with sinister pathology the impact on quality of life can be considerable.

Prevalence and epidemiology

The prevalence of HMB is difficult to establish due to varying definitions. However, 5% of women aged between 25 and 50 years old consult their GP each year and a third of women describe their periods as heavy. HMB can lead to surgical intervention (hysterectomy), and although the number of operations has declined dramatically nearly 19 000 hysterectomies were performed in 2004/5 due to HMB.

Aetiology

In approximately half of cases no identifiable cause can be found for HMB. Identifiable causes can result from uterine and pelvic pathology (e.g. fibroids, polyps and carcinoma), systemic disorders (e.g. hypothyroidism) and iatrogenic factors (e.g. medication and IUDs).

Arriving at a differential diagnosis

The main consideration of the community pharmacist is to exclude sinister pathology and a detailed history of the patient's menstrual cycle is essential. Asking symptom-specific questions will help the pharmacist to determine if referral is needed (Table 5.10).

Clinical features of HMB

The key symptom will be blood loss that is perceived to be greater than normal. The patient's bleeding pattern should be the same as during normal menses but heavier.

Table 5.10
Specific questions to ask the patient: HMB

Question	Relevance
Timing of bleeding	Symptoms that might suggest structural or pathological abnormality include bleeding at times other than menses
Effect on quality of life	An assessment should be made to determine what effect menstrual bleeding is having on the patient
Symptoms in relation to normal cycles	Patients will show cycle-to-cycle variation in the amount of blood loss. It is important to discuss with the patient this normal variation and to determine from the patient if she feels blood loss is within the normal range

Table 5.11
Medication that can alter menstrual bleeding

Anticoagulants
Cimetidine
Monoamine oxidase inhibitors
Phenothiazines
Steroids
Thyroid hormones

Table 5.12
Product license restrictions for sale of Cyklo-f

The product should not be used in the following circumstances:

- Mild to moderate renal failure
- Current thromboembolic disease, or a history of a previous thromboembolic event plus previous thrombosis in other family members
- Pregnancy and breast-feeding
- Younger than 18 and over 45 years of age
- In patients with diabetes, obese and nulliparous women
- Women with polycystic ovary syndrome
- Women with a history of endometrial disease in a first-degree relative

Conditions to eliminate

Medicine-induced menstrual bleeding

Occasionally, medicines can change menstrual bleeding patterns (Table 5.11). If an adverse drug reaction is suspected then the pharmacist should contact the prescriber and discuss other treatment options. Additionally, the incidence of menstrual pain is higher in patients who have had an IUD fitted.

Endometrial and cervical carcinoma

This is characterised by inappropriate uterine bleeding, and it usually occurs in postmenopausal women. Bleeding starts as slight and intermittent but over time becomes heavy and continuous. Discharge and pain are rare. Irregular bleeding between periods, especially if associated with postcoital bleeding, is extremely significant and suggests a precancerous/cancerous cervix.

TRIGGER POINTS indicative of referral: Heavy menstrual bleeding

- Intermenstrual bleeding
- Pelvic pain
- Postcoital bleeding or postcoital pain
- Treatment failure

Evidence base for over-the-counter medication

Tranexamic acid has been in clinical use in the UK for approximately 30 years and has established itself as a clinically effective medicine in decreasing menstrual blood loss.

Practical prescribing and product selection

Tranexamic acid is an antifibrinolytic and stops the conversion of plasminogen to plasmin, an enzyme that digests fibrin and thus brings about clot dissolution. NICE guidance states that if the patient history suggests no abnormalities then drug treatment can be given. This is either hormonal (currently still POM) or non-hormonal (tranexamic acid). In common with more recent POM to P deregulations the manufacturer has produced guidance for pharmacy staff and placed certain restrictions on its sale OTC (Table 5.12). The use of Cyklo-f is restricted to HMB that occurs over several cycles in women with regular (every 21–35 days) cycles with no more than 3 days of individual variability in cycle duration.

Tranexamic acid (Cyklo-f)

Cyklo-f can only be used once heavy bleeding has begun. The dose is two tablets three times a day for a maximum of 4 days. The dose can be increased to two tablets four times a day in very heavy menstrual bleeding. The maximum dose is eight tablets (4 g daily). Women can use Cyklo-f every month if needed. It has an excellent safety record and side effects are unusual. Those reported include indigestion, diarrhoea and headaches (affecting fewer than 1% of patients). Visual disturbances and thromboembolic events have been reported but are very rare. The causal relationship of thromboembolic events and tranexamic acid is unclear and NICE guidance states that no increase in the overall rate of thrombosis has been identified with those taking tranexamic acid. Nevertheless, women at high risk of thrombosis have been excluded from pharmacy supply. Tranexamic acid should not be taken in patients on anticoagulants or those taking the combined oral contraceptive, unopposed oestrogen or tamoxifen.

Further reading
Edozien L. Hysterectomy for benign conditions. BMJ 2005;330:1457–8.

Web sites
NICE guidelines – Heavy menstrual bleeding (Jan 2007): http://www.nice.org.uk/guidance/index.jsp?action=byID&o=11002

Prodigy guidance: http://cks.library.nhs.uk/menorrhagia

Self–assessment questions

The following questions are intended to supplement the text. Two levels of questions are provided: multiple choice questions and case studies. The multiple choice questions are designed to test factual recall and the case studies allow knowledge to be applied to a practice setting.

Multiple choice questions

5.1 Primary dysmenorrhoea affects?

a. 10 to 20% of women
b. 20 to 30% of women
c. 30 to 40% of women
d. 40 to 50% of women
e. Over 50% of women

5.2 When do PMS symptoms usually begin?

a. Before ovulation
b. At the start of ovulation
c. Before menstruation
d. At the start of menstruation
e. Following menstruation

5.3 What percentage of women of childbearing age will experience an episode of thrush?

a. 50%
b. 55%
c. 60%
d. 70%
e. 75%

5.4 What medication can precipitate thrush?

a. Aspirin
b. Propranolol
c. Ampicillin
d. Ramipril
e. Levothyroxine

5.5 Which condition predisposes patients to pyelonephritis?

a. Hypertension
b. Rheumatoid arthritis
c. Diabetes mellitus
d. Hyperlipidaemia
e. Asthma

5.6 Dysuria accompanied with fever and flank pain is indicative of?

a. Cystitis
b. Trichomoniasis
c. Pyelonephritis
d. Vaginitis
e. Endometriosis

5.7 What symptoms are commonly associated with primary dysmenorrhoea?

a. Lower abdominal cramping pain that starts 7 to 10 days before onset of period
b. Lower abdominal cramping pain that starts 2 to 3 days before onset of period
c. Lower abdominal cramping pain that starts 6 to 12 hours before onset of period
d. Lower abdominal griping pain that starts 2 to 3 days before onset of period
e. Lower abdominal griping pain that starts 6 to 12 hours before onset of period

5.8 Which of the following medicines can interact with phenytoin?

a. Fluconazole
b. Hyoscine
c. Potassium citrate
d. Paracetamol
e. Codeine

Questions 5.9 to 5.11 concern the following patient groups:

A. Children under 12 years old
B. Women over 30 years old
C. Women between the ages of 12 and 50
D. Women aged over 60 years old
E. Women between the ages of 40 and 60

Select, from A to E, which of the patient groups:

5.9 Are most likely to suffer from endometriosis

5.10 Are unlikely to suffer from cystitis

5.11 Should be referred automatically if they have vaginal discharge

Questions 5.12 to 5.14 concern the following conditions:

A. Vaginal thrush
B. Bacterial vaginosis
C. Trichomoniasis
D. Atrophic vaginitis
E. Cystitis

Select from A to E, which of the conditions

5.12 Has a fishy-smelling discharge

5.13 Is rare in patients aged over 60 years old

5.14 Has a cottage cheese-like discharge

Questions 5.15 to 5.17: for each of these questions *one or more* of the responses is (are) correct. Decide which of the responses is (are) correct. Then choose:

A. If a, b and c are correct
B. If a and b only are correct
C. If b and c only are correct
D. If a only is correct
E. If c only is correct

Directions summarised

A	B	C	D	E
a, b and c	a and b only	b and c only	a only	c only

5.15 A pharmacist should refer patients with vaginal candidiasis when:

   a. They have had more than two attacks in the last 6 months
   b. Women are under 16 years old
   c. Women are taking antibiotics

5.16 Which of the following symptoms are associated with premenstrual syndrome?

   a. Fatigue
   b. Irritability
   c. Breast tenderness

5.17 Which of the following medicines can cause menstrual bleeding?

   a. Levothyroxine
   b. Sertraline
   c. Amoxicillin

Questions 5.18 to 5.20: these questions consist of a statement in the left-hand column followed by a statement in the right-hand column. You need to:

- decide whether the first statement is true or false
- decide whether the second statement is true or false

Then choose:

A. If both statements are true and the second statement is a correct explanation of the first statement
B. If both statements are true but the second statement is NOT a correct explanation of the first statement
C. If the first statement is true but the second statement is false
D. If the first statement is false but the second statement is true
E. If both statements are false

Directions summarised

	1st statement	2nd statement	
A	True	True	2nd statement is a correct explanation of the first
B	True	True	2nd statement is not a correct explanation of the first
C	True	False	
D	False	True	
E	False	False	

	First statement	*Second statement*
5.18	Cystitis is uncommon in men	They have a shorter urethra than women
5.19	Vaginal discharge is uncommon in children under 12	Antibiotic therapy may precipitate attacks in this age group
5.20	Imidazoles have similar cure rates	Symptoms tend to resolve in about 3 days

Case study

Mrs PR, a 26-year-old woman, presents to the pharmacy one Saturday afternoon asking for something for cystitis. The counter assistant finds out that the patient has had the symptoms for about 3 days and has tried no medication to relieve the symptoms. At this point the patient is referred to the pharmacist.

a. What other questions do you need to ask?
  - *Location of the pain*
  - *Nature of the pain*
  - *Severity of the pain*
  - *Associated symptoms*
  - *Previous history*
  - *Any factors that might have precipitated the attack*
  - *Medical history, including any regular medication currently taking*
  - *Presence of any vaginal discharge*

You find out that Mrs PR is suffering from pain on urination, discomfort and she is going to the toilet frequently but has no other symptoms. She has had these symptoms previously about 2 years ago but they went on their own after a day or two. She takes no medicine from her GP.

b. What course of action are you going to take?

Symptoms suggest an uncomplicated acute urinary tract infection and empirical treatment could be instigated but the patient should be told that if treatment fails then she should visit the GP. Advice about adequate fluid intake should also be given.

Mrs PR returns to the pharmacy on Monday evening with a prescription for erythromycin 250 mg qds x 20.

c. Is this an appropriate antibiotic for a urinary tract infection?

Trimethoprim (or nitrofurantoin) is first-line treatment. This is because Escherichia coli *and* Staphylococcus *usually cause cystitis for which trimethoprim has activity. Prodigy guidance (http://cks.library.nhs.uk/uti_lower_women/about_this_topic) recommends cefalexin, co-amoxiclav or a quinolone as suitable alternatives.*

CASE STUDY 5.2

Ms CL, a girl in her late teens/early twenties, asks for some painkillers for period pain. The following questions are asked, and responses received.

Information gathering	Data generated
Presenting complaint (possible questions)	
What symptoms have you got	General aching pain in tummy (if asked where – rub around umbilicus)
How long have you had the symptoms	2 days
Type/severity of pain	4 (1–10) scale
Any other symptoms	Felt a little sick
When is your period due	Any day now
Additional questions asked	No systemic symptoms No discharge or unusual bleeding
Previous history of presenting complaint	Had period pain before but this seems worse than previous times
Past medical history	None
Drugs (OTC, Rx and compliance)	Paracetamol for pain. Helps a little but wanted something a bit stronger
Allergies	None known

Information gathering	Data generated
Social history Smoking Alcohol Drugs Employment Relationships	Student. Drinks, does not smoke
Family history	N/A
On examination	If temperature taken, is slightly elevated

Epidemiology dictates that the most likely cause of period pain seen in primary care is primary dysmenorrhoea. However, other conditions are possible and are noted below:

Probability	Cause
Most likely	Primary dysmenorrhoea
Likely	Secondary dysmenorrhoea (endometriosis)
Unlikely	Pelvic inflammatory disease, medication, dysfunctional uterine bleeding
Very unlikely	Endometrial carcinoma

Diagnostic pointers with regard to symptom presentation

The following page summarises the expected findings for questions when related to the different conditions that can be seen by community pharmacists.

Continued

CASE STUDY 5.2

	Age	Pain timing to period	Nature and severity of pain	Bleeding pattern	Discharge
Primary dysmenorrhoea	Under 30	Just prior	Aching, mild to moderate	Normal	Unusual
Secondary dysmenorrhoea	Over 30	Days before	Cramping, moderate to severe	Possible	Unusual
Pelvic inflammatory disease	Young, sexually active	Not associated with menstruation	Dull and can vary in severity	Irregular	Yes
Medicines	Any	N/A	None	Irregular	N/A
Dysfunctional uterine bleeding	Any	N/A	None	Irregular	No
Carcinoma	Postmenopausal	N/A	No (only in late stage of disease)	Irregular	Rare

When this information is applied to that gained from our patient (below) we see that her symptoms strongly suggest primary dysmenorrhoea. A degree of caution needs to be exercised because her symptoms seem worse than previous episodes and simple analgesia seems to be ineffective. Treat her symptoms this time but review over the next few cycles.

	Age	Pain timing to period	Nature and severity of pain	Bleeding pattern	Discharge
Primary dysmenorrhoea	✓	✓	✓	✓	✓
Secondary dysmenorrhoea	✗	✗	✗?	✓?	✓
Pelvic inflammatory disease	✓	✗	✗	✗	✗
Medicines	N/A (no medicines taken)				
Dysfunctional uterine bleeding	✓	N/A	✗	✗	✗
Carcinoma	✗	N/A	✗	✗	✗

Danger symptoms/signs (trigger points for referral)

As a final double check it might be worth making sure the person has none of the 'referral signs or symptoms'; this is the case with this patient.

Heavy or unexplained bleeding	✗
Pain experienced before menses	✗
Pain that increases at the onset of menses	Not known
Signs of systemic infection (e.g. fever, malaise)	✗
Vaginal bleeding in postmenopausal women	N/A
Women over the age of 30 with new or worsening symptoms	N/A

CASE STUDY 5.3

Ms FP, a female patient in her early forties, presents in the pharmacy complaining of thrush. The following questions are asked, and responses received.

Information gathering	Data generated
Presenting complaint (possible questions)	
What symptoms have you got	Moderate itching
How long have you had the symptoms	Last 1 or 2 days
Any other symptoms	No other symptoms
Additional questions asked	No discharge No changes to feminine hygiene products
Previous history of presenting complaint	Similar to last symptoms, which cleared with Canesten, but finds cost OTC too much so wants a prescription
Past medical history	Diabetic
Drugs (OTC, Rx and compliance)	Insulin. Medical records do not state last HBA1c reading
Allergies	None known
Social history Smoking Alcohol Drugs Employment Relationships	Smokes 10 cigarettes a day. Drinks at weekends. Two teenage children. Divorced. Works for Sainsbury's.

Information gathering	Data generated
Family history	Mum diabetic. Dad died about 5 years ago with MI.
On examination	N/A

Epidemiology dictates that bacterial vaginosis is most prevalent in primary care. However, other conditions, such as thrush are also common and can be managed by pharmacists.

Probability	Cause
Most likely	Bacterial vaginosis
Likely	Thrush, trichomoniasis, medicine-induced thrush
Unlikely	Atrophic vaginitis, cystitis, mixed infection, diabetes, pregnancy, irritants

Diagnostic pointers with regard to symptom presentation

The following page summarises the expected findings for questions when related to the three commonest conditions in which discharge is present.

Continued

CASE STUDY 5.3

	Timing	Discharge	Odour	Itch
Thrush	Acute and onset quick	White curd or cottage cheese-like (1 in 5 patients)	Little or none	Prominent
Bacterial vaginosis	Acute but onset slower	White and thin (1 in 2 patients)	Strong and fishy, which might be worse during menses and after sex	Slight
Trichomoniasis	Acute but onset slower	Green-yellow and can be frothy	Malodorous	Slight

When this information is applied to that gained from our patient (below) we see that her symptoms support a differential diagnosis of thrush. Discharge is least often reported with thrush compared to bacterial vaginosis and trichomoniasis and lends further weight to the diagnosis being thrush. It is worth remembering that certain disease states and actions can precipitate thrush and should be excluded. Symptoms do not appear to be brought on by any changes in toiletries but the patient is diabetic. The patient has had symptoms previously (although questioning did not reveal when the last episode was) and it is possible that the symptoms are as a consequence of her diabetes. Treatment could be given but the patient should be advised to see her doctor to check her diabetic control.

	Timing	Discharge	Odour	Itch
Thrush	✓	✗?	✓	✓
Bacterial vaginosis	✗?	✗?	✗	✗
Trichomoniasis	✗?	✗?	✗	✗

Chapter 6

Gastroenterology

Background

The main function of the gastrointestinal (GI) tract is to break food down into a suitable energy source to allow normal physiological function of cells. Needless to say, the process is complex and involves many different organs. Consequently, there are many conditions that affect the GI tract, some of which are acute and self-limiting and respond well to OTC medication and others that are serious and require referral.

General overview of the anatomy of the GI tract

It is vital that pharmacists have a sound understanding of GI tract anatomy. Many conditions will present with similar symptoms and from similar locations, for example abdominal pain, and the pharmacist will need a basic knowledge of GI tract anatomy – and in particular of where each organ of the GI tract is located – to facilitate a correct differential diagnosis.

Oral cavity

The oral cavity comprises the cheeks, hard and soft palates and tongue.

Stomach

The stomach is roughly 'J' shaped and receives food and fluid from the oesophagus. It empties into the duodenum. It is located slightly left of midline and anterior (below) to the rib cage. The lesser curvature of the stomach sits adjacent to the liver.

Liver

The liver is located below the diaphragm and mostly right of midline in the upper right quadrant of the abdomen. The liver performs many functions, including carbohydrate, lipid and protein metabolism and the processing of many medicines.

Gall bladder

The gall bladder is a pear-shaped sac that lies deep to the liver and hangs from the lower front margin of the liver. Its function is to store and concentrate bile made by the liver.

Pancreas

The pancreas lies behind the stomach. It is essential for producing digestive enzymes transported to the duodenum via the pancreatic duct and secretion of hormones such as insulin.

History taking and physical exam

A thorough patient history is essential as physical examination of the GI tract in a community pharmacy is limited to inspection of the mouth. This should allow confirmation of the diagnoses for conditions such as mouth ulcers and oral thrush. A description of how to examine the oral cavity appears in the following section.

Conditions affecting the oral cavity

Background

The process of digestion starts in the oral cavity. The tongue and cheeks position large pieces of food so that the teeth can tear and crush food into smaller particles. Saliva moistens, lubricates and begins the process of digesting carbohydrates (by secreting amylase enzymes) prior to swallowing,

The physical exam

The oral cavity can easily be observed in the pharmacy provided the mouth can be viewed with a good light source, preferably a pen torch (Fig. 6.1). The patient will usually present with some form of oral lesion and/or pain in a particular part of the mouth. The pharmacist should examine this area carefully, but the rest of the oral cavity should also be inspected. Checks for periodontal disease (bleeding gums) and other sites of mouth soreness should be performed. The floor of the mouth and underside of

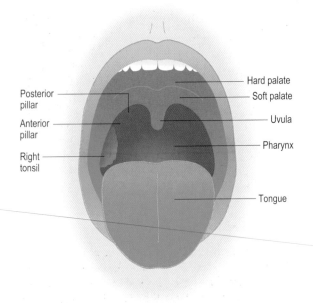

Posterior pillar

Anterior pillar

Right tonsil

Hard palate

Soft palate

Uvula

Pharynx

Tongue

Fig. 6.1 The oral cavity

the tongue can be viewed by asking the patient to curl the tongue towards the roof of the mouth; the buccal mucosa is best observed when the patient half opens the mouth.

Mouth ulcers

Background

Aphthous ulcers, more commonly known as mouth ulcers, is a collective term used to describe various different clinical presentations of superficial painful oral lesions that occur in recurrent bouts at intervals between a few days to a few months. The majority of patients (80%) who present in a community pharmacy will have minor aphthous ulcers (MAU). It is the community pharmacists' role to exclude more serious pathology, for example, systemic causes and carcinoma.

Prevalence and epidemiology

The prevalence and epidemiology of MAU is poorly understood. They occur in all ages but it has been reported that they are more common in patients aged between 20 and 40, and up to 66% of young adults give a history consistent with MAU. Lifetime prevalence is estimated to affect one in five of the general population.

Aetiology

The cause of MAU is unknown. A number of theories have been put forward to explain why people get MAU, including stress, trauma, food sensitivities, nutritional deficiencies (iron, zinc and vitamin B_{12}) and infection, but none have so far been proven.

Arriving at a differential diagnosis

There are three main clinical presentations of ulcers: minor, major or herpetiform. Although it is likely the patient will be suffering from MAU it is essential that these and other causes are recognised and referred to the GP for further evaluation. A number of ulcer-specific questions should always be asked of the patient to aid in diagnosis (Table 6.1). After questioning the patient, the oral cavity should be inspected to confirm the diagnosis.

Clinical features of minor aphthous ulcers

The ulcers of MAU are roundish, grey-white in colour and painful. They are small – usually less than 1 cm in diameter – and shallow with a raised red rim. Pain is the key presenting symptom and can make eating and drinking difficult, although pain subsides after 3 or 4 days. They rarely occur on the gingival mucosa and occur

Table 6.1
Specific questions to ask the patient: Mouth ulcers

Question	Relevance
Number of ulcers	• MAU occur singly or in small crops. A single large ulcerated area is indicative of more serious pathology • Patients with numerous ulcers are more likely to be suffering from other forms of ulceration such as major or herpetiform ulcers rather than MAU
Location of ulcers	• Ulcers on the side of the cheeks, tongue and inside of the lips are likely to be MAU • Ulcers located towards the back of the mouth are more consistent with major or herpetiform ulcers
Size and shape	• Irregular-shaped ulcers tend to be caused by trauma. If trauma is not the cause then referral is necessary to exclude sinister pathology • If ulcers are large or very small they are unlikely to be caused by MAU
Painless ulcers	• Any patient presenting with a painless ulcer in the oral cavity must be referred. This can indicate sinister pathology such as leukoplakia or carcinoma
Age	• MAU in young children (<10 years old) is not common and other causes such as primary infection with herpes simplex should be considered. If MAU is suspected, and it is the first time the patient has had ulcers, then referral should be considered to confirm the diagnosis • If ulcers appear for the first time after adolescence then the diagnostic probability is increased for them to be caused by things other than MAU

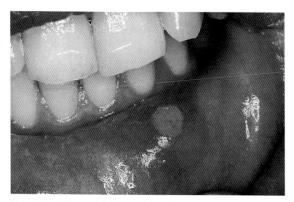

Fig. 6.2 Minor aphthous ulcer. Reproduced from *Essentials of Oral Pathology and Oral Medicine* by R Cawson et al, 2002, Churchill Livingstone, with permission

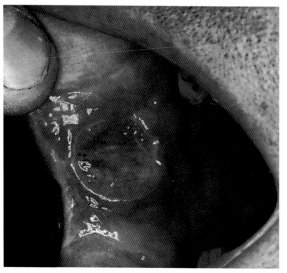

Fig. 6.3 Major aphthous ulcer. Reproduced from *Essentials of Oral Pathology and Oral Medicine* by R Cawson et al, 2002, Churchill Livingstone, with permission

singly or in small crops of up to five ulcers. It normally takes 7 to 14 days for the ulcers to heal but recurrence typically occurs after an interval of 1 to 4 months (Fig. 6.2).

Conditions to eliminate

Major aphthous ulcers

Characterised by large (greater than 1 cm in diameter) numerous ulcers, in crops of 10 or more. The ulcers often coalesce to form one large ulcer. The ulcers heal slowly and can persist for many weeks (Fig. 6.3).

Herpetiform ulcers

Herpetiform ulcers are pinpoint and occur in large crops of up to 100 at a time. They usually heal within a month and often occur in the posterior part of the mouth, an unusual location for MAU (Fig. 6.4). Both herpetiform and major aphthous ulcers are approximately ten times less common than MAU.

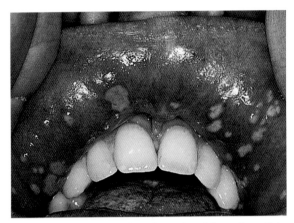

Fig. 6.4 Herpetiform ulcer. Reproduced from *Essentials of Oral Pathology and Oral Medicine* by R Cawson et al, 2002, Churchill Livingstone, with permission

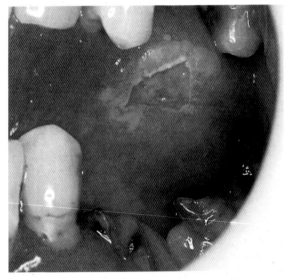

Fig. 6.5 Ulcer caused by trauma. Reproduced from *Textbook of General and Oral Medicine* by D Wray et al, 1999, Churchill Livingstone, with permission

Trauma

Trauma to the oral mucosa will result in damage and ulceration. Trauma may be mechanical (e.g. tongue biting) or thermal resulting in ulcers with an irregular border. Patients should be able to recall the traumatic event and have no history of ulceration or signs of systemic infection (Fig. 6.5).

Oral thrush

Oral thrush usually presents as creamy-white soft elevated patches. It is covered in more detail in the next section and the reader is referred to pages 129–131 for differential diagnosis of thrush from other oral lesions.

Herpes simplex

Herpes simplex virus is a common cause of oral ulceration in children. Primary infection results in ulceration of any part of the oral mucosa, especially the gums, tongue and cheeks. The ulcers tend to be small and discrete and many in number. Prior to the eruption of ulcers the person might show signs of systemic infection such as fever and pharyngitis.

Medicine-induced ulcers

A number of case reports have been received of medication causing ulcers. These include: cytotoxic agents, nicorandil, alendronate, NSAIDs and beta-blockers.

Squamous cell carcinoma

Squamous cell carcinoma is the most common oral malignant lesion in the UK, with approximately 2000 people diagnosed each year and 800 deaths. It is twice as common in men than women, and 90% of people are aged over 40 years when diagnosed; the average age at diagnosis is 64 for men and 61 for women. Smokers are at increased risk and account for 75% of cases; therefore, patients should always be asked about their smoking history.

The majority of cancers are noted on the side of the tongue, mouth and lower lip. Initial presentation ranges from painless spots, lumps or ulcers in the mouth or lip area that fail to resolve. Over time these become painful, change colour or bleed. The painless nature of early symptoms leads people to seek help only when other symptoms become apparent. Symptoms therefore can be present for a number of weeks before the patient presents to a healthcare practitioner. Urgent referral is needed as survival rates increase dramatically if the disease is diagnosed in its early stages.

Erythema multiforme

Infection or drug therapy can cause erythema multiforme, although in about 50% of cases no cause can be found. Symptoms are sudden in onset causing widespread ulceration of the oral cavity. In addition, the patient can have annular and symmetric erythematous skin lesions located towards the extremities. Conjunctivitis and eye pain are also common.

Behcet's syndrome

Most patients will suffer from recurrent, painful major aphthous ulcers that are slow to heal. Lesions are also observed in the genital region and eye involvement (iridocyclitis) is common.

Figure 6.6 will aid the differentiation between serious and non-serious conditions that cause mouth ulcers.

6

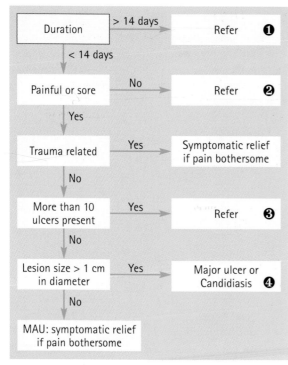

Fig. 6.6 Primer for differential diagnosis of mouth ulcers

❶ Duration
MAU normally resolve in 7 to 14 days. Ulcers that fail to heal within this time need referral to exclude other causes.

❷ Painless ulcers
These can indicate sinister pathology, especially if the patient is over 50 years old. In addition, it is likely that the ulcer will have been present for some time before the patient presented to the pharmacy.

❸ Numerous ulcers
Crops of 5 to 10 or more ulcers are rare in MAU. Referral is necessary to determine the cause.

❹ Major ulcer or candidiasis
See Fig. 6.9 for primer for differential diagnosis of oral thrush.

> **❶ TRIGGER POINTS indicative of referral: Mouth ulcers**
>
> - Children under 10
> - Duration longer than 14 days
> - Painless ulcer
> - Signs of systemic illness, e.g. fever
> - Ulcers greater than 1 cm in diameter
> - Ulcers in crops of five to ten, or more

Evidence base for over-the-counter medication

A wide range of products are marketed for the temporary relief and treatment of mouth ulcers. These products contain corticosteroids, local anaesthetics, antibacterials, astringents and antiseptics.

Corticosteroids

Very few random controlled trials have been conducted using topical corticosteroids. Those conducted involved small patient numbers or products that are not commercially available OTC. A review by Porter and Scully in *Clinical Evidence* (http://clinicalevidence.bmj.com/ceweb/index.jsp) concluded that corticosteroids did heal ulcers more quickly than control preparations. However, this review included products not available OTC in the UK. Specific trial data for commercially available products in the UK are therefore discussed.

Triamcinolone acetonide 0.1% in Orabase

Triamcinolone acetonide was deregulated from POM to P status in 1994. It has been suggested as a useful preparation to treat MAU by a number of authors, although there is a lack of clinical evidence from trial data. A study by Browne et al (1968) failed to demonstrate statistically significant improvement in the time it took to heal ulcers, although subjective improvements were noted by patients using triamcinolone in Orabase and not by those using Orabase alone. The improvements were minor and the authors suggest that triamcinolone in Orabase should not be used for routine use and reserved for severe episodes. A further trial, which evaluated triamcinolone, Orabase, betametasone 0.1 mg tablets and carbenoxolone gel failed to demonstrate statistical improvement for any of the treatments.

Hydrocortisone sodium succinate (Corlan) pellets

Only one trial conducted by Truelove et al (1958) could be found that investigated the efficacy of hydrocortisone sodium succinate pellets. At the request of the authors, a specific tablet formulation of hydrocortisone was made, which could be placed on the surface of the ulcer. The request was made because attempts using hydrocortisone ointment were largely unsuccessful as oral fluids washed the ointment away. The authors recruited 52 patients suffering from various forms of oral ulceration; 23 of the patients were suffering from minor aphthous ulceration. The authors stated that 22 of the 23 patients obtained rapid relief of pain and the healing rate of the ulcers was accelerated. However, the study lacked randomisation, a placebo or blinding. Owing to the limited data and poor trial design it is difficult to say whether hydrocortisone succinate pellets are effective, better than placebo or indeed have any effect at all.

Antibacterial agents (e.g. chlorhexidine)

A number of random controlled trials have investigated antibacterial mouthwashes containing chlorhexidine

Table 6.2
Practical prescribing: Summary of medicines for ulcers

Name of medicine	Use in children	Likely side effects	Drug interactions of note	Patients in whom care should be exercised	Pregnancy and breast-feeding
Adcortyl in Orabase	Yes but manufacturers do not state a lower age limit	None	None	None	Inadequate evidence, best to avoid use
Corlan	>12 years	None			
Choline salicylate	>10 years*				OK
Lidocaine		Can cause sensitisation reactions			
Benzocaine					
Carmellose	Yes	None			
Chlorhexidine	Yes but manufacturers do not state a lower age limit	None			

*Age limit is arbitrarily set by author. Marketed products do have licences for use in younger people

gluconate. Data from some, but not all studies, have found that they reduced the pain and severity of each episode of ulceration.

Products containing anaesthetic or analgesics

There are very little trial data to support the pain-relieving effect of anaesthetics or analgesics in MAU, apart from choline salicylate. However, these preparations are clinically effective in other painful oral conditions. It is therefore not unreasonable to expect some relief of symptoms to be shown when using these products to treat MAU.

Choline salicylate

Choline salicylate has been shown to exert an analgesic effect in a number of small studies. However, only one study by Reedy (1970) involving 27 patients evaluated choline salicylate in the treatment of oral aphthous ulceration. No significant differences were found between choline salicylate and placebo in ulcer resolution but choline salicylate was found to be significantly superior to placebo in relieving pain.

Protectants

Orabase is a paste of gelatin, pectin and carmellose sodium, which sticks when it comes in contact with wet mucosal surfces. There is a paucity of data to support its efficacy. However, it has no known side effects, and

HINTS AND TIPS BOX 6.1: ULCERS

Application of Adcortyl	Apply after food, as food is likely to rub off the paste

can be used in any patient population. It should be noted that Orabase contains no pain-relieving agents, and only protects the ulcer from further abrasion. Therefore, it is often used in combination with anaesthetics or analgesics.

Practical prescribing and product selection

Prescribing information relating to the medicines used for ulcers reviewed in the section 'Evidence base for over-the-counter medication' is discussed and summarised in Table 6.2; useful tips relating to patients presenting with ulcers are given in Hints and Tips Box 6.1.

Triamcinolone acetonide 0.1% in Orabase (Adcortyl in Orabase 0.1%)

Adcortyl should be applied between two and four times a day for up to 5 days. All patient groups can use the product and it is well tolerated with no side effects reported. Because it is locally applied there are no drug interactions.

Hydrocortisone sodium succinate pellets (Corlan pellets)

Each pellet contains 2.5 mg hydrocortisone in the form of the ester hydrocortisone sodium succinate. The dose for adults and children over 12 years is one pellet to be dissolved in close proximity to the ulcers four times a day for up to 5 days. It does not interact with any medicines, can be taken by all patient groups and has no side effects.

(Note: For both products, triamcinolone and hydrocortisone sodium succinate, there is inadequate evidence of safety in pregnancy and breast-feeding and therefore manufacturers advise avoidance.)

Choline salicylate (Bonjela)

Choline salicylate is licensed from 4 months upwards for the treatment of soreness in the mouth (e.g. teething pain); however, it would be good practice to refer children under 10 years old presenting with MAU for the first time. Adults and children over 10 years old should apply the gel, using a clean finger, over the ulcer every 3 hours or when needed. It is a very safe medicine and can be given to all patient groups. It is not known to interact with any medicines or cause any side effects.

Local anaesthetics (lidocaine, e.g. the Anbesol range, Calgel, Medijel and benzocaine, e.g. Rinstead Adult Gel)

All local anaesthetics have a short duration of action; frequent dosing is therefore required to maintain the anaesthetic effect. They are thus best used on a when-needed basis although, depending on the concentration of anaesthetic included in products, the upper limit on the number of applications allowed does vary. In most instances the products should not be used more than eight times in a day. They appear to be free from any drug interactions, have minimal side effects and can be given to most patients. A small percentage of patients might experience a hypersensitivity reaction with lidocaine or benzocaine; this appears to be more common with benzocaine.

Antibacterial agents (e.g. chlorhexidine)

Chlorhexidine (Corsodyl) mouthwash is indicated as an aid in the treatment and prevention of gingivitis and in the maintenance of oral hygiene, which includes the management of aphthous ulceration. Ten millilitres of the mouthwash should be rinsed around the mouth for about 1 minute twice a day. It can be used by all patient groups, including during pregnancy and breast-feeding. Side effects associated with its use include reversible tongue and tooth discolouration, burning of the tongue and taste disturbance.

Carmellose sodium (Orabase Protective Paste)

Orabase can be applied as frequently as required. It is important that it is dabbed on, and not rubbed on, for it to stick correctly. Also, patients should be discouraged from putting too much on as the excess can peel off leaving the lesion exposed. There are no apparent interactions and Orabase can be used in all patient groups.

Further reading

Browne RM, Fox EC, Anderson RJ. Topical triamcinolone acetonide in recurrent aphthous stomatitis. A clinical trial. Lancet 1968;1:565-7.

Davis G. CPPE distance learning. Oral health, vol 2. Recognition and treatment of orofacial problems. London: Outset Publishing Ltd, 1996.

MacPhee IT, Sircus W, Farmer ED, et al. Use of steroids in treatment of aphthous ulceration. Br Med J 1968;2(598):147-9.

Reedy BL. A topical salicylate gel in the treatment of oral aphthous ulceration. Practitioner 1970;204:846-50.

Scully C. Aphthous ulceration. N Engl J Med 2006;355: 165-72.

Truelove SC, Morris-Owen RM. Treatment of aphthous ulceration of the mouth. BMJ 1958;1:603-7.

Zakrzewska JM. Fortnightly review: oral cancer. BMJ 1999;318:1051-4.

Web sites

General site on oral health: http://www.nlm.nih.gov/medlineplus/mouthandteeth.html

The Behcet's Syndrome Society: http://www.behcets-society.fsnet.co.uk/looklike.html

The British Dental Health Foundation: http://www.dentalhealth.org.uk/

Oral thrush (candidiasis)

Background

Oropharyngeal candidiasis (oral thrush) is an opportunistic mucosal infection and is unusual in healthy adults. If oral thrush is suspected in this population, community pharmacists should determine if any identifiable risk factors exist or, if not, suspect potential underlying sinister pathology.

Prevalence and epidemiology

The very young (neonates) and the very old are most likely to suffer from oral thrush. It has been reported that 5% of newborn infants and 10% of debilitated elderly patients suffer from oral thrush. Most other cases will be associated with underlying pathology such as diabetes, xerostomia (dry mouth), patients who are immunocompromised or be attributable to identifiable risk factors such as recent antibiotic therapy, inhaled corticosteroids and ill-fitting dentures.

Aetiology

It is reported that *Candida albicans* is found in the oral cavity of 30 to 60% of healthy people in developed countries (Gonsalves et al 2007). It is transmitted directly between infected people or via objects that can hold the organism. Prevalence in denture wearers is even higher. Changes to the normal environment in the oral cavity will allow *C. albicans* to proliferate.

Arriving at a differential diagnosis

Oral thrush is not difficult to diagnose with the aid of a careful history and an oral examination. It is the role of the pharmacist to eliminate underlying pathology and exclude risk factors. A number of oral thrush specific questions should always be asked of the patient (Table 6.3). After questioning the pharmacist should inspect the oral cavity to confirm the diagnosis.

Clinical features of oral thrush

The classical presentation of oral thrush is of creamy-white soft elevated patches that can be wiped off revealing underlying erythematous mucosa (Fig. 6.7). Pain, soreness, altered taste and a burning tongue can be present. Lesions can occur anywhere in the oral cavity but usually affect the tongue, palate, lips and cheeks. Patients sometimes complain of malaise and loss of appetite. In neonates, spontaneous resolution usually occurs but can take a few weeks.

Table 6.3 **Specific questions to ask the patient: Oral thrush**	
Question	**Relevance**
Size and shape of lesion	• Typically, patients with oral thrush present with 'patches'. They tend to be irregularly shaped and vary in size from small to large
Associated pain	• White, painless patches, especially in people aged over 50, should be referred to exclude sinister pathology such as leukoplakia
Location of lesions	• Oral thrush often affects the tongue and cheeks, although if precipitated by inhaled steroids the lesions appear on the pharynx

Conditions to eliminate

Leukoplakia

Leuloplakia is a predominantly white lesion of the oral mucosa that cannot be characterised as any other definable lesion and is therefore a diagnosis based on exclusion (Fig. 6.8). It is often associated with smoking and is a precancerous lesion, although epidemiological data suggest that annual transformation rate to squamous cell carcinoma is approximately 1%. Patients present with a symptomless white patch that develops over a period of weeks on the tongue or cheek. The lesion cannot be wiped off, unlike oral thrush. Most cases are

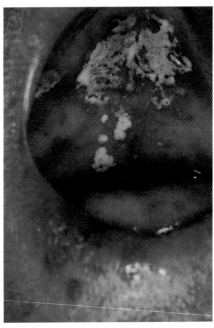

Fig. 6.7 Oral candidiasis. Reproduced from *Illustrated Pocket Guide to Clinical Medicine* by C D Forbes and W F Jackson, 2004, Mosby, with permission

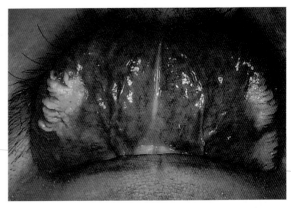

Fig. 6.8 Leukoplakia. Reproduced from *Illustrated Pocket Guide to Clinical Medicine* by C D Forbes and W F Jackson, 2004, Mosby, with permission

seen in people over the age of 40 years and it is more common in men. All suspected cases require referral.

Mouth ulcers and squamous cell carcinoma

Mouth ulcers and squamous cell carcinoma are covered in more detail on pages 124–126 and the reader is referred to this section for differential diagnosis of these from oral thrush.

Lichen planus

Lichen planus is a dermatological condition with lesions similar in appearance to plaque psoriasis. In about 50% of people the oral mucous membranes are affected. The cheeks, gums or tongue develop white, slightly raised painless lesions that look a little like a spider's web. Other symptoms can include soreness of the mouth and a burning sensation. Occasionally, lichen planus of the mouth occurs without any skin rash.

Figure 6.9 will aid the differentiation of thrush from other oral lesions.

TRIGGER POINTS indicative of referral: Oral thrush

- Diabetic
- Duration greater than 3 weeks
- Immunocompromised patients
- Painless lesions

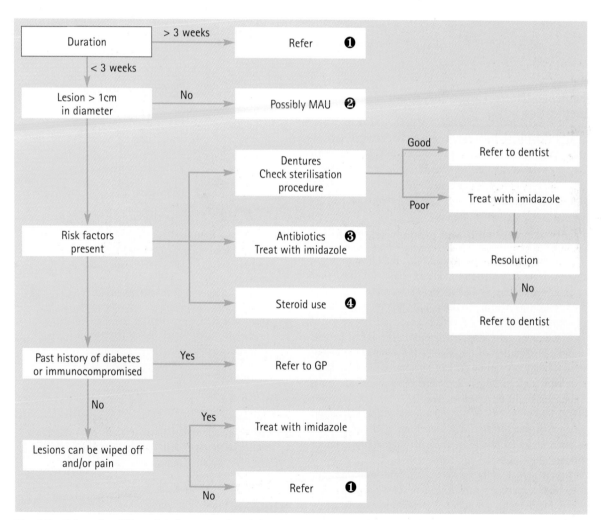

Fig. 6.9 Primer for differential diagnosis of oral thrush

❶ Duration
Any lesion lasting more than 3 weeks must be referred to exclude sinister pathology.

❷ MAU
See Fig. 6.6 for primer for differential diagnosis of mouth ulcers.

❸ Antibiotics
Broad-spectrum antibiotics, e.g. amoxicillin and macrolides, can precipitate oral thrush by altering normal flora of the oral cavity.

❹ Inhaled corticosteroids
High-dose inhaled corticosteroids can cause oral thrush. Patients should be encouraged to use a spacer and wash their mouth out after inhaler use to minimise this problem.

Table 6.4
Practical prescribing: Summary of medicines for oral thrush

Name of medicine	Use in children	Likely side effects	Drug interactions of note	Patients in whom care should be exercised	Pregnancy and breast-feeding
Daktarin	Infants upwards	Nausea and vomiting	Warfarin	None	OK

HINTS AND TIPS BOX 6.2: DAKTARIN

Application of Daktarin	Patients should be advised to hold the gel in the mouth for as long as possible to increase contact time between the medicine and the infection
Duration of treatment	Treatment should be continued for up to 2 days after the symptoms have cleared to prevent relapse and reinfection
Patient acceptability	Gel is flavoured orange to make retention in the mouth more acceptable to patients

Evidence base for over-the-counter medication

Only Daktarin oral gel (miconazole) is available OTC to treat oral thrush. It has proven efficacy and appears to have clinical cure rates between 80 to 90%. In comparative trials, Daktarin appears to have superior cure rates than the POM Nystatin.

Practical prescribing and product selection

Prescribing information relating to Daktarin oral gel reviewed in the section 'Evidence base for over-the-counter medication' is discussed and summarised in Table 6.4; useful tips relating to the application of Daktarin are given in Hints and Tips Box 6.2.

The dose of gel varies dependent on the age of patient and the distribution of the lesions. If lesions are localised then a small amount of gel can be applied directly to the area with a clean finger. For more generalised infections the dose should be given by way of a 5 mL spoon. For adults and children over 6 years, 5 mL of the gel should be applied four times a day and 5 mL used twice a day in children under 6 years. For infants and children under 2 years the dose is 2.5 mL twice a day.

It can occasionally cause nausea and vomiting, but these side effects are rare. The manufacturers state that it can interact with a number of medicines, namely mizolastine, cisapride, triazolam, midazolam, quinidine, pimozide, HMG-CoA reductase inhibitors and anticoagulants. However, there is a lack of published data to determine how clinically significant these interactions are except with warfarin. Co-administration of warfarin with miconazole increases warfarin levels markedly and the patient's international normalised ratio (INR) should be monitored closely. The manufacturers also state that Daktarin should be avoided in pregnancy but published data do not support an association between miconazole and congenital defects.

Further reading

Gonsalves WC, Chi A, Neville BW. Common oral lesions: Part I. Superficial mucosal lesions. Am Fam Phys 2007;75:501–7.

Hoppe JE, Hahn H. Randomized comparison of two nystatin oral gels with miconazole oral gel for treatment of oral thrush in infants. Antimycotics Study Group. Infection 1996;24:136–9.

Hoppe JE. Treatment of oropharyngeal candidiasis in immunocompetent infants: a randomized multicenter study of miconazole gel vs. nystatin suspension. The Antifungals Study Group. Pediatr Infect Dis J 1997;16:288–93.

Parvinen T, Kokko J, Yli-Urpo A. Miconazole lacquer compared with gel in treatment of denture stomatitis. Scand J Dent Res 1994;102:361–6.

Web sites

General information: http://www.netdoctor.co.uk/diseases/facts/oralthrush.htm and http://www.patient.co.uk/

Gingivitis

Background

Gingivitis simply means inflammation of the gums and is usually caused by an excess build-up of plaque on the teeth. The condition is entirely preventable if regular tooth brushing is undertaken. Despite this, dental caries and gum disease still affect almost everyone.

Prevalence and epidemiology

It is estimated that 50% of the UK population are affected by gum disease and that more than 85% of people over 40 years will experience gingival disease. Men more than women tend to suffer from severe gingivitis, which might be due to women practising better oral hygiene.

Aetiology

Following tooth brushing, the teeth soon become coated in a mixture of saliva and gingival fluid, known as pellicle. Oral bacteria and food particles adhere to this coating and begin to proliferate forming plaque; subsequent brushing of the teeth removes this plaque build-up. However, if plaque is allowed to build up for 3 or 4 days, bacteria begin to undergo internal calcification producing calcium phosphate better known as tartar (or calculus). This adheres tightly to the surface of the tooth and retains bacteria in situ. The bacteria release enzymes and toxins that invade the gingival mucosa, causing inflammation of the gingiva (gingivitis). If the plaque is not removed the inflammation travels downwards, involving the periodontal ligament and associated tooth structures (periodontitis). A pocket forms between the tooth and gum and, over a period of years, the root of the tooth and bone are eroded until such time that the tooth becomes loose and lost. This is the main cause of tooth loss in people over 40 years of age.

A number of risk factors are associated with gingivitis and periodontitis; these include diabetes mellitus, cigarette smoking, poor nutritional status and poor oral hygiene.

Arriving at a differential diagnosis

Gingivitis often goes unnoticed because symptoms can be very mild and painless. This often explains why a routine check-up at the dentist reveals more severe gum disease than patients thought they had. A dental history needs to be taken from the patient, in particular details of their tooth brushing routine and technique, as well as the frequency of visits to their dentist. The mouth should be inspected for tell-tale signs of gingival inflammation. A number of gingivitis-specific questions should always be asked of the patient to aid in diagnosis (Table 6.5).

Clinical features of gingivitis

Gingivitis is characterised by swelling and reddening of the gums, which bleed easily with slight trauma, for example when brushing teeth. Plaque might be visible; especially on teeth that are difficult to reach when tooth brushing. Halitosis might also be present.

Table 6.5	Specific questions to ask the patient: Gingivitis
Question	**Relevance**
Tooth brushing technique	• Overzealous tooth brushing can lead to bleeding gums and gum recession. Make sure the patient is not 'over cleaning' their teeth. An electric toothbrush might be helpful for people who apply too much force when brushing teeth
Bleeding gums	• Gums that bleed without exposure to trauma and is unexplained or unprovoked need referral to exclude underlying pathology

Conditions to eliminate

Periodontitis

If gingivitis is left untreated it will progress into periodontitis. Symptoms are similar to gingivitis but the patient will experience spontaneous bleeding, taste disturbances, halitosis and difficulty while eating. Periodontal pockets might be visible and the patient might complain of loose teeth. Referral to a dentist is needed for evaluation and removal of tartar.

Spontaneous bleeding

A number of conditions can produce spontaneous gum bleeding, for example agranulocytosis and leukaemia. Other symptoms should be present, for example, progressive fatigue, weakness and signs of systemic illness such as fever. Immediate referral to the GP is needed.

Medicine-induced gum bleeding/hypertrophy

Medicines such as warfarin, heparin and NSAIDs might produce gum bleeding. Consultation with the prescriber to suggest alternative medication would be needed. Gum hypertrophy is very common in people taking phenytoin, ciclosporin and nifedipine and patients must be told about these adverse events when they are first prescribed them.

TRIGGER POINTS indicative of referral: Gingivitis

- Foul taste associated with gum bleeding
- Loose teeth
- Signs of systemic illness
- Spontaneous gum bleeding

Evidence base for over-the-counter medication

Put simply, there is no substitute for good oral hygiene. Prevention of plaque build-up is the key to healthy gums and teeth. Once-daily brushing is adequate to maintain oral hygiene at adequate levels. If the patient brushes more regularly than this then this should not be discouraged. Brushing teeth with a fluoride toothpaste, to prevent tooth decay, should preferably take place after eating, and flossing is recommended to access areas that a toothbrush might miss. A recent Cochrane review (Robinson et al 2005) concluded that powered toothbrushes (with rotation oscillation action – where brush heads rotate in one direction and then the other) are more effective than manual brushing at plaque removal.

However, there are a plethora of oral hygiene products marketed for general sale to the public, whether through a pharmacy outlet or a general store. These products should be reserved for established gingivitis or those patients who are unable to use a toothbrush.

Mouthwashes contain chlorhexidine, hexetidine, hydrogen peroxide, sodium perborate and povidone-iodine. Of these, chlorhexidine in concentrations of either 0.1 or 0.2% has been proven the most effective antibacterial in reducing plaque formation and gingivitis (Ernst et al 1998). In clinical trials it has been shown to be consistently more effective than placebo and comparator medicines, and there appears to be no difference in effect between concentrations. It has even been used as a positive control.

Povidone-iodine has antiseptic properties and is beneficial in oral infection but has failed to show a significant effect in decreasing gingivitis and plaque formation except when combined with hydrogen peroxide. Hydrogen peroxide and povidone-iodine might therefore work synergistically because both products alone have failed to demonstrate effectiveness in inhibition of plaque formation.

Practical prescribing and product selection

Prescribing information relating to the medicines used for gingivitis reviewed in the section 'Evidence base for over-the-counter medication' is discussed and summarised in Table 6.6; useful tips relating to products for oral care are given in Hints and Tips Box 6.3.

All mouthwashes, except those containing iodine, appear to be free from any drug interactions, have minimal side effects and can be used by all patient groups. They are rinsed around the mouth for between 30 seconds and 1 minute then spat out.

Chlorhexidine gluconate (e.g. Corsodyl 0.2%, Eludril 0.1%)

The standard dose for adults and children is 10 mL twice a day. Although it is free from side effects, patients should be warned that prolonged use may stain the tongue and teeth brown. This can be reduced or removed by brushing teeth before use. If this fails to remove the staining then it can be removed by a dentist. Corsodyl is also available as a spray (0.2%) and gel (1%) and used twice a day.

Povodine-iodine (Betadine)

Adults and children over 6 years of age should use a 10 mL dose four times a day, either undiluted or diluted with an equal volume of water. Because of its iodine content it should not be used for periods longer than 14 days because a significant amount of iodine is absorbed. Pregnant and breast-feeding women and patients with thyroid disorders should avoid its use.

Table 6.6
Practical prescribing: Summary of medicines for gingivitis

Name of medicine	Use in children	Likely side effects	Drug interactions of note	Patients in whom care should be exercised	Pregnancy and breast-feeding
Chlorhexidine	No age limit stated	Staining of teeth and tongue. Mild irritation	None	None	OK
Povidone-iodine	>6 years	None		Patients with thyroid disease	Avoid if possible
Hexetidine		Mild irritation or numbness of tongue		None	OK
Hydrogen peroxide		None			

HINTS AND TIPS BOX 6.3: IODINE MOUTHWASH

Regular use of iodine-containing mouthwashes	Regular use in pregnant women should be avoided because prolonged use can lead to iodine crossing the placental barrier and absorption by the foetus of a significant amount of iodine. This can result in hypothyroidism and goitre in the foetus and newborn
Dental flossing	Ideally people should floss once a day to remove plaque from between teeth. Correct technique is important otherwise gums can be traumatised. A piece of floss about eight inches long should be wrapped around the ends of the middle fingers of each hand leaving two to three inches between the first finger and thumb. The floss should be placed between two teeth and curved in to a 'C' shape around one tooth and slid up between the gum and tooth until resistance is felt then moved vertically up and down several times to remove plaque
Using fluoride	Fluoride has shown to reduce dental caries. In some parts of the UK drinking water contains measurable concentrations of fluoride and the need for fluoride toothpastes or supplementation is not needed. However, most people in Britain require fluoride supplementation, which is normally through toothpaste. Most packs of toothpaste state how many parts per million of fluoride the toothpaste contains; 500 ppm is a low level, 1000–1500 ppm is a high level. A low-dose toothpaste should be used for children under 7 to avoid dental fluorosis, which causes tooth discolouration. Oral fluoride supplements can also be given where fluoride in water is less than 0.7 parts per million

Hexetidine (Oraldene)

Adults and children over 6 years of age should use a 15 mL dose two or three times a day.

Hydrogen peroxide (e.g. Peroxyl)

Adults and children over 6 years of age should use 10 mL rinsed around the mouth up to four times a day.

Further reading

Brecx M, Brownstone E, MacDonald L, et al. Efficacy of Listerine, Meridol and chlorhexidine mouthrinses as supplements to regular tooth cleaning measures. J Clin Periodontol 1992;19:202–7.

Ernst CP, Prockl K, Willershausen B. The effectiveness and side effects of 0.1% and 0.2% chlorhexidine mouthrinses: a clinical study. Quintessence Int 1998;29:443–8.

Greenstein G. Povidone-iodine's effects and role in the management of periodontal diseases: a review. J Periodontol 1999;70:1397–405.

Hase JC, Ainamo J, Etemadzadeh H, et al. Plaque formation and gingivitis after mouthrinsing with 0.2% delmopinol hydrochloride, 0.2% chlorhexidine digluconate and placebo for 4 weeks, following an initial professional tooth cleaning. J Clin Periodontol 1995;22:533–9.

Jones CM, Blinkhorn AS, White E. Hydrogen peroxide, the effect on plaque and gingivitis when used in an oral irrigator. Clin Prev Dent 1990;12:15–8.

Kelly M. Adult Dental Health Survey: Oral Health in the United Kingdom 1998. London: TSO, 2000.

Lang NP, Hase JC, Grassi M, et al. Plaque formation and gingivitis after supervised mouthrinsing with 0.2% delmopinol hydrochloride, 0.2% chlorhexidine digluconate and placebo for 6 months. Oral Dis 1998;4:105–13.

Maruniak J, Clark WB, Walker CB, et al. The effect of 3 mouthrinses on plaque and gingivitis development. J Clin Periodontol 1992;19:19–23.

Robinson PG, Deacon SA, Deery C, et al. Manual versus powered toothbrushing for oral health. Cochrane Database of Systematic Reviews 2005, issue 2.

Web sites

The British Dental Association: http://www.bda.org/
The British Fluoridation Society: http://www.bfsweb.org/
The British Dental Health Foundation: http://www.dentalhealth.org.uk/
The American Academy of Periodontology: http://www.perio.org/

Dyspepsia

Background

Confusion surrounds the terminology associated with upper abdominal symptoms and the term dyspepsia is used by different authors to mean different things. For example, the Rome II definition simply states: 'dyspepsia refers to pain or discomfort centred (that is around the midline) in the upper abdomen' (https://www.degnon.org/secure/romecriteria/romeii/). This should be compared with the British Society of Gastroenterology criteria, which are broader, and define dyspepsia as: 'any symptom referable to the upper gastrointestinal tract . . . including upper abdominal pain or discomfort, heartburn, acid reflux, nausea and vomiting'.

It is therefore an umbrella term generally used by healthcare professionals to refer to a group of upper abdominal symptoms that arise from five main conditions:

- non-ulcer dyspepsia/functional dyspepsia (indigestion)
- gastro-oesophageal reflux disease (GORD)
- gastritis
- duodenal ulcers
- gastric ulcers

These five conditions represent 90% of dyspepsia cases presented to the GP.

In August 2004, The National Institute for Health and Clinical Excellence (NICE) issued clinical guidance on the management of dyspepsia in adults in primary care (http://www.nice.org.uk/page.aspx?o=CG017). In this section, specific reference is made to NICE guidance, especially in the management of dyspepsia.

Prevalence and epidemiology

The exact prevalence of dyspepsia is unknown. This is largely because of the number of people who self-medicate or do not report mild symptoms to their GP. However, it is clear that dyspepsia is extremely common. Between 25 and 40% of the general population in Western society are reported to suffer from dyspepsia and virtually everyone at some point in their lives will experience an episode of dyspepsia. Estimates suggest that 10% of people suffer on a weekly basis and that 5% of all GP consultations are for dyspepsia. The prevalence of dyspepsia is modestly higher in women than men.

Aetiology

The aetiology of dyspepsia differs depending on which condition the patient is suffering from. Lower oesophageal sphincter incompetence is the principal cause of GORD and is often caused by decreased muscle tone via medicines or overeating. Increased acid production results in inflammation of the stomach (gastritis) and is usually attributable to *Helicobacter pylori* infection, NSAIDs or acute alcohol indigestion. The presence of *H. pylori* is central to duodenal and gastric ulceration – *H. pylori* is present in 95% of duodenal ulcers and 70% of gastric ulcers. The mechanism by which it affects the aetiology of ulcers is still unclear but the bacteria is thought to secrete certain chemical factors resulting in gastric mucosal damage. Finally, when no specific cause can be found for a patient's symptoms the complaint is said to be non-ulcer dyspepsia. (Some authorities do not advocate the use of this term, preferring the term 'functional dyspepsia'.)

Arriving at a differential diagnosis

Overwhelmingly, patients who present with dyspepsia are likely to be suffering from GORD, gastritis or non-ulcer dyspepsia. Research has shown that even those patients who meet NICE guidelines for endoscopical investigation are found to have either gastritis/hiatus hernia (30%), oesphagitis (10 to 17%) or no abnormal findings (30%). It has also been reported that a medical practitioner with an average list size will only see one new case of oesophageal cancer and one new case of stomach cancer every 4 years. Despite this, a thorough medical and drug history should be taken to enable the community pharmacist to rule out serious pathology and diagnose dyspepsia. Alarm symptoms (see Trigger points indicative of referral) that would warrant further investigation are surprisingly common and it is important that these are referred to rule out serious pathology. A number of dyspepsia-specific questions should always be asked of the patient to aid in diagnosis (Table 6.7).

Clinical features of dyspepsia

Patients with dyspepsia present with a range of symptoms commonly involving:

- vague abdominal discomfort (aching) above the umbilicus associated with belching
- bloating
- flatulence
- a feeling of fullness
- nausea and/or vomiting
- heartburn

Although, dyspeptic symptoms are a poor predictor of disease severity or underlying pathology, retrosternal heartburn is the classic symptom of GORD.

Conditions to eliminate

Peptic ulceration

Ruling out peptic ulceration is probably the main consideration for community pharmacists when assessing patients with symptoms of dyspepsia. Ulcers are classed as either gastric or duodenal. They occur most commonly in patients aged between 30 and 50, although patients over the age of 60 account for 80% of deaths even though they only account for 15% of cases. Typically the patient will have well localised mid-epigastric pain described as 'constant', 'annoying' or 'gnawing/boring'. In gastric ulcers the pain comes on whenever the stomach is empty, usually 30 minutes after eating and is generally relieved by antacids or food and aggravated by alcohol and caffeine. Gastric ulcers are also more commonly associated with weight loss and GI bleeds than duodenal ulcers. Patients can experience weight loss of 5 to 10 kg and although this could indicate carcinoma, especially in

Table 6.7
Specific questions to ask the patient: Dyspepsia

Question	Relevance
Age	• The incidence of dyspepsia decreases with advancing age and therefore young adults are likely to suffer from dyspepsia with no specific pathological condition, unlike patients over 50 years of age, in whom a specific pathological condition becomes more common
Location	• Dyspepsia is experienced as pain above the umbilicus and centrally located (epigastric area). Pain below the umbilicus will not be due to dyspepsia • Pain experienced behind the sternum (breastbone) is likely to be heartburn • If the patient can point to a specific area of the abdomen then it is unlikely to be dyspepsia and could be caused by another GI condition, or could be musculoskeletal in origin
Nature of pain	• Pain associated with dyspepsia is described as aching or discomfort. Pain described as gnawing, sharp or stabbing is unlikely to be dyspepsia
Radiation	• Pain that radiates to other areas of the body is indicative of more serious pathology and the patient must be referred. The pain might be cardiovascular in origin, especially if the pain is felt down the inside aspect of the left arm
Severity	• Pain described as debilitating or severe must be referred to exclude more serious conditions
Associated symptoms	• Persistent vomiting with or without blood is suggestive of ulceration or even cancer and must be referred • Black and tarry stools indicate a bleed in the GI tract and must be referred
Aggravating or relieving factors	• Pain shortly after eating can indicate a gastric ulcer whereas pain 2 to 3 hours after eating can indicate a duodenal ulcer • Symptoms of dyspepsia are often brought on by certain types of food, for example, caffeine-containing products and spicy food
Social history	• Bouts of excessive drinking are commonly implicated in dyspepsia. Likewise, eating food on the move or too quickly is often the cause of the symptoms. A person's job is often a good clue to whether these are contributing to their symptoms

people aged over 40, on investigation a benign gastric ulcer is found most of the time. NSAID use is associated with a three- to four-fold increase in gastric ulcers.

Duodenal ulcers tend to be more consistent in symptom presentation. Pain occurs 2 to 3 hours after eating and pain that wakes a person at night is highly suggestive of duodenal ulcer. If ulcers are suspected referral to the GP is necessary as peptic ulcers can only be conclusively diagnosed by endoscopy.

Medicine-induced dyspepsia

A number of medicines can cause gastric irritation leading to or provoking GI discomfort or a decrease in oesophageal sphincter tone resulting in reflux. Patients should be questioned about medication, especially the use of aspirin and NSAIDs, which provoke dyspepsia in 25% of patients. Table 6.8 lists other medicines commonly implicated in causing dyspepsia.

Irritable bowel syndrome

Patients younger than 45 years who have uncomplicated dyspepsia and also lower abdominal pain and altered

Table 6.8
Medicines that commonly cause dyspepsia

Antibiotics, e.g. macrolides and tetracyclines
ACE inhibitors
Alcohol (in excess)
Bisphosphonates
Calcium antagonists
Iron
Metformin
Metronidazole
Nitrates
Oestrogens
Potassium supplements
Sibutramine
Steroids
Theophylline

bowel habits are likely to have irritable bowel syndrome (IBS). For further details on IBS see page 155.

Gastric carcinoma

Gastric carcinoma is the third most common GI malignancy after colorectal and pancreatic cancer. However, only 2% of patients who are referred by their GP for an endoscopy have malignancy. It is therefore a rare condition and community pharmacists are extremely unlikely to encounter a patient with carcinoma. One or more ALARM symptoms should be present plus symptoms such as nausea and vomiting.

Oesophageal carcinoma

In its early stages, oesophageal carcinoma might go unnoticed. Over time, however, as the oesophagus becomes constricted, patients will complain of difficulty in swallowing and experience a sensation of food sticking in the oesophagus. As the disease progresses weight loss becomes prominent despite the patient maintaining a good appetite.

Atypical angina

Not all cases of angina have classical textbook presentation of pain in the retrosternal area with radiation to the neck, back or left shoulder that is precipitated by temperature changes or exercise. Patients can complain of dyspepsia-like symptoms and feel generally unwell. These symptoms might be brought on by a heavy meal. In such cases antacids will fail to relieve symptoms and referral is needed.

Figure 6.10 will aid differentiation of the causes of dyspepsia.

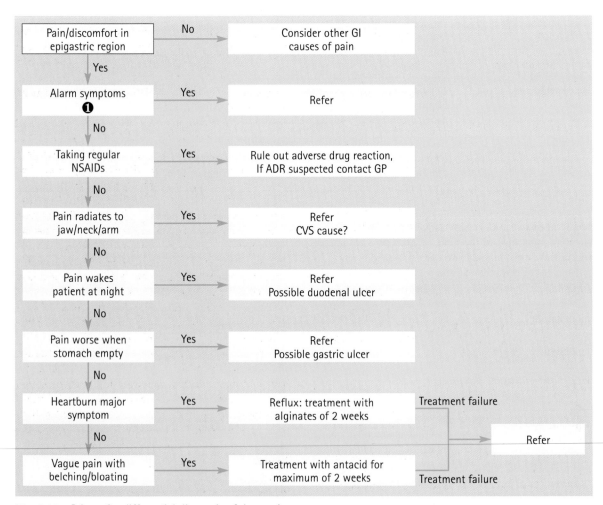

Fig. 6.10 Primer for differential diagnosis of dyspepsia

❶ **Alarm symptoms**
These include, anaemia (signs can include tiredness and pale complexion), loss of weight, anorexia, dark stools, difficulty in swallowing, vomiting blood.

Evidence base for over-the-counter medication

In accordance with NICE guidelines the group of patients that should be treated by pharmacists are classed as having 'uninvestigated dyspepsia' (i.e. those that have not had endoscopical investigation). OTC treatment options consist of antacids, H_2 antagonists and proton pump inhibitors. Before treatment is instigated lifestyle advice should be given where appropriate. Although there is no strong evidence that dietary changes will lessen dyspepsia symptoms, a general healthier lifestyle will have wider health benefits. The patient should be assessed in terms of diet and physical activity:

1. Move to a lower fat diet
2. Alcohol intake to recommended levels (14 and 21 units/week for women and men, respectively)
3. Smoking cessation
4. Decrease weight
5. Reduce caffeine intake

It might also be possible to identify factors that precipitate or worsen symptoms. Commonly implicated foods that precipitate dyspepsia are spicy or fatty food, caffeine, chocolate and alcohol. Bending is also said to worsen symptoms.

Antacids

Antacids have been used for many decades to treat dyspepsia and have proven efficacy in neutralising stomach acid. However, the neutralising capacity of each antacid varies dependent on the metal salt used. In addition, the solubility of each metal salt differs, which affects their onset and duration of action. Sodium and potassium salts are the most highly soluble, which makes them quick but short-acting. Magnesium and aluminium salts are less soluble so have a slower onset but greater duration of action. Calcium salts have the advantage of being quick-acting yet have a prolonged action.

It is therefore commonplace for manufacturers to combine two or more antacid ingredients together to ensure a quick onset (generally sodium salts, e.g. sodium bicarbonate) and prolonged action (aluminium, magnesium or calcium salts).

Alginates

For patients suffering from heartburn and reflux an alginate product should be first-line treatment. When in contact with gastric acid the alginate precipitates out, forming a sponge-like matrix that floats on top of the stomach contents. Alginate preparations are also commonly combined with antacids (e.g. Gaviscon Advance) to help neutralise stomach acid. In clinical trials alginate-containing products have demonstrated superior symptom control compared to placebo and antacids. However, proton pump inhibitors and H_2 antagonists do have superior efficacy to alginates.

H_2 antagonists

Two H_2 antagonists are currently available OTC in the UK: ranitidine and famotidine. Cimetidine was also available OTC but was withdrawn by the manufacturer, presumably because of poor sales, and nizatidine has exemption from POM control but currently there is no product on the market.

H_2 antagonists are effective at POM doses but OTC licensed indications use lower doses. The question is, at these lower doses are they still effective? There is a paucity of publicly available trial data supporting their use at non-prescription doses. Famotidine appears to have the greatest body of accessible trial data. A number of trials have been conducted in patients suffering from heartburn and who regularly self-medicate with antacids. Famotidine was shown to be more effective than placebo and equally effective to antacids. No trials involving ranitidine could be found on public databases that involved patients taking OTC doses.

However, the inhibitory effects of OTC doses of ranitidine on gastric acid have been investigated in healthy volunteers. Trials showed conclusively that ranitidine, and its comparator drug famotidine, did significantly raise intragastric pH compared to placebo, although antacids (calcium carbonates) had a significantly quicker onset of action but with shorter duration. Despite ranitidine appearing to have no trial data relating to OTC doses, it is assumed that the product licence holders had enough evidence for their product to be granted a licence.

Proton pump inhibitors

Omeprazole is the first proton pump inhibitor (PPI) in the UK to be deregulated from POM control, although it is likely, in time, that others will follow suit. No specific OTC trials have been carried out with omeprazole.

However, a number of studies have used omeprazole 10 mg in head-to-head trials with antacid/alginate combinations and ranitidine for symptoms of dyspepsia/heartburn. Trials have shown omeprazole to be significantly more effective than both antacids and H_2 antagonists. The manufacturer's dosage schedule for OTC omeprazole is in line with current Prodigy guidelines for uninvestigated dyspepsia.

Summary

Antacids will work for the majority of people presenting at the pharmacy with mild dyspeptic symptoms. They can be used as first-line therapy unless heartburn predominates then an alginate or alginate/antacid combination can be used. H_2 antagonists appear to be equally effective to antacids but are considerably more expensive. Omeprazole has greater efficacy than all other OTC medicines for dyspepsia and should be considered first-line for those patients that suffer from moderate to severe or recurrent symptoms. Like H_2 antagonists it is expensive in com-

parison to simple antacids and might influence patient choice or pharmacist recommendation.

Practical prescribing and product selection

Prescribing information relating to the medicines used for dyspepsia reviewed in the section 'Evidence base for over-the-counter medication' is discussed and summarised in Table 6.9.

Antacids

The majority of marketed antacids are combination products containing two, three or even four constituents. The rationale for combining different salts together appears to be two-fold. First, to ensure the product has quick onset (containing sodium or calcium) and a long duration of action (containing magnesium, aluminium or calcium). Second, to minimise any side effects that might be experienced from the product. For example, magnesium salts tend to cause diarrhoea and aluminium salts con-

Table 6.9
Practical prescribing: Summary of medicines for dyspepsia

Name of medicine	Use in children	Likely side effects	Drug interactions of note	Patients in whom care should be exercised	Pregnancy and breast-feeding
Antacids Sodium only	>12 years	None	None	Patients with heart disease	OK
Calcium only		Constipation	Tetracyclines, quinolones, imidazoles, phenytoin, penicillamine and bisphosphonates	None	OK
Magnesium only		Diarrhoea			
Aluminium only		Constipation			
Alginates e.g. Gaviscon range, Gastrocote, Topal, Rennie liquid relief	>12 years*	None	None	Patients with heart disease	OK
H_2 antagonists Pepcid AC	>16 years	Diarrhoea, constipation, headache or rash	None	None	Experience has shown them to be OK
Zantac, Gavilast, Ranzac					
PPIs Omeprazole	>18 years	Headache, diarrhoea, constipation, nausea and vomiting, abdominal pain, flatulence	Azole antifungals, diazepam, fluvoxamine, cilostazol	None	Avoid

*Certain products such as Gaviscon, Gastrocote and Topal can be given to children but dyspepsia is unusual in children and it might be prudent to refer such patients to their GP.

HINTS AND TIPS BOX 6.4: ANTACIDS

Type of formulation?	Ideally, antacids should be given in the liquid form because the acid-neutralising capacity and speed of onset is greater than that of tablet formulations
Overuse of antacids	Misuse and chronic use of antacids will result in significant systemic absorption leading to various unwanted medical conditions. Milk-alkali syndrome has been reported with chronic abuse of calcium-containing antacids, as has osteomalacia with aluminium-containing products
	Antacid therapy should ideally not be longer than 2 weeks. If symptoms have not resolved in this time then other treatments and/or evaluation from the GP should be recommended
When is the best time to take antacids?	Antacids should be taken after food because gastric emptying is delayed in the presence of food. This allows antacids to exert their effect for up to 3 hours
Salt content	Be aware that some antacid preparations do contain significant amounts of salt – for example, Gaviscon Advance contains 4.6 mmol of sodium per 10 mL
The elderly	Avoid constipating products, as the elderly are prone to constipation
Possible solutions to minimise symptoms	Simple suggestions such as eating less but more often or eating smaller meals might help control symptoms. Eating late at night and lying flat at night should be avoided – a pillow should be used to prop the person up

stipation; however, if both are combined in the same product then neither side effect is noticed. Useful tips relating to antacids are given in Hints and Tips Box 6.4.

Antacids can affect the absorption of a number of medications via chelation and adsorption. Commonly affected medicines include tetracyclines, quinolones, imidazoles, phenytoin, penicillamine and bisphosphonates. In addition, the absorption of enteric-coated preparations can be affected due to antacids increasing the stomach pH. The majority of these interactions are easily overcome by leaving a minimum gap of 1 hour between the respective doses of each medicine.

Most patient groups can take antacids, although patients on salt-restricted diets (e.g. patients with coronary heart disease) should ideally avoid sodium-containing antacids. In addition, antacids should not be recommended in children because dyspepsia is unusual in children under 12 years. Indeed, most products are licensed for use only for children aged 12 and over. However, there are a few exceptions (e.g. Acidex, Gaviscon Advance, Topal), which have product licences for use in children.

Alginates (e.g. the Gaviscon range, Algicon)

Products containing alginates are combination preparations that contain an alginate with antacids. They are best given after each main meal and before bedtime, although they can be taken on a when-needed basis. They can be given during pregnancy and breast-feeding and to most patient groups but, as with antacids, patients on salt-restricted diets should ideally avoid sodium-containing alginate preparations. They are reported not to have any side effects or interactions with other medicines.

H₂ antagonists

Sales of H_2 antagonists are restricted to adults and children over the age of 16. They possess no clinically important drug interactions and side effects are rare. Safety concerns were raised on deregulation of H_2 antagonists about the potential to mask serious underlying conditions and the possibility of increased adverse reactions. These fears appear to have been unfounded as follow-up studies and post marketing surveillance has not shown any increase in risk associated with greater availability. Indeed, H_2 antagonists are now available as general sales list medicines. They have been used in pregnancy and breast-feeding, with ranitidine having been used most. Data suggest that there are no significant increases in any major malformations in pregnancy and they can be used while breast-feeding, and manufacturers of OTC products advise patients to speak to the doctor or pharmacist before taking.

Famotidine (PepcidTwo)

The dose for famotidine is 10 mg (one tablet) at the onset of symptoms; however, if symptoms persist an additional dose can be repeated after 1 hour. The maximum dose is 20 mg (two tablets) in 24 hours. A dose can be taken 1 hour prior to consuming food or drink that are known to bring on symptoms. PepcidTwo is a combination of famotidine, calcium carbonate and magnesium hydroxide. The antacid component of the product provides quick onset of action helping to relieve symptoms before famotide exerts its action, which can take 2 hours.

Ranitidine (Zantac 75, Zantac Relief, Gavilast and Gavilast P, Ranzac)

Dosing for ranitidine is similar to famotidine in that one tablet should be taken straight away but if symptoms persist then a further tablet should be taken 1 hour later. The maximum dose is 300 mg (four tablets) in 24 hours. The General Sales List version of ranitidine, Zantac 75 Relief (and Ranzac), has a slightly different licence in that it cannot be used for prevention of heartburn and the maximum dose is only two tablets in 24 hours.

Omeprazole (Zanprol)

Zanprol is licensed for the relief of reflux-like symptoms (e.g. heartburn) associated with acid-related dyspepsia in patients aged over 18 years of age. The initial dose is two 10 mg tablets once daily. Once symptoms improve the dose can be reduced to one tablet (10 mg). If symptoms return then the dose can be stepped back up to 20 mg. Patients should be referred to their GP if symptoms do not resolve in 2 weeks or they need to use omeprazole for more than 4 weeks continuously. Omeprazole can cause a number of common side effects (>1 in 100), which include headache, diarrhoea, constipation, abdominal pain, nausea and vomiting and flatulence. Drug interactions with omeprazole are possible because it is metabolised in the liver by cytochrome P450 isoenzymes. These include 'azole' antifungals (decrease in azole bioavailability), diazepam (enhanced diazepam side effects), fluvoxamine (increased omeprazole levels) and cilostazol (increased cilostazol levels – UK manufacturers advise against co-administration). Other interactions listed in the manufacturer's literature include phenytoin and warfarin but their clinical significance appears low.

It appears to be safe in pregnancy and is excreted in only small amounts in breast milk. It is not contraindicated when used as a POM medicine; however, for pharmacy use it is not recommended.

Further reading

Castell DO, Dalton CB, Becker D, et al. Alginic acid decreases postprandial upright gastroesophageal reflux. Comparison with equal-strength antacid. Dig Dis Sci 1992;37:589–93.

Drake D, Hollander D. Neutralizing capacity and cost effectiveness of antacids. Ann Intern Med 1981;94:215–7.

Feldman M. Comparison of the effects of over-the-counter famotidine and calcium carbonate antacid on postprandial gastric acid. A randomized controlled trial. JAMA 1996;275:1428–31.

Halter F. Determination of neutralization capacity of antacids in gastric juice. Z Gastroenterol 1983;21:S33–40.

Li Wan Po A. H2 antagonists for the relief of dyspepsia. Pharm J 1994;252:84–7.

Moayyedi P, Soo S, Deeks J, et al. Pharmacological interventions for non-ulcer dyspepsia. Cochrane Database of Systematic Reviews 2006, issue 4.

Netzer P, Brabetz-Hofliger A, Brundler R, et al. Comparison of the effect of the antacid Rennie versus low dose H2 receptor antagonists (ranitidine, famotidine) on intragastric acidity. Ailment Pharmacol Ther 1998;12:337–42.

Rao SSC. Belching, bloating and flatulence. Postgrad Med 1997;101:263–78.

Reilly TG, Singh S, Cottrell J, et al. Low dose famotidine and rantidine as single post-prandial doses: a three-period placebo-controlled comparative trial. Ailment Pharmacol Ther 1996;10:749–55.

Smart HL, Atkinson M. Comparison of a dimethicone/antacid (Asilone gel) with an alginate/antacid (Gaviscon liquid) in the management of reflux oesophagitis. J R Soc Med 1990;83:554–6.

Web sites

British Society of Gastroenterology: http://www.bsg.org.uk/

NPC Resource on dyspepsia: http://www.npc.co.uk/dyspepsia_addtl_resources.htm

CORE: http://www.corecharity.org.uk/

American Gastroenterological Association: http://www.gastro.org/

NICE Guidance on dyspepsia: http://www.nice.org.uk/page.aspx?o=218381

On-line article on GORD from The Prescriber (August 2004): http://www.escriber.com/Prescriber/Features.asp?ID=854&GroupID=6&Action=View

Diarrhoea

Background

Diarrhoea can be defined as an increase in frequency of the passage of soft or watery stools relative to the usual bowel habit for that individual. It is not a disease but a sign of an underlying problem such as an infection or gastrointestinal disorder. It can be classed as acute (less than 7 days), persistent (more than 14 days) or chronic (lasting longer than a month). Most patients will present to the pharmacy with a self-diagnosis of acute diarrhoea. It is necessary to confirm this self-diagnosis because patients' interpretations of their symptoms might not match up with the medical definition of diarrhoea.

Prevalence and epidemiology

The exact prevalence and epidemiology of diarrhoea is not well known. This is probably due to the number of patients who do not seek care or who self-medicate.

However, acute diarrhoea does generate high GP consultation rates. For example, diarrhoeal illness has been reported as being the second most common medical problem in American households. It has been reported that children under the age of 5 years have between one and three bouts of diarrhoea per year and adults, on average, just under one episode of diarrhoea per year. Many of these cases are thought to be food related.

Aetiology

The aetiology of diarrhoea depends on its cause. Acute gastroenteritis, the most common cause of diarrhoea in all age groups, is usually viral in origin. In the UK rotavirus and small round structured virus (SRSV) are the most commonly identified causes of gastroenteritis in children, and in adults, *Campylobacter* followed by rotavirus are the most common. Other pathogens identified include *E. coli*, *Salmonella*, *Shigella*, viruses such as adenovirus and the protozoa *Cryptosporidium* and *Giardia*. Viral causes tend to cause diarrhoea by blunting of the villi of the upper small intestine decreasing the absorptive surface. Bacterial causes of diarrhoea are normally a result of eating contaminated food or drink and cause diarrhoea by a number of mechanisms. For example, enterotoxigenic *E. coli* produce enterotoxins that affect gut function with secretion and loss of fluids; enteropathogenic *E. coli* interferes with normal mucosal func-

tion; and enteroinvasive *E. coli*, *Shigella* and *Salmonella* species cause injury to the mucosa of the small intestine and deeper tissues.

Other organisms, for example *Staphylococcus aureus* and *Bacillus cereus*, produce preformed enterotoxins, which on ingestion stimulate the active secretion of electrolytes into the intestinal lumen.

Arriving at a differential diagnosis

Acute diarrhoea is rarely life-threatening. The most common causes of diarrhoea are viral or bacterial infection and the community pharmacist can appropriately manage the vast majority of cases. The main priority is identifying those patients that need referral and how quickly they need to be referred. Dehydration is the main complicating factor, especially in the very young and very old. Questions aimed at establishing the frequency, fluidity and nature of the stools should enable a patient self-diagnosis to be rejected or confirmed. A number of diarrhoea-specific questions should always be asked of the patient to aid in diagnosis (Table 6.10).

Clinical features of acute diarrhoea

Symptoms are normally rapid in onset, with the patient having a history of prior good health. Nausea and vomiting might be present prior to or during the bout of acute

Table 6.10
Specific questions to ask the patient: Diarrhoea

Question	Relevance
Frequency and nature of the stools	• Patients with acute self-limiting diarrhoea will be passing watery stools more frequently than normal • Diarrhoea associated with blood and mucus (dysentery) requires referral to eliminate invasive infection such as *Shigella*, *Campylobacter*, *Salmonella* or *E. coli* O157 • Bloody stools are also associated with conditions such as inflammatory bowel disease
Periodicity	• A history of recurrent diarrhoea of no known cause should be referred for further investigation
Duration	• A person who presents with a history of chronic diarrhoea should be referred. The most frequent causes of chronic diarrhoea are IBS, inflammatory disease and colon cancer
Onset of symptoms	• Ingestion of bacterial pathogens can give rise to symptoms in a matter of a few hours (toxin-producing bacteria) after eating contaminated food or up to 3 days later. It is therefore important to ask about food consumption over the last few days, establish if anyone else ate the same food and to check the status of his or her health
Timing of diarrhoea	• Patients who experience diarrhoea first thing in the morning might well have underlying pathology such as IBS • Nocturnal diarrhoea is often associated with inflammatory bowel disease
Recent change of diet	• Changes in diet can cause changes to bowel function, for example, when away on holiday. If the person has recently been to a non-Western country then giardiasis is a possibility
Signs of dehydration	• Mild (<5%) dehydration can be vague but may include tiredness, anorexia, nausea and light-headedness • Moderate (5 to 10%) dehydration is characterised by dry mouth, sunken eyes, decreased urine output, moderate thirst and decreased skin turgor (pinch test of 1 to 2 seconds or longer)

diarrhoea. Abdominal cramping, flatulence and tenderness are also often present. If rotavirus is the cause the patient might also experience viral prodromal symptoms such as cough and cold. Acute infective diarrhoea is usually watery in nature with no blood present. Complete resolution of symptoms should be observed in 2 to 4 days. However, diarrhoea caused by the rotavirus can persist for longer.

Conditions to eliminate

Giardiasis

Giardiasis, a protozoan infection of the small intestine, is contracted through drinking contaminated water. It is an uncommon cause of diarrhoea in Western society. However, with more people taking exotic foreign holidays, enquiry about recent travel should be made. The patient will present with watery and foul-smelling diarrhoea accompanied by symptoms of bloating, flatulence and epigastric pain. If giardiasis is suspected the patient must be referred to the GP quickly for confirmation and appropriate antibiotic treatment.

Irritable bowel syndrome

Patients younger than 45 with lower abdominal pain and a history of alternating diarrhoea and constipation are likely to have IBS. For further details on IBS see page 155.

Medicine-induced diarrhoea

Many medicines – both POM and OTC – can induce diarrhoea (Table 6.11). If medication is suspected as the cause of the diarrhoea the GP should be contacted and an alternative suggested.

Ulcerative colitis and Crohn's disease

Both conditions are characterised by chronic inflammation at various sites in the GI tract and follow periods of remission and relapse. They can affect any age group, although peak incidence is between 20 and 30 years of age. In mild cases of both conditions, diarrhoea is one of the major presenting symptoms, although blood in the stool is usually present. Patients might also find that they have urgency, nocturnal diarrhoea and early morning rushes. In the acute phase patients will appear unwell and have malaise.

Malabsorption syndromes

Lactose intolerance is often diagnosed in infants under 1 year old. In addition to more frequent loose bowel movements symptoms such as fever, vomiting, perianal excoriation and a failure to gain weight might occur.

Coeliac disease has a bimodal incidence: first, in early infancy when cereals become a major constituent of the diet, and second, during the fourth and fifth decades. Steatorrhoea (fatty stools) is common and might be observed by the patient as frothy or floating stools in the toilet pan. Bloating and weight loss in the presence of a normal appetite might also be observed.

Faecal impaction

Faecal impaction is most commonly seen in the elderly and those with poor mobility. Patients might present with continuous soiling as a result of liquid passing around hard stools and mistakenly believe they have diarrhoea. On questioning, the patient might describe the passage of regular poorly formed hard stools that are difficult to pass. Referral is needed as manual removal of the faeces is often necessary.

Colorectal cancer

Any middle-aged patient presenting with a long-standing change of bowel habit must be viewed with suspicion. Persistent diarrhoea accompanied by a feeling that the bowel has not really been emptied is suggestive of neoplasm. This is especially true if weight loss is also present.

Figure 6.11 will aid differentiation of diarrhoeal cases that require referral.

> **❗ TRIGGER POINTS indicative of referral: Diarrhoea**
>
> - Change in bowel (long term) habit in patients over 50
> - Diarrhoea following recent travel to tropical or subtropical climate
> - Duration longer than 2 to 3 days in children and elderly
> - Patients unable to drink fluids
> - Presence of blood or mucous in the stool
> - Signs of dehydration
> - Severe abdominal pain
> - Steatorrhoea
> - Suspected faecal impaction in the elderly

Evidence base for over-the-counter medication

Acute infectious diarrhoea still remains one of the leading causes of death in developing countries, despite advances in its treatment. In developed and Western countries diarrhoeal disease is primarily of economic and socially disruptive significance. Goals of OTC treatment in the UK are therefore concentrated on relief of symptoms.

Table 6.11
Medicines known to cause diarrhoea (defined as >1% from manufacturers' data)

α-blocker	Prazosin
ACEI & angiotension II antagonist	Lisinopril, perindopril, telmisartan
Acetylcholinesterase inhibitor	Donepezil, galantamine, rivastigmine
Antacid	Magnesium salts
Antibacterial	All
Antidiabetic	Metformin, acarbose
Antidepressant	SSRIs, clomipramine, venlafaxine
Anti-emetic	Aprepitant, dolasetron
Anti-epileptic	Carbamazepine, oxcarbamazepine, tiagabine, zonisamide, pregabalin, levtiracetam
Antifungal	Caspofungilin, fluconazole, flucytosine, nystatin (in large doses), terbinafine, voriconazole
Antimalarial	Mefloquine
Antiprotozoal	Metronidazole, sodium stibogluconate
Antipsychotic	Arirpiprazole
Antiviral	Abacavir, emtricitabine, stavudine, tenofovir, zalcitabine, zidovudine, amprenavir, atazanavir, indinavir, lopinavir, nelfinavir, saquinavir, efavirinez, ganciclovir, valganciclovir, adefovir, oseltamivir, ribavrin, fosamprenavir
β-blocker	Bisoprolol, carvedilol, nebivolol
Bisphosphonate	Alendronic acid, disodium etidronate, ibandronic acid, risedronate, sodium clodronate, disodium pamidronate, tiludronic acid
Cytokine inhibitor	Adalimumab, infliximab
Cytotoxic	All classes of cytotoxics
Dopaminergic	Levodopa, entacapone
Growth hormone antagonist	Pegvisomant
Immunosuppressant	Ciclosporin, mycophenolate, leflunomide
NSAID	All
Ulcer healing	Proton pump inhibitors
Vaccines	Pediacel, haemophilus, meningococcal
Miscellaneous	Calcitonin, strontium ranelate, colchicines, dantrolene, olsalazine, anagrelide, nicotinic acid, pancreatin, eplerenone, acamprosate

Oral rehydration solution (ORS)

ORS represents one of the major advances in medicine. It has proven to be a simple highly effective treatment, which has decreased mortality and morbidity associated with acute diarrhoea in developing countries. The formula recommended by the World Health Organization (WHO) contains glucose (75 mmol/L), sodium (75 mmol/L), potassium (20 mmol/L), chloride (65 mmol/L) and citrate (10 mmol/L) in an almost isotonic fluid. Until recently, the WHO oral rehydration solution contained 90 mmol/L sodium but a systematic review (Hahn et al 2002) concluded that ORSs with a reduced osmolarity compared to the standard WHO formula were associated with fewer

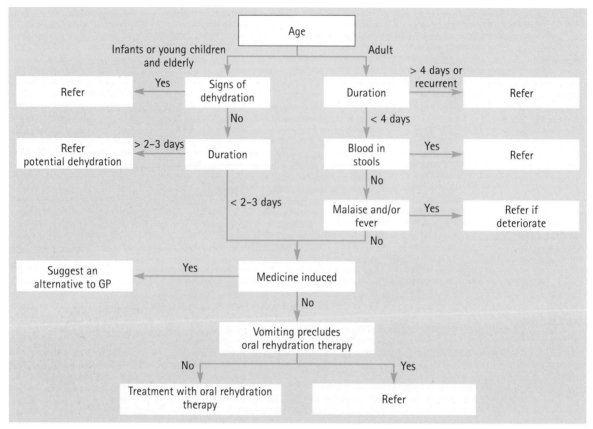

Fig. 6.11   Primer for differential diagnosis of diarrhoea

complications in children with mild to moderate diarrhoea. Based on this, and other findings, the WHO oral rehydration solution now has a reduced osmolarity of 245 mm/L, which contains 75 mmol of sodium. A number of similar preparations are available commercially in the form of sachets that require reconstitution in clean water before use; however, commercially available solutions in the UK still contain lower sodium concentrations as diarrhoea tends to be isotonic and therefore replacement of large quantities of sodium is less important.

Rice-based ORS

In many developing countries a glucose substitute was added to electrolytes because of glucose unavailability. These products were found to be quite successful. Clinical trials have subsequently shown rice-based ORS to be highly efficacious, well tolerated and potentially more effective than conventional ORS.

Loperamide

Loperamide is a synthetic opioid analogue and is thought to exert its action via opiate receptors slowing intestinal tract time and increasing the capacity of the gut. It has been extensively researched, with many published trials investigating its effectiveness in acute infectious diarrhoea. The majority of well-designed double-blind placebo-controlled trials have consistently shown it to be significantly better than placebo and comparable to diphenoxylate.

Bismuth subsalicylate

Bismuth-containing products have been used for many decades. The use of bismuth subsalicylate has declined over time as other products have become more popular. However, it has been shown to be effective in treating traveller's diarrhoea. A review paper by Steffen (1990) concluded that bismuth subsalicylate was clinically superior to placebo, decreasing the number of unformed stools and increasing the number of patients who were symptom-free. However, two of the trials reviewed showed bismuth subsalicylate to be significantly slower in symptom resolution than its comparator drug loperamide.

Kaolin and morphine

The constipating side effect of opioid analgesics can be used to treat diarrhoea. However, kaolin and morphine products have no evidence of efficacy and should not be recommended. This remains a popular home remedy, especially with the elderly.

Rotavirus vaccine

In 2006, two new oral vaccines (Rotarix and RotaTeq) were licensed by the European Medicines Agency and the US Food and Drug Administration. Clinical trials have shown them to protect against the most common circulating strains of rotavirus (G1 and G3) and the emerging G9 strain. The vaccine can be co-administered with other childhood vaccinations according to manufacturers but currently it is not part of the UK childhood vaccination programme.

Summary

As diarrhoea results in fluid and electrolyte loss it is important to re-establish normal fluid balance and so ORS is first-line treatment for all age groups, especially children and the frail elderly. Loperamide is a useful adjunct in reducing the number of bowel movements but should be reserved for those patients who will find it inconvenient to have to go to the toilet.

Practical prescribing and product selection

Prescribing information relating to the medicines used for diarrhoea reviewed in the section 'Evidence base for over-the-counter medicine' is discussed and summarised in Table 6.12; useful tips relating to patients presenting with diarrhoea are given in Hints and Tips Box 6.5.

ORS (Dioralyte, Dioralyte Relief (rice-based), Electrolade, Rapolyte)

ORS can be given to all patient groups and has no side effects or drug interactions. The volume of solution

Table 6.12
Practical prescribing: Summary of medicines for diarrhoea

Name of medicine	Use in children	Likely side effects	Drug interactions of note	Patients in whom care should be exercised	Pregnancy and breast-feeding
ORS	Infant upwards	None	None	None	OK
Loperamide	>12 years	Abdominal cramps, nausea, vomiting, tiredness	None	None	OK
Bismuth	>16 years	Black stools or tongue	Quinolone antibiotics	None	Avoid if possible
Morphine salts Kaolin and morphine	>12 years	None	None	None	OK
Diocalm	>6 years				

HINTS AND TIPS BOX 6.5: DIARRHOEA

Reconstitution of ORS	All proprietary sachets require 200 mL of water per sachet to reconstitute Different brands come in different flavours, e.g. Dioralyte – blackcurrant and citrus Dioralyte Relief – apricot, raspberry or blackcurrant Rapolyte – blackcurrant or raspberry Electrolade – banana, blackcurrant, lemon and lime and orange Once reconstituted ORS must be stored in the fridge and drunk within 24 hours
Rough guidelines for referral for children	<1 year old: refer if duration >1 day <3 years old: refer if duration >2 days >3 years old: refer if duration >3 days
Kaolin and morphine	Subject to abuse. Store out of sight
Alternative to ORS	Patients can be advised to increase their intake of fluids, particularly fruit juices with their glucose and potassium content, and soups because of their sodium chloride content

given is dependent on how much fluid is lost. As infants and the elderly are more at risk of developing dehydration they should be encouraged to drink as much ORS as possible. In adults, 2 L of ORS should be given in the first 24 hours, followed by unrestricted normal fluids with 200 mL of rehydration solution per loose stool or vomit. The solution is best sipped every 5 to 10 minutes rather than drunk in large quantities less frequently. In infants, 1 to $1\frac{1}{2}$ times the usual feed volume should be given.

Loperamide (e.g. Arret, Diocalm Ultra, Diah–Limit, Imodium)

The dose is two capsules immediately, followed by one capsule after each further bout of diarrhoea. It has minimal CNS side effects, although CNS depressant effects and respiratory depression have been reported at high doses. OTC doses are therefore limited to 16 mg a day and cannot be used in children under 12. The excellent safety record of loperamide has seen it granted General Sales List status, although abdominal cramps, nausea, vomiting, tiredness, drowsiness, dizziness and dry mouth have been reported. Loperamide is also available as dispersible tablets, melt-tabs and liquid (the Imodium range of products).

Bismuth (Pepto–Bismol 87.6 mg/5 mL bismuth subsalicylate)

Pepto-Bismol should only be given to people over the age of 16. This age limit has been set by the company due to the association of taking aspirin and Reye's syndrome. The dose is 30 mL taken every 30 minutes to 1 hour when needed, with a maximum of eight doses in 24 hours. Bismuth subsalicylate is well tolerated and has a favourable side effect profile, although black stools are commonly observed (caused by unabsorbed bismuth compound). Occasional use is not known to cause problems during pregnancy but the manufacturers state it should not be taken during pregnancy. Bismuth can decrease the bioavailability of quinolone antibiotics therefore a minimum 2-hour gap should be left between doses of each medicine.

Morphine (e.g. kaolin and morphine, Diocalm Dual Action)

Morphine is generally well tolerated at OTC doses, with no side effects reported. The products can be given to all patient groups, including pregnant women. There are no drug interactions of note.

Kaolin and morphine

If kaolin and morphine is prescribed then it can only be given to adults and children over the age of 12. The normal dose is 10 mL every 4 hours.

Diocalm Dual Action

Adults and children over the age of 12 should take two tablets every 2 to 4 hours as required and children aged 6 to 12 years should take half the adult dose.

Further reading

American Academy of Pediatrics (AAP) Committee on Quality Improvement SoAG. Practice parameter. The management of acute gastroenteritis in young children. Pediatrics 1996;97:4224–433.

Amery W, Duyck F, Polak J, et al. A multicentre double-blind study in acute diarrhoea comparing loperamide (R 18553) with two common antidiarrhoeal agents and a placebo. Curr Ther Res Clin Exp 1975;17:263–70.

Chassany O, Michaux A, Bergman JF. Drug-induced diarrhoea. Drug Safety 2000;22:53–72

Cornett JWD, Aspeling RL, Mallegol D. A double blind comparative evaluation of loperamide versus diphenoxylate with atropine in acute diarrhea. Curr Ther Res 1977;21:629–37.

De Bruyn G, Hahn S, Borwick A. Antibiotic treatment for travellers' diarrhoea. Cochrane Database of Systematic Reviews 2000, issue 3.

Gavin N, Merrick N, Davidson B. Efficacy of glucose-based oral rehydration therapy. Pediatrics 1996;98:45–51.

Hahn S, Kim Y, Garner P. Reduced osmolarity oral rehydration solution for treating dehydration due to diarrhoea in children. Cochrane Database of Systematic Reviews 2002, issue 1.

Islam A, Molla AM, Ahmed MA, et al. Is rice based oral rehydration therapy effective in young infants? Arch Dis Child 1994;71:19–23.

Molla AM, Sarker SA, Hossain M, et al. Rice-powder electrolyte solution as oral-therapy in diarrhoea due to *Vibrio cholerae* and *Escherichia coli*. Lancet 1982;1(8285):1317–9.

Nelemans FA, Zelvelder WG. A double-blind placebo controlled trial of loperamide (Imodium) in acute diarrhea. J Drug Res 1976;2:54–9.

Patra FC, Mahalanabis D, Jalan KN, et al. Is oral rice electrolyte solution superior to glucose electrolyte solution in infantile diarrhoea? Arch Dis Child 1982;57:910–2.

Selby W. Diarrhoea-differential diagnosis. Aust Fam Physician 1990;19:1683–6.

Steffen R. Worldwide efficacy of bismuth subsalicylate in the treatment of travelers' diarrhea. Rev Infect Dis 1990;12:S80–6.

Web sites

General information on diarrhoea: http://www.diarrhoea.org/index.html

National Association for Colitis and Crohn's disease (NACC): http://www.nacc.org.uk

Clinical signs and diagnosis of dehydration: http://www.pediatrics.org/cgi/content/full/99/5/e6.

Constipation

Background

Constipation, like diarrhoea, means different things to different people. Constipation arises when the patient experiences a reduction in their normal bowel habit accompanied with more difficult defecation and/or hard stools. In Western populations 90% of people defecate between three times a day and once every three days. However, many people still believe that anything other than one bowel movement a day is abnormal.

Prevalence and epidemiology

Constipation is very common. It occurs in all age groups but is especially common in the elderly. It has been estimated that 25 to 40% of all people over the age of 65 have constipation. The majority of the elderly have normal frequency of bowel movements but strain at stool. This is probably a result of sedentary lifestyle, a decreased fluid intake, poor nutrition, avoidance of fibrous foods and chronic illness. Women are two to three times more likely to suffer from constipation than men and 40% of women in late pregnancy experience constipation.

Aetiology

The normal function of the large intestine is to remove water and various salts from the colon, drying and expulsion of the faeces. Any process that facilitates water resorption will generally lead to constipation. The commonest cause of constipation is an increase in intestinal tract transit time of food, which allows greater water resorption from the large bowel leading to harder stools that are more difficult to pass. This is most frequently caused by a deficiency in dietary fibre, a change in lifestyle and/or environment and medication. Occasionally, patients ignore the defactory reflex as it may be inconvenient for them to defecate.

Arriving at a differential diagnosis

The first thing a pharmacist should do is to establish the patient's current bowel habit compared to normal. This should establish if the patient is suffering from constipation. Questioning should then concentrate on determining the cause because constipation is a symptom and not a disease and can be caused by many different conditions. Constipation does not usually have sinister pathology and the commonest cause in the vast majority of non-elderly adults will be a lack of dietary fibre. However, constipation can be caused by medication and many disease states including neurological disorders (e.g. multiple sclerosis, Parkinson's disease), metabolic and endocrine conditions (diabetes, hypothroidism) and neoplasm. A number of constipation-specific questions should always be asked of the patient to aid in diagnosis (Table 6.13).

Clinical features of constipation

Besides the inability to defecate, patients might also have abdominal discomfort and bloating. In children, parents might also notice the child is more irritable and have a decreased appetite. Specks of blood in the toilet pan might be present and are usually due to straining at stool.

Table 6.13
Specific questions to ask the patient: Constipation

Question	Relevance
Change of diet or routine	Constipation usually has a social or behavioural cause. There will usually be some event that has precipitated the onset of symptoms
Pain on defecation	Associated pain when going to the toilet is usually due to a local anorectal problem. Constipation is often secondary to the suppression of defecation because it induces pain. These cases are best referred for physical examination
Presence of blood	Bright red specks in the toilet or smears on toilet tissue suggest haemorrhoids or a tear in the anal canal (fissure). However, if blood is mixed in the stool (melaena) then referral to the GP is necessary. A stool that appears black and tarry is suggestive of an upper GI bleed
Duration (chronic or recent?)	Constipation lasting 6 weeks or more is said to be chronic. If a patient suffers from long-standing constipation and has been previously seen by the GP then treatment could be given. However, cases of more than 14 days with no identifiable cause or previous investigation by the GP should be referred
Lifestyle changes	Changes in job or marital status can precipitate depressive illness that can manifest with physiological symptoms such as constipation

In the vast majority of cases blood in the stool does not indicate sinister pathology. Those patients presenting with acute constipation with no other symptoms apart from very small amounts of bright red blood can be managed in the pharmacy; however, if blood loss is substantial (stools appear tarry, red or black) or the patient has other associated symptoms such as malaise and abdominal distension and is over 40 years old then referral is needed.

Conditions to eliminate

Medicine-induced constipation

Many medicines are known to cause constipation. Most exert their action by decreasing gut motility, although opioids tend to raise sphincter tone and reduce sensitivity to rectal distension. A detailed medication history should always be sought from the patient and Table 6.14 lists the commonly implicated medicines that cause constipation.

Irritable bowel syndrome

Patients younger than 45 with lower abdominal pain and a history of alternating diarrhoea and constipation are likely to have IBS. For further details on IBS see page 155.

Pregnancy

Constipation is common in pregnancy, especially in the third trimester. A combination of increased circulating progestogen, displacement of the uterus against the colon by the foetus, decreased mobility and iron supplementation all contribute to an increased incidence of constipation whilst pregnant. Most patients complain of hard stools rather than a decrease in bowel movements. If a laxative is used a bulk-forming laxative should be recommended.

Functional causes in children

Constipation in children is common and the cause can be varied. Constipation is not normally a result of organic disease but stems from poor diet or a traumatic experience associated with defecation, for example, unwillingness to defecate due to association of prior pain on defecation.

Depression

Upwards of 20% of the population will suffer from depression at some time. Many will present with physical rather than emotional symptoms. It has been reported that a third of all patients suffering from depression present with gastrointestinal complaints in a primary care setting. It is important to ensure that a social history is taken.

Colorectal cancer

Colorectal carcinomas are rare in patients under the age of 40. However, the incidence of carcinoma increases with increasing age and any patient over the age of 40 presenting for the first time with a marked change in bowel habit should be referred. Sexes appear to be equally affected. The patient might complain of abdominal pain, rectal bleeding and tenesmus. Weight loss – a classical textbook sign of colon cancer – is common but observed only in the latter stages of the disease. Therefore, a patient is unlikely to have noticed marked weight loss when visiting a pharmacy early in disease progression.

Hypothyroidism

The signs and symptoms of hypothyroidism are often subtle and insidious in onset. Patients might experience weight gain, lethargy, cold intolerance, coarse hair and dry skin as well as constipation. Hypothyroidism affects ten times more women than men and peak incidence is in the fifth or sixth decade. Constipation is often less pronounced than lethargy and cold intolerance.

Figure 6.12 will aid differentiation between common causes of constipation and more serious causes.

TRIGGER POINTS indicative of referral: Constipation

- Blood in stool
- Greater than 14 days' duration with no identifiable cause
- Pain on defecation causing patient to suppress defecatory reflex
- Patients aged over 40 with sudden change in bowel habits with no obvious cause
- Suspected depression
- Tiredness

Evidence base for over-the-counter medication

For uncomplicated constipation, non-drug treatment is advocated as first-line treatment for all patient groups as simple dietary and lifestyle modifications (increasing exercise) will relieve the majority of acute cases of constipation. Advice includes increasing fluid and fibre intake. Dietary fibre increases stool bulk, stool water content and colonic bacterial load. Fibre intake should be increased to approximately 30 g day in the form of fruit, vegetables, cereals, grain foods and wholemeal bread. It is important to remind patients that adequate fluid intake (2 L per day) is needed when following a high-fibre diet and patients might experience excessive gas production, colicky abdominal pain and bloating. Effects of a high-fibre diet are usually seen in 3 to 5 days.

Table 6.14
Medicines known to cause constipation (defined as >1% from manufacturers' data)

α-blocker	Prazosin
Antacid	Aluminium and calcium salts
Anticholinergic	Trihexyphenidyl, hyoscine, oxybutynin, procyclidine, tolterodine
Antidepressant	Tricyclics, SSRIs, reboxetine, venlafaxine, duloxetine, mirtazepine
Anti-emetic	Palonosetron, dolasetron, aprepitant
Anti-epileptic	Carbamazepine, oxcarbazepine
Antipsychotic	Phenothiazines, haloperidol, pimozide and atypical antipsychotics such as amisulpride, arirpiprazole, olanzapine, quetiapine, risperidone, zotepine, clozapine
Antiviral	Foscarnet
β-blocker	Oxprenolol, bisoprolol, nebivolol; other β-blockers tend to cause constipation more rarely
Bisphosphonate	Alendronic acid
CNS stimulant	Atomoxetine
Calcium channel blocker	Diltiazem, verapamil
Cytotoxic	Bortezomib, buserelin, cladribine, docetaxel, doxorubicin, exemestane, gemcitabine, irinotecan, mitozantrone, pentostatin, temozolomide, topotecan, vinblastine, vincristine, vindesine, vinorelbine
Dopaminergic	Amantadine, bromocriptine, carbegolide, entacapone, tolcapone, levodopa, pergolide, pramipexole, quinagolide
Growth hormone antagonist	Pegvisomant
Immunosuppressant	Basiliximab, mycophenolate, tacrolimus
Lipid-lowering agent	Colestyramine, colestipol, rosuvastatin, atorvastatin (other statins reported as uncommon), gemfibrozil
Iron	Ferrous sulphate
Metabolic disorders	Miglustat
Muscle relaxant	Baclofen
NSAID	Meloxicam; other NSAIDs, e.g. aceclofenac, and Cox-2 inhibitors reported as uncommon
Smoking cessation	Bupropion
Opioid analgesic	All opioid analgesics and derivatives
Ulcer healing	Proton pump inhibitors, sucralfate

If medication is required, four classes of OTC laxatives are available: bulk-forming agents, stimulants, osmotic laxatives and stool softeners. Despite their widespread use surprisingly few well-designed trials have substantiated clinical efficacy.

A systematic review by Tramonte in 1997 identified 36 trials involving 1815 participants that met their inclusion criteria and involved 25 different laxatives representing all four classes of laxative. Twenty of the trials compared laxative against placebo or regular diet, 13 of which demonstrated statistically significant increases in bowel movement. The remaining 16 trials compared different types of laxatives with each other. The review concluded that laxatives do increase the number of bowel movements and in 9 of 11 trials studying overall symptom control, laxatives did perform significantly better than placebo. Unfortunately, because of a lack of comparative trial data, the review could not conclude which laxative was most efficacious. A further review of laxative effect in elderly patients suffering with chronic constipation

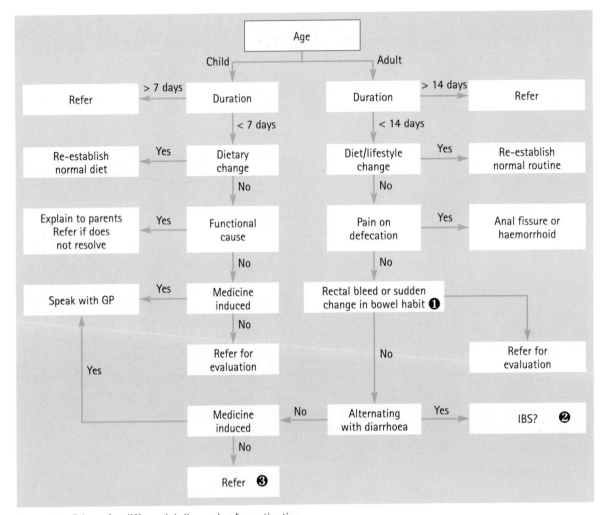

Fig. 6.12 Primer for differential diagnosis of constipation

❶ Patients with unexplained constipation of recent onset accompanied with rectal bleeding should be referred for further investigation; most likely a colonoscopy or sigmoidoscopy and stool culture to eliminate carcinoma

❷ See Fig. 6.13 for primer for differential diagnosis of IBS.

❸ If no obvious cause of constipation can be found referral to the GP is needed for further evaluation.

also failed to determine superior clinical effect between laxative classes. The findings from the Tramonte paper were reviewed in 2005 by the Centre for Reviews and Dissemination, which supported them.

Summary

It appears from the evidence that laxatives do work, but deciding on which laxative to give a patient cannot be made on an evidence-based approach. Other factors will need to be considered such as the patients' status, side effect profile of the medicine and its cost.

Practical prescribing and product selection

Prescribing information relating to the medicines used for constipation reviewed in the section 'Evidence base for over-the-counter medication' is discussed and sum-

marised in Table 6.15; useful tips relating to these medicines are given in Hints and Tips Box 6.6.

The BNF (edition 55) recommends that laxatives should be prescribed by healthcare professionals experienced in the management of constipation in children. Products OTC can be used in younger age groups but in accordance with good practice those children younger than 6 years old who have failed to respond to dietary intervention should be referred to their GP. The text below does, however, make reference to dosing in children younger than 6.

Bulk-forming laxatives (e.g. ispaghula husk, methylcellulose and sterculia)

Bulk-forming laxatives exert their effect by mimicking increased fibre consumption swelling in the bowel and increasing faecal mass. In addition, they also encourage

Table 6.15
Practical prescribing: Summary of medicines for constipation

Name of medicine	Use in children	Likely side effects	Drug interactions of note	Patients in whom care should be exercised	Pregnancy and breast-feeding
Bulk-forming laxatives					
Ispaghula husk	>6 years	Flatulence and abdominal bloating	None	None	OK
Methylcellulose	Not recommended				
Sterculia	>6 years				
Stimulant laxatives					
Senna	>2 years	Abdominal pain	None	None	OK, but use other laxatives in preference to stimulants in pregnancy
Glycerol	Infant upwards				
Sodium picosulphate	>4 years				
Bisacodyl	>4 years				
Osmotic laxatives					
Lactulose	Infant upwards	Flatulence, abdominal pain and colic	None	None	OK
Magnesium hydroxide	Not recommended				
Stool softeners					
Docusate	>6 months	None reported	None	None	OK

the proliferation of colonic bacteria and this helps further increase faecal bulk and stool softness. Patients should be advised to increase their fluid intake while taking bulk-forming medicines. Their effect is usually seen in 12 to 36 hours but can take as long as 72 hours. Side effects commonly experienced include flatulence and abdominal distension. They are well tolerated in pregnancy and breast-feeding and have no teratogenic effects. They appear to have no drug interactions of any note.

Ispaghula husk

Ispaghula husk is widely available as either granules (Fibrelief, Fybogel, Isogel, Ispagel and Senokot Hi-fibre) or powder (Regulan). All have to be reconstituted with water prior to taking. The dose for adults and children over 12 years old can range from one to six sachets a day depending on the brand used and the severity of the condition. Fybogel is probably the most familiar branded product used OTC in the UK – adults should take one sachet or two level 5 mL spoonfuls twice a day and for children aged between 6 and 12 years, a half to one 5 mL spoonful.

Methylcellulose (Celevac)

Methylcellulose is only available as Celevac tablets. The product is only recommended for adults and the dose is

three to six tablets twice daily. Each dose should be taken with at least 300 mL of liquid.

Sterculia (Normacol and Normacol Plus granules or sachets)

Both products contain 62% sterculia but Normacol Plus also contains 8% frangula. The dose for both products is the same. Adults and children over 12 should take either one or two sachets or heaped 5 mL spoonfuls, once or twice daily after meals. For children aged between 6 and 12 the dose is half that of the adult dose.

The granules should be placed dry on the tongue and swallowed immediately with plenty of water or a cool drink. They can also be sprinkled onto, and taken with, soft food such as yoghurt.

Stimulant laxatives (e.g. bisacodyl, glycerol, senna, sodium picosulfate)

Stimulant laxatives increase GI motility by directly stimulating colonic nerves. It is this action that, presumably, causes abdominal pain and is the main side effect associated with stimulant laxatives. Additionally, stimulant laxatives are associated with the possibility of nerve damage in long-term use and are the most commonly abused laxatives. Their onset in action is quicker than

HINTS AND TIPS BOX 6.6: CONSTIPATION

Administration of suppositories	1. Wash your hands 2. Lie on one side with your knees pulled up towards your chest 3. Gently push the suppository, pointed end first, into your back passage with your finger 4. Push the suppository in as far as possible 5. Lower your legs, roll over onto your stomach and remain still for a few minutes 6. If you feel your body trying to expel the suppository, try to resist this. Lie still and press your buttocks together 7. Wash your hands
Sachets containing ispaghula husk	Once the granules have been mixed with water the drink should be taken as soon as the effervescence subsides because the drink 'sets' and becomes undrinkable
Prolonged use of lactulose	In children this can contribute to the development of dental caries. Patients should be instructed to pay careful attention to dental hygiene
Lactulose taste	The sweet taste is unpalatable to many patients, especially if high doses need to be taken
Bisacodyl	Bisacodyl tablets are enterically coated and therefore patients should be told to avoid taking antacids and milk at the same time because the coating can be broken down leading to dyspepsia and gastric irritation
Laxative abuse	Some people, especially young women, use laxatives as a slimming aid. Any very slim person who is regularly purchasing laxatives should be politely asked about why they are taking the laxatives. An opening question could be phrased 'We've noticed that you have been buying quite a lot of these and we are concerned that you should be better by now, is there anything we can do for you to help?'
Onset of action	Stimulants are the quickest acting laxative, usually within 6 to 12 hours. Lactulose and bulk-forming laxatives may take 48 to 72 hours before an effect is seen
Which laxative to use in pregnancy?	Fibre supplementation and bulk-forming agents are considered to be safe and should therefore be first-line treatments wherever possible. Stimulant laxatives and macrogols also appear to be safe in pregnancy. Stimulant laxatives are more effective than bulk-forming laxatives but are more likely to cause diarrhoea and abdominal pain
Avoid drinks with caffeine	These can act as a diuretic and serve to make constipation worse
Combining laxatives	There is little evidence on the beneficial effect of combining different classes of laxatives. However, in refractory cases this approach might be justifiable

other laxative classes, with patients experiencing a bowel movement in 8 to 12 hours. They can be taken by all patient groups, have no drug interactions and are safe in pregnancy and breast-feeding. However, because of their stimulant effect on uterine contractions they are best avoided in pregnancy if possible.

Bisacodyl (Dulcolax)

Bisacodyl is available as either tablets or suppositories and can be given to patients aged over 4 years old. The dose should be taken at bedtime. For children aged between 4 and 10 years the dose is 5 mg (one tablet or one paediatric suppository) and for adults and children over 10 years the dose is 5 to 10 mg (one to two tablets or one Dulcolax 10 mg suppository).

Glycerol suppositories

Glycerol suppositories are normally used when a bowel movement is needed quickly. The patient should experi-ence a bowel movement in 15 to 30 minutes. Varying sizes are made and can be used by all ages. The 1 g suppositories are designed for infants, the 2 g for children and the 4 g for adults.

Senna (e.g. Senokot, Nylax)

Senna is available as syrup, tablets or granules. All products deliver 7.5 mg of sennoside per dose except granules and Senokot Max, which deliver 15 mg per dose, and Ex-Lax Senna Pills (20 mg per dose) and Ex-Lax Senna (25 mg per dose). Adults and children over 12 should take 15 to 30 mg each day, preferably at bedtime. For children over 6 the dose is half that of the adult dose (7.5 to 15 mg) and for children over the age of 2 the dose is 3.75 to 7.5 mg (half to one 5 mL spoonful) each day.

Sodium picosulphate (e.g. Laxoberal liquid)

Adults and children over 10 years old should take one to two 5 mL spoonfuls (5 to 10 mg) at night. Children aged

6

between 4 and 10 years old can take half the adult dose (half to one 5 mL spoonful (2.5 to 5 mg)) at night. Children aged under 4 can take Laxoberal but the dose must be based on the child's weight (250 μg/kg). Sodium picosulphate is also available in a solid dose form (Dulcolax perles) for children aged over 10 years.

Osmotic laxatives (e.g. Lactulose, macrogols and magnesium salts)

These act by retaining fluid in the bowel by osmosis or by changing the pattern of water distribution in the faeces. Flatulence, abdominal pain and colic are frequently reported. They can be taken by all patient groups, have no drug interactions and can be safely used in pregnancy and breast-feeding.

Lactulose

Lactulose is given twice daily for all ages. The dose for adults is 15 mL, for children aged between 5 and 10 the dose is 10 mL, those aged between 1 and 5 the dose is 5 mL and children under 1 year is 2.5 mL. The dose for all ages can be reduced according to the need of the patient after 2 to 3 days. It has been reported that up to 20% of patients experience troublesome flatulence and cramps, although these often settle after a few days. It may take 48 hours or longer for it to work.

Macrogols (Idrolax, Movicol)

Macrogols are available as powders that are reconstituted with water. They are licensed for chronic constipation and should therefore not be routinely recommended by pharmacists because treatment should be only instigated in those presenting with acute constipation. The BNF highlights doses for the respective products.

Magnesium salts

Magnesium, when used as a laxative, is usually given as magnesium hydroxide. The adult dose ranges between 20 and 50 mL when needed. It is generally not recommended for use in children but is commonly prescribed in the elderly.

Stool softeners (liquid paraffin and docusate sodium)

Liquid paraffin has been traditionally used to treat constipation. However, the adverse side effect profile of liquid paraffin now means it should never be recommended because other, safer and more effective medications are available.

Docusate sodium

Docusate sodium is a non-ionic surfactant that has stool-softening properties that allow penetration of intestinal fluids into the faecal mass. It also has weak stimulant properties. Docusate is available as either capsules (Dioctyl, DulcoEase) or solution (Docusal). It can be given

to children aged 6 months and over. Children between the age of 6 months and 2 years should take 12.5 mg (5 mL of Docusal paediatric solution) three times a day. For children aged between 2 and 12 the dose is 12.5 to 25 mg (5 to 10 mL) three times a day. Adults and children over 12 years old should take up to 500 mg daily in divided doses. In contrast to liquid paraffin, docusate sodium seems to be almost free of any side effects. Docusate sodium can be given to all patients.

Further reading

Borum ML. Constipation: evaluation and management. Primary Care 2001;28:577–90

Gattuso JM, Kamm MA. Adverse effects of drugs used in the management of constipation and diarrhoea. Drug Saf 1994;10:47–65.

Gerber PD, Barrett JE, Barrett JA, et al. The relationship of presenting physical complaints to depressive symptoms in primary care patients. J Gen Intern Med 1992;170–3.

Herz MJ, Kahan E, Zalevski S, et al. Constipation: a different entity for patients and doctors. Fam Pract 1996;13:156–9.

Higgins PDR, Johnson JF. Epidemiology of constipation in North America: a systemic review. Am J Gastroenterol 2004;99:750–9.

Jewell DJ, Young G. Interventions for treating constipation in pregnancy. Cochrane Database of Systematic Reviews 2001, issue 2.

Leng-Peschlow E. Senna and its rational use. Pharmacology 1992;44:S1–52.

Marshall JB. Chronic constipation in adults. How far should evaluation and treatment go? Postgrad Med 1990;88:49–51, 54, 57–9, 63.

Petticrew M, Watt I, Brand M. What's the 'best buy' for treatment of constipation? Results of a systematic review of the efficacy and comparative efficacy of laxatives in the elderly. Br J Gen Pract 1999;49:387–93.

Paraskevaides EC. Fatal lipid pneumonia and liquid paraffin. Br J Clin Pract 1990;44:509–10.

Talley NJ, Fleming KC, Evans JM, et al. Constipation in an elderly community: a study of prevalence and potential risk factors. Am J Gastroenterol 1996;9:19–25.

Tramonte SM, Brand MB, Mulrow CD, et al. The treatment of chronic constipation in adults. A systematic review. J Gen Intern Med 1997;12:15–24.

Web sites

Prodigy guidance: http://cks.library.nhs.uk/constipation

Irritable bowel syndrome

Background

Irritable bowel syndrome (IBS) is one of the commonest GI tract conditions seen in primary care. Approximately 25% of GP consultations for GI conditions are finally diagnosed as IBS. It can be defined as a functional bowel disorder (i.e. absence of abnormality) in which abdominal pain and bloating is associated with a change in bowel habit. The diagnosis is suggested by the presence of long-standing colonic symptoms without any deterioration in the patient's general condition. Diagnostic criteria (e.g. Rome II criteria) have been developed to define IBS but these are little used in a clinical setting and are more applicable for research purposes.

Prevalence and epidemiology

IBS is common. Adult prevalence rates in Western countries are reported to be between 10 and 15%, with approximately twice as many women than men affected. It most commonly affects people between 20 and 30 years old but recent trends indicate that there is a significant prevalence of IBS in older people.

Aetiology

No anatomic cause can be found to explain the aetiology of IBS but it is now clearly understood to be multifactorial. Many factors can contribute to disease expression and include motility dysfunction, diet and genetics. In a small proportion of cases symptoms appear after bacterial gastroenteritis. Psychological factors also influence symptom reporting and consultation and some studies have shown patients who suffer from higher levels of stress or depression experience worse symptoms when compared to other patients. Flare-up of symptoms has also been associated with periods of increased stress. Symptoms of diarrhoea and constipation appear to be linked with hyperactivity of the small intestine and colon in response to food ingestion and parasympathomimetic drugs. Excessive parasympathomimetic activity might account for mucus associated with the stool.

Arriving at a differential diagnosis

As only 20 to 30% of people with IBS symptoms consult their doctor the pharmacist has a pivotal role to play in establishing a diagnosis. A diagnosis of IBS relies almost exclusively on taking a thorough history as physical examination and diagnostic tests such as rectal examination and biopsy are of limited use. A number of IBS-specific questions should always be asked of the patient to aid in diagnosis (Table 6.16).

Clinical features of IBS

IBS is characterised by abdominal pain or discomfort, located especially in the left lower quadrant of the abdomen, which is sometimes relieved by defecation or the passage of wind. Altered defecation, either constipation or diarrhoea, with associated bloating is also normally present. People with IBS can present with 'diarrhoea-predominant', 'constipation-predominant' or alternating symptom profiles. During bouts of diarrhoea,

Table 6.16
Specific questions to ask the patient: IBS

Question	Relevance
Age	• IBS usually affects people under the age of 45 • Particular care is required in labelling middle-aged (over 45 to 50 years old) and elderly patients with IBS when presenting with bowel symptoms for the first time. Such patients are best referred for further evaluation to eliminate organic bowel disease
Periodicity	• IBS tends to be episodic. The patient might have a history of being well for a number of weeks or months in between bouts of symptoms. Often patients can trace their symptoms back many years, even to childhood
Presence of abdominal pain	• The nature of pain experienced by patients with IBS is very varied, ranging from localised and sharp to diffuse and aching. It is therefore not very discriminatory; however, the patient will probably have experienced similar abdominal pain in the past. Any change in the nature and severity of the pain is best referred for further evaluation
Location of pain	• Pain from IBS is normally located in the left lower quadrant. For further information on other conditions that cause pain in the lower abdomen see pages 171–172
Diarrhoea and constipation	• Patients with IBS experience altered defecation. They do not have textbook definitions of constipation or diarrhoea but bowel function will be different from normal • Constipation-predominant IBS is more common in women • The presence of blood in the stool is not usual in IBS and can suggest inflammatory bowel disease

mucus tends to be visible on the stools. Patients might also complain of increased stool frequency but pass normal or pellet-like stools. Diarrhoea on wakening and shortly after meals is also observed in many patients. Patients will normally have a long-standing history of symptoms (NICE Guidance, August 2007 states primary care clinicians should consider assessment for IBS if the patient reports having had change in bowel habit, abdominal pain/discomfort or bloating for at least 6 months).

Conditions to eliminate

Constipation and diarrhoea

As the major presenting symptom of IBS is an alteration in defecation, it is necessary to differentiate IBS from acute and chronic causes of constipation and diarrhoea. For further information on differentiating these conditions from IBS please refer to page 149 (for constipation) and page 143 (for diarrhoea).

Figure 6.13 will aid differentiation of IBS from other abdominal conditions.

> **TRIGGER POINTS** indicative of referral:
> Irritable bowel syndrome

- Blood in the stool
- Children under 16
- Fever
- Nausea and/or vomiting
- Patients over 45 with recent change to bowel habit
- Patients with no previous history of IBS and no precipitating factors
- Severe abdominal pain
- Steatorrhoea

Evidence base for over-the-counter medication

Before medicines are recommended it might be useful to discuss if stress is a factor and if this can be avoided. In addition, dietary modification has shown to be effective

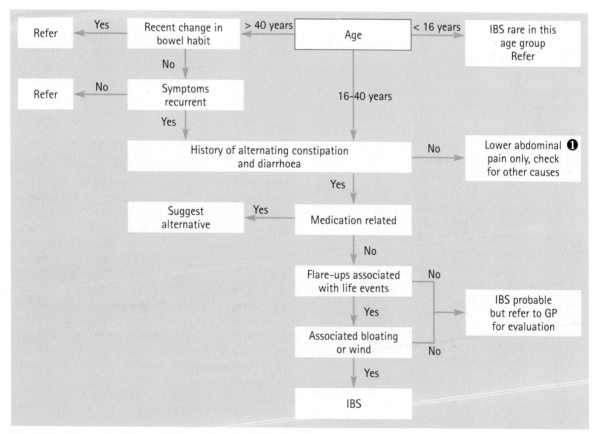

Fig. 6.13   Primer for differential diagnosis of irritable bowel syndrome

❶ **Lower abdominal pain**
See Fig. 6.29 for primer for differential diagnosis of abdominal pain.

for some patients. Suspected food products must be excluded from the diet for a minimum of 2 weeks and then gradually reintroduced to determine if the food item triggers symptoms.

Medicines are generally needed but those with a specific licence for IBS have a poor evidence base. These include mebeverine, alverine, hyoscine and peppermint oil and are generally used to treat abdominal pain and discomfort. In addition, bulk-forming and stimulant laxatives can be used to treat constipation-predominant IBS and loperamide for diarrhoea-predominant IBS. Both laxatives and diarrhoeals can be taken on a regular basis using the lowest effective dose. The following text only concentrates on the evidence for those products specifically marketed for the treatment of IBS.

Hyoscine

A number of trials have investigated the effectiveness of hyoscine in the treatment of IBS. However, only three trials of sufficient methodological quality allow conclusions to be drawn regarding its effectiveness. Each of the three trials demonstrated partial symptomatic improvement in some of the patients, although no trial proved hyoscine to be significantly better than placebo. A recent meta-analysis conducted by Poynard et al (2001) confirmed these findings and suggested that hyoscine was the least effective of the six smooth muscle relaxant medicines reviewed.

Antispasmodics (mebeverine, alverine and peppermint oil)

Mebeverine has been available as a POM for many years and as a pharmacy medicine since 1996, yet trial data to support its effectiveness are mixed. Conclusions drawn from five well-designed trials (two published in non-English) are conflicting. Of the three papers written in English, two studies appear to show a significant effect and one no effect. The meta-analysis by Poynard et al suggests a significant difference exists between mebeverine and placebo when data from all trials (including the two non-English trials) are combined.

Even fewer trials appear to have been conducted with alverine than mebeverine. One study by Tudor (1986) compared alverine to mebeverine in 45 patients; the authors concluded that alverine had similar efficacy to mebeverine. However, no placebo group was included in this study and it is therefore unclear to what extent alverine is effective.

Peppermint oil is the major constituent of several OTC remedies yet it has little evidence to support its effectiveness. Pittler & Ernst (1998) evaluated eight randomised controlled trials involving peppermint oil. Collectively, they indicate that peppermint oil could be efficacious for symptom relief in IBS but study design limitations meant that definitive judgement about efficacy was not possible.

Summary

A recent Cochrane review by Quartero et al (2005) concluded that antispasmodics were beneficial for abdominal pain and global assessment scores but it could not be shown whether antispasmodic subgroups were individually effective. It must also be noted that the majority of trials in this review were for products not available OTC. Based on the available evidence for OTC products, mebeverine should be first-line choice.

Alternative treatments

Herbal remedies for IBS have been subject to a Cochrane review (Liu et al 2006). Seventy-five trials were reviewed involving 71 different herbal medicines, although most trials were deemed to be of poor methodological quality. Nonetheless, the review concluded that certain remedies, in particular STW5, Padma Lax and Tongxie Yaofang, improved IBS symptoms.

Practical prescribing and product selection

Prescribing information relating to the medicines used for IBS reviewed in the section 'Evidence base for over-the-counter medication' is discussed and summarised in Table 6.17; useful tips relating to the treatment of patients with IBS are given in Hints and Tips Box 6.7.

All marketed products can be given to children (see individual entries) but anyone aged under 16 suspected of having IBS for the first time should be referred to a GP.

Hyoscine butylbromide (Buscopan IBS Relief)

The recommended starting dose for adults is one tablet three times a day, although this can be increased to two tablets four times a day if necessary. It is not recommended for children under the age of 12. It is a quaternary derivative of hyoscine so it does not readily cross the blood–brain barrier and therefore sedation is not normally encountered, although it might cause dry mouth and constipation. Because of its anticholinergic effects it is best avoided with other medicines that also have anticholinergic effects, for example, antihistamines, tricyclic antidepressants, neuroleptics and disopyramide. It can be given during pregnancy and breast-feeding but should be avoided if possible. It should also be avoided in patients with glaucoma, myasthenia gravis and prostate enlargement.

Mebeverine (Colofac IBS)

Adults and children 10 years and over should take one tablet three times a day, preferably 20 minutes before meals. Mebeverine is not known to interact with other medicines, has no cautions in its use and can be given in pregnancy and breast-feeding although there is a lack

Table 6.17
Practical prescribing: Summary of IBS medicines

Name of medicine	Use in children	Likely side effects	Drug interactions of note	Patients in whom care should be exercised	Pregnancy and breast-feeding
Hyoscine (Buscopan)	>12 years	Constipation and dry mouth	Tricyclic antidepressants, neuroleptics, antihistamines and disopyramide	Glaucoma, myasthenia gravis and prostate enlargement	Avoid if possible
Mebeverine Colofac IBS	>10 years	None	None	None	OK
Peppermint oil Colpermin	>15 years	Heartburn	None	None	OK in pregnancy; try to avoid in breast-feeding
Mintec	>18 years				
Equilon herbal	Not recommended				
Alverine	>12 years	Rash	None	None	OK

HINTS AND TIPS BOX 6.7:
IRRITABLE BOWEL SYNDROME

Non-drug treatment	Hypnotherapy has been reported as being effective for some patients. A register of IBS therapists specialising in hypnotherapy can be found at http://www.ibs-register.co.uk

of detailed studies. It is associated with very few side effects, although allergic reactions have been reported.

Alverine (Spasmonal)

Adults and children over 12 years should take one or two capsules three times a day before food. Like mebeverine, it is not known to interact with other medicines, has no cautions in its use and can be given in pregnancy and breast-feeding, although there is a lack of detailed studies. It has no interactions with other medicines and can be used by all patient groups. It can cause nausea, headache, dizziness, itching, rash and allergic reactions.

Peppermint oil (e.g. Mintec, Colpermin, Equilon herbal)

Adults and children aged over 15 years can take peppermint oil. The dose is one capsule three times a day before food, which can be increased to two capsules three

times a day in severe symptoms. It often causes heartburn and rarely allergic rashes have been reported. It is safe to use in pregnancy but can decrease breast milk production. It has no drug interactions and can be used by all patient groups.

Further reading

Agrawal A, Whorwell PJ. Irritable bowel syndrome: diagnosis and management. BMJ 2006;332:280–83.

Jamieson DJ, Steege JF. The prevalence of dysmenorrhea, dyspareunia, pelvic pain, and irritable bowel syndrome in primary care practices. Obstet Gynecol 1996;87:55–8.

Kruis W, Weinzierl M, Schussler P, Holl J. Comparison of the therapeutic effect of wheat bran, mebeverine and placebo in patients with the irritable bowel syndrome. Digestion 1986;34:196–201.

Liu JP, Yang M, Liu YX, et al. Herbal medicines for treatment of irritable bowel syndrome. Cochrane Database of Systematic Reviews 2006, issue 1.

Pittler MH, Ernst E. Peppermint oil for irritable bowel syndrome: a critical review and metaanalysis. Am J Gastroenterol 1998;93:1131–5.

Poynard T, Regimbeau C, Benhamou Y. Meta-analysis of smooth muscle relaxants in the treatment of irritable bowel syndrome. Aliment Pharmacol Ther 2001; 5:355–61.

Quartero AO, Meineche-Schmidt V, Muris J, et al. Bulking agents, antispasmodic and antidepressant medication for the treatment of irritable bowel syndrome. Cochrane Database of Systematic Reviews 2005, issue 2.

Ritchie JA, Truelove SC. Treatment of irritable bowel syndrome with lorazepam, hyoscine butylbromide, and ispaghula husk. Br Med J 1979;1(6160):376–8.

Saito YA, Schoenfeld P, Locke GR. The epidemiology of irritable bowel syndrome in North America: a systematic review. Am J Gastroenterol 2002;97:1910–5.

Tasmin-Jones C. Mebeverine in patients with the irritable colon syndrome: double blind study. N Z Med J 1973;77:232–5.

Tudor GJ. A general practice study to compare alverine citrate with mebeverine hydrochloride in the treatment of irritable bowel syndrome. Br J Clin Pract 1986;40:276–8.

Whitehead WE, Crowell MD, Robinson JC, et al. Effects of stressful life events on bowel symptoms: subjects with irritable bowel syndrome compared with subjects without bowel dysfunction. Gut 1992;33:825–30.

Web sites

IBS Self-help groups and associations: http://www.ibsgroup.org, http://www.ibsnetwork.org.uk and http://www.ibsassociation.org/

Articles: Thomas L. Current management options for irritable bowel syndrome. Available at http://www.escriber.com/Prescriber/Features.asp?ID=1042&GroupID=6&Action=View

Prodigy guidance: http://cks.library.nhs.uk/irritable_bowel_syndrome

NICE guidelines (draft): http://www.nice.org.uk/page.aspx?o=291060 (accessed 30 Nov 2007).

Haemorrhoids

Background

Haemorrhoids (piles) are the most common problem affecting the anorectal region. Patients might feel embarrassed talking about symptoms and it is therefore important that any requests for advice are treated sympathetically and away from others to avoid embarrassment.

Prevalence and epidemiology

The exact prevalence of haemorrhoids is unknown but it is estimated that one in two people will experience at least one episode at some point during their lives. Haemorrhoids can occur at any age but are rare in children and adults under the age of 20. It affects both sexes equally and is more common with increasing age, especially in people aged between 40 and 65 years of age. There is a high incidence of haemorrhoids in pregnant women.

Aetiology

The cause of haemorrhoids is probably multifactorial with anatomical (degeneration of elastic), physiological (increased anal canal pressure) and mechanical (straining at stool) processes implicated. Haemorrhoids have been traditionally described as engorged veins of the haemorrhoidal plexus. The analogy of varicose veins of the anal canal is often used but is misleading. Current thinking favours the theory of prolapsed anal cushions. Anal cushions maintain fine continence and are submucosal vascular structures suspended in the canal by a connective tissue framework derived from the internal anal sphincter and longitudinal muscle. Within each of the three cushions is a venous plexus that is fed by arteriovenous blood supply. Veins in these cushions fill with blood when sphincters inside them relax and empty when the sphincters contract. Fragmentation of the connective tissue supporting the cushions leads to their descent and is due to anatomical, physiological and mechanical processes. The prolapsed anal cushion has impaired venous return resulting in venous stasis and inflammation of the cushion's epithelium.

Haemorrhoids are classified as either internal or external. This distinction is an anatomical one. Superior to the anal sphincter there is an area known as the dentate line. At this junction epithelial cells change from squamous to columnar epithelial tissue. Above the dentate line haemorrhoids are classed as internal and below, external. Furthermore internal haemorrhoids are graded according to severity: grade I – do not prolapse out of the anal canal; grade II – prolapse on defecation but reduce spontaneously; grade III – require manual reduction; and grade IV – cannot be reduced.

Arriving at a differential diagnosis

In the first instance most patients with anorectal symptoms will self-diagnose haemorrhoids and often self-treat due to embarrassment about symptoms. Requests for advice need to be treated sympathetically, away from others, and importantly this gives the pharmacist the opportunity to confirm the patient's self diagnosis. Bleeding tends to cause the greatest concern and often instigates the patient to seek help. Invariably, rectal bleeding is of little consequence but should be thoroughly investigated to exclude sinister pathology. A number of haemorrhoid-specific questions should always be asked (Table 6.18).

Clinical features of haemorrhoids

Symptoms experienced by the patient are dependent upon the severity or type of haemorrhoid and can include bleeding, perianal itching, mucus discharge and pain. Often patients are asymptomatic until the haemorrhoid prolapses. Any blood associated is bright red and is most commonly seen as spotting around the toilet pan, streaking on toilet tissue or visible on the surface of the stool. Symptoms are often intermittent and each episode usually lasts from a few days to a few weeks

Internal haemorrhoids are rarely painful whereas external haemorrhoids often cause pain due to the

Table 6.18
Specific questions to ask the patient: Haemorrhoids

Question	Relevance
Duration	• Patients with haemorrhoids tend to have had symptoms for some time before requesting advice. However, patients with symptoms that have been present for more 3 weeks should be referred
Pain	• Pain associated with haemorrhoids tends to occur on defecation and at times other than defecation, for example, when sitting. It is usually described as a dull ache • Sharp or stabbing pain at the time of defecation can suggest an anal fissure or tear
Rectal bleeding	• Slight rectal bleeding is often associated with haemorrhoids. Blood appears bright red and might be visible in the toilet bowl or on the surface of the stool. The presence of blood is usually a direct referral sign but if the cause is haemorrhoids this could be treated unless the patient is unduly anxious in which case referral is appropriate • Blood mixed in the stool has to be referred to eliminate a GI bleed • Large volumes of blood or blood loss not associated with defecation must be referred to eliminate possible carcinoma
Associated symptoms	• Symptoms associated with haemorrhoids are usually localised, for example, anal itching. Other symptoms such as nausea, vomiting, loss of appetite and altered bowel habit should be viewed with caution and underlying pathology suspected. Referral would be needed
Diet	• A lack of dietary fibre that leads to constipation is a contributory factor to haemorrhoids. The passage of hard stools and straining during defecation can cause haemorrhoids. Find out about the patient's diet and current bowel habits

6

cushion becoming thrombosed. Pain is described as a dull ache that increases in severity when the patient defecates leading to patients ignoring the urge to defecate. This can then lead to constipation, which in turn will lead to more difficulty in passing stools and further increase the pain associated with defecation.

Conditions to eliminate

Dermatitis

Localised anal itching can result from dermatitis (or even threadworm infection). If pruritus is the only presenting symptom then the most likely cause is contact dermatitis caused by toiletries.

Medication

As constipation is a contributory factor in the manifestation of haemorrhoids, those medicines that are prone to causing constipation should, if possible, be avoided. Table 6.14 lists those medicines that are commonly known to cause constipation.

Conditions causing rectal bleeding

A number of conditions can present with varying degrees of rectal bleeding. However, other symptoms should be present that will allow them to be excluded.

Anal fissure

Anal fissures are common, with the 20- to 30-year-old age group most affected. Symptoms often follow a period of constipation and are normally caused by straining at stool. Pain can be intense on defecation and can last between a few minutes and a few hours after defecation. Bright red blood is commonly seen. Non-urgent referral is necessary for confirmation of the diagnosis. In the meantime the patient should be instructed to eat more fibre and increase their fluid intake.

Ulcerative colitis and Crohn's disease

Other symptoms besides blood in the stool are usually present with ulcerative colitis and Crohn's disease. These tend to be stools that are watery, abdominal pain in the lower left quadrant, weight loss and fever. Patients will appear unwell and also find that they have urgency, nocturnal diarrhoea and early morning rushes. In the acute phase patients will have malaise.

Upper GI bleeds

Erosion of the stomach wall or upper intestine is normally responsible for GI bleeds and is often associated with NSAID intake. The colour of the stool is related to the rate of bleeding. Stools from GI bleeds can be tarry (indicating a bleed of 100 to 200 mL of blood) or black (indicating a bleed of 400 to 500 mL of blood). Urgent referral is needed.

Colorectal cancer

Rectal carcinoma is most common in the 50- to 70-year-old age group and is characterised by rectal bleeding, a change in bowel habit and tenesmus. Rectal bleeding tends to be persistent and steady though slight for all tumours. Colorectal bleeds depend on the site of tumour, for example, sigmoid tumours lead to bright red blood in or around the stool. Any middle-aged patient presenting with rectal bleeding and a change of bowel habit must be referred. NICE have produced referral guidelines for doctors for suspected cases of colorectal cancer (http://www.nice.org.uk/guidance/CG27).

Figure 6.14 will aid the differentiation of haemorrhoids.

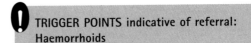

TRIGGER POINTS indicative of referral: Haemorrhoids

- Abdominal pain
- Blood mixed in the stool
- Fever
- Patients who have to reduce their haemorrhoids manually
- Persistent change in bowel habit in middle-aged patients
- Severe pain associated with defecation
- Unexplained rectal bleeding

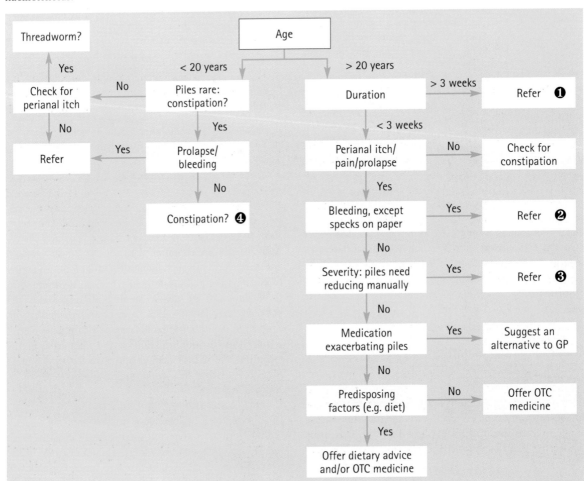

Fig. 6.14 Primer for differential diagnosis of haemorrhoids

❶ **Duration**
Patients with long-standing symptoms that have not been seen previously by the GP should be referred to eliminate any underlying pathology. In the vast majority of cases no sinister findings will result.

❷ **Rectal bleeding**
In the majority of cases rectal bleeding is a sign of referral. However, in cases where sinister pathology has been excluded and only mild local bleeding has occurred the pharmacist could instigate treatment.

❸ **Severity**
Medication is unlikely to help any patient who has to manually reduce haemorrhoids. Referral for other treatments is recommended.

❹ **Constipation**
See Fig. 6.12.

Evidence base for over-the-counter medication

Diet

Reviews by Alonso-Coelle et al (2005, 2006) have concluded that general measures to prevent constipation will help to decrease straining during defecation, ease the symptoms of haemorrhoids and reduce recurrence. Patients should therefore be asked about their normal diet to determine fibre intake. Those with diets low in fibre should be encouraged to increase their fibre and fluid intake; this will help produce softer stools and reduce constipation. Patients should try to eat more fruit, vegetables, bran and wholemeal bread. If this is not possible then fibre supplementation with a bulk-forming laxative could be recommended. Bulk-forming laxatives will take 2–3 days to relieve constipation and may take up to 6 weeks to improve symptoms of haemorrhoids.

Pharmacological intervention

Numerous products are marketed for the relief and treatment of haemorrhoids. These include a wide range of therapeutic agents and commonly include anaesthetics, astringents, anti-inflammatories and protectorants. Most products contain a combination of these agents with some having three or more different agents included.

The inclusion of such a diverse range of chemical entities appears to be based largely on theoretical grounds rather than any evidence base. Extensive literature searching found only one published trial regarding the efficacy of any marketed product (Ledward 1980); however, this trial suffered from serious methodological flaws.

Anaesthetics (lidocaine, benzocaine and cinchocaine)

No trials appear to have been conducted using local anaesthetics in the treatment and relief of symptoms for haemorrhoids. However, anaesthetics have proven efficacy when used on other mucosal surfaces; their use could therefore be justifiably recommended. Their action is short-lived and will produce temporary relief from perianal itching and pain. They require frequent application and might therefore cause skin sensitisation.

Astringents (allantoin, bismuth, zinc, Peru balsam)

Astringents are included in haemorrhoid preparations on the theoretical basis that they precipitate surface proteins thus producing a protective coat over the haemorrhoid. There appears to be no evidence to support this theory. Certain proprietary products only contain astringents and at best will provide a placebo effect.

Anti-inflammatories (hydrocortisone)

Steroids have proven effectiveness in reducing inflammation and would therefore be useful in reducing haemorrhoidal swelling. Trials with OTC products containing hydrocortisone appear not to have taken place. It must be assumed that manufacturers have incorporated hydrocortisone into haemorrhoid products on the assumption that they will have an effect. Recommendation of a steroid-containing product is probably justified.

Protectorants (e.g. shark liver oil)

Protectorants are claimed to provide a protective coating over the skin and thus produce temporary relief from pain and perianal itch. These claims cannot be substantiated and, as with astringents, any benefit conveyed by a protectorant is probably a placebo effect. In addition, there is also an ethical dimension to using a product with no efficacy sourced from sharks.

Other agents

Sclerosing agents (lauromacrogol) and wound-healing agents (yeast cell extract) can also be found in some products. There is no evidence supporting their effectiveness.

Flavanoids

Dietary supplementation with flavanoids is a common alternative treatment that is popular in continental Europe and the Far East. As an adjunct, their use has been shown to reduce acute symptoms and secondary haemorrhage after haemorrhoidectomy.

Summary

With so little data available on their effectiveness it is impossible to say whether any product is a credible treatment for haemorrhoids, and many medical authorities regard them as little more than placebos. However, products containing a local anaesthetic or hydrocortisone will probably confer some benefit, and they do have proven effectiveness in other similar conditions. It would therefore seem most prudent if recommending a product that it should contain one or both of these chemical entities.

Treatment should only be recommended to patients with mild haemorrhoids. Any person complaining of prolapsing haemorrhoids, which need reducing by the patient, should be referred because these patients require non-surgical intervention with sclerotherapy or rubber band ligation. If these fail to cure the problem then a haemorrhoidectomy might be performed.

Practical prescribing and product selection

Prescribing information relating to the medicines used for haemorrhoids reviewed in the section 'Evidence base for over-the-counter medication' is discussed and summarised in Table 6.19.

Table 6.19
Practical prescribing: Summary of haemorrhoid products

	Form	Anaesthetics	Astringents	Steroids	Protectorant
Anacal*	Cream or suppository	No	No	No	No
Anodesyn	Ointment or suppository	Yes	Yes	No	No
Anusol	Cream, ointment or suppository	No	Yes	No	No
Anusol Plus HC	Ointment or suppository	No	Yes	Yes	No
Germoloids	Cream, ointment or suppository	Yes	Yes	No	No
Germoloids HC	Spray	Yes	No	Yes	No
Hemocane	Cream	Yes	No	No	No
Nupercainal	Ointment	Yes	No	No	No
Perinal	Spray	Yes	No	Yes	No
Preparation H**	Ointment or suppository	No	No	No	Yes
Preparation H	Gel	No	Yes	No	No

*Contains a sclerosing agent
**Contains yeast cell extract

The product licences of products for haemorrhoids allow all patient groups, except children under 12 years, to use them. (Note – good practice dictates that people under 20 years old with suspected haemorrhoids should be referred.) They do not interact with any other medicines and can be used in pregnancy. The standard dose for any formulation is twice daily, plus application after each bowel movement. Minimal side effects have been reported and are usually limited to slight irritation. Products that contain hydrocortisone are subject to several licensing restrictions: they are restricted to use in patients over a certain age (Perinal spray 14 years, Germoloids spray 16 years and Anusol Plus products 18 years); they should be used for no longer than a week's duration; and they should not be used by pregnant or lactating women.

Further reading

Alonso-Coello P, Guyatt G, Heels-Ansdell D, et al. Laxatives for the treatment of hemorrhoids. The Cochrane Database of Systematic Reviews 2005, issue 4.

Alonso-Coello P, Mills E, Heels-Ansdell D, et al. Fiber for the treatment of hemorrhoids complications: a systematic review and meta-analysis. Am J Gastroenterol 2006;101:181–8.

Alonso-Coello P, Zhou Q, Martinez-Zapata MJ, et al. Meta-analysis of flavonoids for the treatment of haemorrhoids. Br J Surg 2006;93:909–20.

Nisar PJ, Scholefield JH. Managing haemorrhoids. Br Med J 2003:327;847–51.

Ledward RS. The management of puerperal haemorrhoids: A double blind clinical trial of Anacal rectal ointment. Practitioner 1980;224:660–1.

Web sites

Prodigy guidance: http://cks.library.nhs.uk/haemorrhoids
Chemist and Druggist: http://www.dotpharmacy.com/upmain.html (August 2006 update).

Abdominal pain

Background

Abdominal pain is a symptom of many different conditions, ranging from acute self-limiting problems to life-threatening conditions such as ruptured appendicitis and bowel obstruction. However, the overwhelming majority of cases will be of a non-serious nature, self-limiting and not require medical referral. The most common conditions that present to community pharmacies are dyspepsia affecting the upper abdomen and IBS affecting the lower abdomen. These are covered in more detail on pages 167 and 170. However, other conditions will present with abdominal pain (Fig. 6.15 and Table 6.20) and these are covered in this chapter.

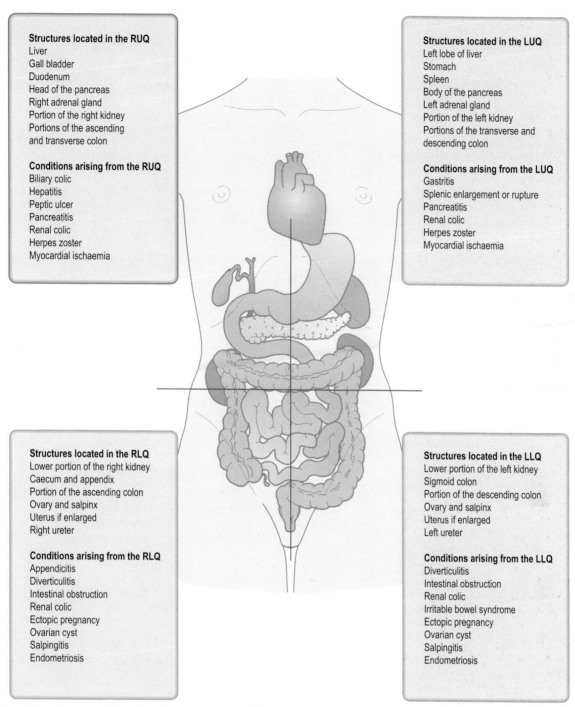

Structures located in the RUQ
Liver
Gall bladder
Duodenum
Head of the pancreas
Right adrenal gland
Portion of the right kidney
Portions of the ascending
and transverse colon

Conditions arising from the RUQ
Biliary colic
Hepatitis
Peptic ulcer
Pancreatitis
Renal colic
Herpes zoster
Myocardial ischaemia

Structures located in the LUQ
Left lobe of liver
Stomach
Spleen
Body of the pancreas
Left adrenal gland
Portion of the left kidney
Portions of the transverse and
descending colon

Conditions arising from the LUQ
Gastritis
Splenic enlargement or rupture
Pancreatitis
Renal colic
Herpes zoster
Myocardial ischaemia

Structures located in the RLQ
Lower portion of the right kidney
Caecum and appendix
Portion of the ascending colon
Ovary and salpinx
Uterus if enlarged
Right ureter

Conditions arising from the RLQ
Appendicitis
Diverticulitis
Intestinal obstruction
Renal colic
Ectopic pregnancy
Ovarian cyst
Salpingitis
Endometriosis

Structures located in the LLQ
Lower portion of the left kidney
Sigmoid colon
Portion of the descending colon
Ovary and salpinx
Uterus if enlarged
Left ureter

Conditions arising from the LLQ
Diverticulitis
Intestinal obstruction
Renal colic
Irritable bowel syndrome
Ectopic pregnancy
Ovarian cyst
Salpingitis
Endometriosis

Fig. 6.15 Anatomical location of organs and conditions that can cause abdominal pain

Prevalence and epidemiology

The prevalence and epidemiology of abdominal pain within the population is determined by those conditions that cause it. As so many conditions can give rise to abdominal pain it is likely that the majority of the population will, at some point, suffer from abdominal pain. For example, one study found that 40% of the UK population had suffered from dyspepsia during the previous 12 months and gastroenteritis, which is commonly associated with abdominal pain, is extremely common.

Aetiology

Abdominal pain does not only arise from the GI tract but also from the cardiovascular and musculoskeletal system. Therefore, the aetiology of abdominal pain is dependent on its cause. For example, GI tract causes include poor

Table 6.20
Causes of abdominal pain

Probability	Cause		
	Upper abdomen	Lower abdomen	Diffuse
Most likely	Dyspepsia	Irritable bowel syndrome	Gastroenteritis
Likely	Peptic ulcers	Diverticulitis (elderly)	Not applicable
Unlikely	Cholecystitis, cholelithiasis, renal colic	Appendicitis, endometriosis, renal colic	Not applicable
Very unlikely	Splenic enlargement, hepatitis, myocardial infarction	Ectopic pregnancy, salpingitis, intestinal obstruction	Pancreatitis, peritonitis

Table 6.21
Specific questions to ask the patient: Abdominal pain

Question	Relevance
Location of pain	• Knowing the anatomical location of abdominal structures is helpful in the differential diagnosis of abdominal pain (Fig. 6.15)
Presence only of abdominal pain/ discomfort	• In general, patients without other symptoms rarely have serious pathology. The symptoms are usually self-limiting and often no cause can be determined
Nature of the pain	• Heartburn is classically associated with a retrosternal burning sensation • Cramp-like pain is seen in diverticulitis, IBS, salpingitis and gastroenteritis • Colicky pain (pain that comes and goes) has been used to describe the pain of appendicitis, biliary and renal colic and intestinal obstruction • Gnawing pain is associated with pancreatitis and pancreatic cancer, and boring pain with ulceration
Radiating pain	• Abdominal pain that moves from its original site should be viewed with caution • Pain that radiates to the jaw, face and arm could be cardiovascular in origin • Pain that moves from a central location to the right lower quadrant could suggest appendicitis • Pain radiating to the back may suggest peptic ulcer or pancreatitis
Severity of pain	• Non-serious causes of abdominal pain generally do not give rise to severe pain. Pain associated with pancreatitis, biliary and renal colic and peritonitis tends to be severe (subjective scores higher than 6 out of 10)
Age of patient	• With increasing age, abdominal pain is more likely to have an identifiable and serious organic cause. Appendicitis is the only serious abdominal condition that is much more common in young patients
Onset & duration	• Onset can be gradual or sudden. In general, if no identifiable cause can be found, abdominal pain with sudden onset is generally a symptom of more serious conditions. For example, peritonitis, appendicitis, ectopic pregnancy, renal and biliary colic • Pain that lasts more than 6 hours is suggestive of underlying pathology
Aggravating or ameliorating factors	• The presence of food can aggravate gastric ulcers and antacids can relieve symptoms • Biliary colic can be aggravated by fatty foods • Vomiting tends to relieve pain in gastric ulcers • Pain in duodenal ulcer is relieved after ingestion of food • Pain in salpingitis, pancreatitis and appendicitis is often made worse by movement
Associated symptoms	• Vomiting, weight loss, melaena, altered bowel habit and haematemesis are all symptoms that suggest more serious pathology and require referral

muscle tone leading to reflux (e.g. lower oesophageal sphincter incompetence), infections that cause peptic ulcers (from *H. pylori*) and mechanical blockages causing renal and biliary colic. Cardiovascular causes include angina and myocardial infarction whereas musculoskeletal problems often involve tearing of abdominal muscles.

Arriving at a differential diagnosis

The main role of the community pharmacist is to identify patients in whom symptoms suggest more serious pathology, so that they can be further evaluated. This is not easy, as many abdominal conditions do not present with classical textbook symptoms in a primary care setting.

Patients tend to present to the pharmacist early in the course of the disease, often before the presenting symptoms have assumed the more usual description. The low prevalence of serious disease and overlapping symptoms with minor illness makes the task even more difficult. Single symptoms are poor predictors of final diagnosis (except for reflux oesophagitis, in which the presence of heartburn is highly suggestive). It is therefore important to look for 'symptom clusters' and to use knowledge of the incidence and prevalence of conditions to determine if referral is needed. This necessitates taking a very careful history and not relying on a single symptom to label a patient with a particular problem. Specific questions relating to abdominal pain should be asked (Table 6.21).

Conditions affecting the upper abdomen

Left upper quadrant pain

Dyspepsia/gastritis

Patients with dyspepsia present with a range of symptoms that commonly involve vague abdominal discomfort (aching) above the umbilicus (Fig. 6.16) associated with belching, bloating, flatulence, feeling of fullness and heartburn. It is normally relieved by antacids and aggravated by spicy foods or excessive caffeine. Vomiting is unusual. For further information on dyspepsia see page 135.

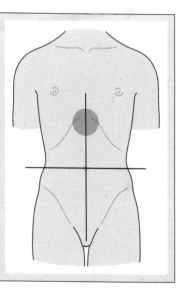

Fig. 6.16   The position of pain in gastritis and dyspepsia

Splenic enlargement or rupture

If the spleen is enlarged, generalised left upper quadrant pain associated with abdominal fullness and early feeding satiety is observed (Fig. 6.17). The condition is rare and is nearly always secondary to another primary cause, which might be an infection, a result of inflammation or haematological in origin.

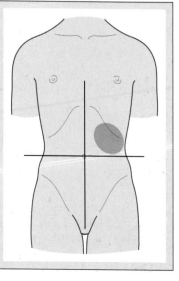

Fig. 6.17   The position of pain associated with splenic enlargement

Right upper quadrant pain

Acute cholecystitis and cholelithiasis

Acute cholecystitis (inflammation of the gall bladder) and cholelithiasis (presence of gall stones in the bile ducts, also called biliary colic) are characterised by persistent, steady severe pain (Fig. 6.18). Classically, the onset is sudden and starts a few hours after a meal, frequently waking the patient in the early hours of the morning. The pain can also be felt in the epigastric area and radiates to the tip of the right scapula in cholelithiasis. Fatty foods often aggravate the pain. The incidence increases with increasing age and is most common in people aged over 50. It is also more prevalent in women than men.

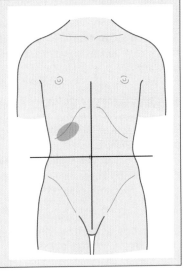

Fig. 6.18 The position of pain associated with acute cholecystitis and cholelithiasis

Hepatitis

Liver enlargement from any type of hepatitis will cause discomfort or dull pain (Fig. 6.19). Associated symptoms of general malaise, nausea, vomiting, jaundice and pruritus should be present. The most common causes of acute hepatitis are alcohol abuse and viral infection.

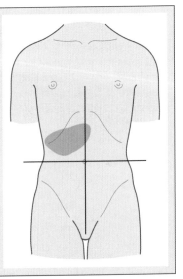

Fig. 6.19 The position of pain associated with hepatitis

Ulcers

Ulcers are classed as either gastric or duodenal. They occur most commonly in patients aged 30 to 50 years and are more common in men than women. Symptoms are variable but typically the patient will have localised mid-epigastric pain (Fig. 6.20) described as 'constant', 'annoying' or 'gnawing/ boring'.

With gastric ulcers, symptoms are inconsistent but the pain usually comes on whenever the stomach is empty – usually 15 to 30 minutes after eating – and is generally relieved by antacids or food and aggravated by alcohol and caffeine. NSAID use is associated with a three- to four-fold increase in gastric ulcers.

Duodenal ulcers tend to be more consistent in symptom presentation. Pain occurs 2 to 3 hours after eating and pain that wakes a person at night is highly suggestive of duodenal ulcer.

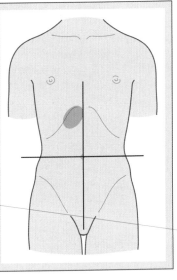

Fig. 6.20 The position of pain associated with ulcers

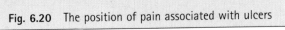

Pain affecting both right and left upper quadrants

Acute pancreatitis

Pain of pancreatitis develops suddenly and is described as agonising with the pain being centrally located that often radiates into the back (Fig. 6.21). Pain reaches its maximum intensity within minutes and can last hours or days. Vomiting is common but does not relieve the pain. Early in the attack patients might get relief from the pain by sitting forwards. It is commonly seen in alcoholics and it is likely that the patient will have a history of long-term heavy drinking. Patients are very unlikely to present in a community pharmacy due to the severity of the pain but a mild attack could present with steady epigastric pain sometimes centred close to the umbilicus and can be difficult to distinguish from other causes of upper quadrant pain.

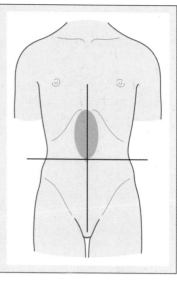

Fig. 6.21 The position of pain associated with pancreatitis

Renal colic

Urinary calculi (stones) can occur anywhere in the urinary tract, although most frequently stones get lodged in the ureter. Pain begins in the loin, radiating round the flank into the groin and sometimes down the inner side of the thigh (Fig. 6.22). Pain is severe and colicky in nature. Attacks tend to last minutes to hours and often leave the person prostrate with pain. Symptoms of nausea and vomiting might also be present. Men aged between 20 and 40 years are most likely to suffer from renal colic.

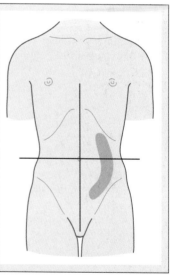

Fig. 6.22 The position of pain in renal colic

Myocardial ischaemia

Angina and myocardial infarction (MI) cause chest pain that can be difficult to distinguish initially from epigastric/retrosternal pain caused by dyspepsia (Fig. 6.23). However, pain of cardiovascular origin often radiates to the neck, jaw and inner aspect of the left arm. Typically, angina pain is precipitated by exertion and subsides after a few minutes once at rest. Pain associated with MI will present with characteristic deep crushing pain. The patient will appear pale, display weakness and be tachycardic. Cardiovascular pain should respond to sublingual glyceryl trinitrate therapy.

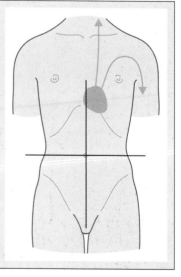

Fig. 6.23 The position of pain associated with myocardial ischaemia

Herpes zoster (shingles)

Pain associated with herpes zoster typically occurs once the rash has erupted, although it can precede the rash by several days. Pain that precedes the rash and is right-sided can be confused with appendicitis (Fig. 6.24).

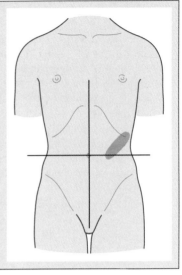

Fig. 6.24 The position of pain in herpes zoster

Conditions affecting the lower abdomen

The most common causes of lower abdominal pain are muscle strains, IBS, appendicitis and salpingitis in women. Apart from appendicitis, all these conditions can present in either quadrant.

Irritable bowel syndrome

Pain is most often observed in the left lower quadrant (Fig. 6.25); however, the discomfort can be vague and diffuse and about one-third of patients exhibit upper abdominal pain. The pain is described as 'cramp-like' and is recurrent. Alternating diarrhoea and constipation and mucus coating the stools is also often present. For further information on IBS see page 155.

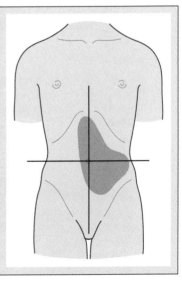

Fig. 6.25 The position of pain associated with irritable bowel syndrome

Diverticulitis

The incidence of diverticulitis increases with increasing age. It is most prevalent in the elderly and is characterised by constant pain and local tenderness. Pain is more commonly seen in the left lower quadrant (Fig. 6.26) but can be suprapubic and occasionally in the right lower quadrant. Pain tends to be cramp-like in nature. Fever is a prominent feature and altered bowel habit is usual with diarrhoea more common than constipation.

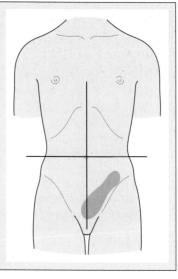

Fig. 6.26 The position of pain associated with diverticulitis

Intestinal obstruction

Intestinal obstruction is most prevalent in people over the age of 50. It has sudden and acute onset. The pain is described as colicky and can be experienced anywhere in the lower abdomen. Constipation and vomiting are prominent features. A patient with lower abdominal pain in the absence of constipation and vomiting is very unlikely to have an intestinal obstruction.

Appendicitis

Classically, the pain starts in the mid-abdomen region, around the umbilicus, before migrating to the right lower quadrant after a few hours (Fig. 6.27), although right-sided pain is experienced from the outset in about 50% of patients. The pain of appendicitis is described as colicky or cramp-like but after a few hours becomes constant. Movement tends to aggravate the pain and vomiting might also be present. Appendicitis is most common in young adults, especially young men. The absence of right lower quadrant pain and a history that the person has suffered similar pain previously should eliminate appendicitis from any differential diagnosis.

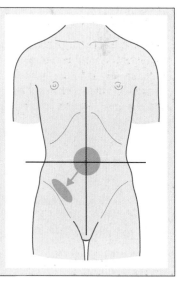

Fig. 6.27 The position of pain associated with appendicitis

Conditions affecting women

Generalised lower abdominal pain can be experienced in a number of gynaecological conditions (Fig. 6.28):

- Ectopic pregnancy: patients suffer from persistent moderate to severe pain that is sudden in onset. A menstrual history will reveal that the patient's last period is late. Additionally, 80% of patients will experience bleeding ranging from spotting to the equivalent of a menstrual period. Any patient who is sexually active, with abdominal pain whose period is late should be referred.
- Salpingitis (inflammation of the fallopian tubes): occurs predominantly in young, sexually active women, especially those fitted with an IUD. Pain is usually bilateral and cramping. Pain starts shortly after menstruation and can worsen with movement.
- Endometriosis: patients experience lower abdominal aching pain that usually starts 5 to 7 days before menstruation begins and can be constant and severe. The pain often worsens at the onset of menstruation. Referred pain into the back and down the thighs is also possible.

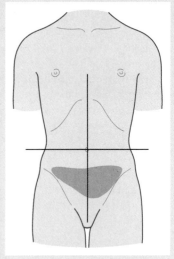

Fig. 6.28 The position of pain associated with women's conditions

Diffuse abdominal pain

A number of conditions will present with diffuse abdominal pain over the four quadrants. The most common cause of diffuse pain that will be seen by the pharmacist is gastroenteritis. Other causes include peritonitis and pancreatitis.

Gastroenteritis

Other symptoms of nausea, vomiting and diarrhoea will be more prominent in gastroenteritis than abdominal pain. The patient might also have a fever and suffer from general malaise.

Peritonitis

Although the pain of acute peritonitis can be diffuse, severe pain in the upper abdomen is often present. This is accompanied by intense rigidity of the abdominal wall producing a 'board-like' appearance; vomiting might also be present.

Figure 6.29 will aid in the differentiation of the different types of abdominal pain.

> **! TRIGGER POINTS indicative of referral: Abdominal pain**
>
> - Abdominal pain with fever
> - ALARM signs and symptoms:
>   - Anaemia
>   - Loss of weight
>   - Anorexia
>   - Recent onset of progressive symptoms
>   - Melaena, dysphagia and haematemesis
> - Elderly
> - Pregnancy or suspected pregnancy
> - Trauma
> - Severe pain or pain that radiates
> - Vomiting

Evidence base for over-the-counter medication and practical prescribing and product selection

The two conditions that have abdominal pain/discomfort as one of the major presenting symptoms and can be treated OTC are dyspepsia and IBS. For further information on products used to treat these conditions, please refer to pages 139–142 and 157–159.

6

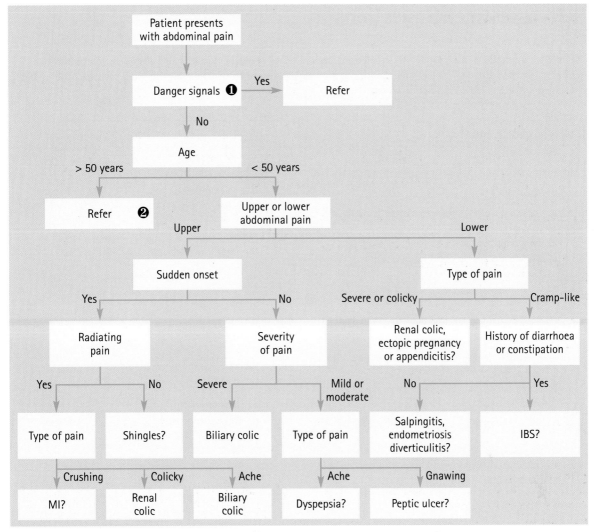

Fig. 6.29   Primer for differential diagnosis of abdominal pain

❶ Danger signals are significant bleeding, vomiting and fever.

❷ Organic disease is more likely to be the cause of abdominal pain in patients aged over 50, especially if symptoms are new or more severe than normal.

Further reading

Bagshaw EJ. Abdominal pain protocol: right upper quadrant pain. Lippincotts Prim Care Pract 1999;3:486–92.

Guthrie E, Thompson D. Abdominal pain and functional gastrointestinal disorders. BMJ 2002;325:701–3.

Kalloo AN, Kantsevoy SV. Gallstones and biliary disease. Prim Care 2001;28:591–606.

Lucenti MJ, Nadel ES, Brown DF. Right lower quadrant pain. J Emerg Med 2001;21:431–4.

Web sites

Prodigy guidance on renal colic: http://cks.library.nhs.uk/renal_colic_acute

The Pancreatitis Supporters' Network: http://www.pancreatitis.org.uk/

Self–assessment questions

The following questions are intended to supplement the text. Two levels of questions are provided: multiple choice questions and case studies. The multiple choice questions are designed to test factual recall and the case studies allow knowledge to be applied to a practice setting.

Multiple choice questions

6.1 Which one of the following statements about gastric ulcers is false?

 a. The pain is often aggravated by caffeine
 b. The pain is localised
 c. Symptoms tend to be episodic
 d. Endoscopical findings are usually positive for *H. pylori*
 e. Weight loss is common

6.2 In the treatment of constipation which one of the following statements is true?

 a. Bulk-forming laxatives usually act within 12 to 24 hours
 b. Senna tablets should be avoided in nursing mothers
 c. Fybogel is not suitable for a patient with coeliac disease
 d. Lactulose should not be taken by diabetic patients
 e. Liquid paraffin has been linked with causing lipid pneumonia

6.3 A man asks for the best thing to stop diarrhoea as he is going on holiday and he doesn't want to be caught short. Which of the following is the first-line treatment to be recommended?

 a. Kaolin and morphine
 b. Rehydration solution
 c. Antibiotics
 d. Antispasmodics
 e. Loperamide

6.4 Antacids that contain aluminium, calcium or magnesium salts inhibit the intestinal absorption of which of the following?

 a. Chloramphenicol
 b. Cephalexin
 c. Erythromycin
 d. Tetracycline
 e. Phenoxymethylpenicillin

6.5 What condition predisposes patients to oral thrush?

 a. Heart failure
 b. Asthma

 c. Diabetes mellitus
 d. Hyperlipidaemia
 e. Parkinson's disease

6.6 Abdominal pain that starts centrally then moves to the right lower quadrant is indicative of?

 a. Irritable bowel syndrome
 b. Pancreatitis
 c. Pyelonephritis
 d. Appendicitis
 e. Renal colic

6.7 Which condition is least likely to cause rectal bleeding?

 a. Haemorrhoids
 b. Crohn's disease
 c. Colorectal cancer
 d. IBS
 e. Anal fissure

6.8 Which one of the following preparations would not be used for the treatment of pain-free gingivitis?

 a. Corsodyl mouthwash
 b. Eludril mouthwash
 c. Corsodyl gel
 d. Bocasan
 e. Difflam mouthwash

Questions 6.9 to 6.11 concern the following conditions:

A. Irritable bowel syndrome
B. Constipation
C. Diarrhoea
D. Haemorrhoids
E. Dyspepsia

Select, from A to E, which statement best relates to the conditions above

6.9 Is characterised with epigastric pain

6.10 Can be treated with antispasmodics

6.11 Is associated with left lower quadrant pain

Questions 6.12 to 6.14 concern the following OTC medications:

A. Gaviscon liquid
B. Asilone suspension
C. Milk of magnesia
D. Sodium bicarbonate powder
E. Aludrox liquid

6.12 Is most suitable for treating heartburn, which tends to get worse when lying down A

6.13 Is most suitable to treat abdominal discomfort caused by trapped gas B

6.14 Could be used to relieve constipation, as well as indigestion C

Questions 6.15 to 6.17: for each of these questions *one or more* of the responses is (are) correct. Decide which of the responses is (are) correct. Then choose:

A. If a, b and c are correct
B. If a and b only are correct
C. If b and c only are correct
D. If a only is correct
E. If c only is correct

Directions summarised

A	B	C	D	E
a, b and c	a and b only	b and c only	a only	c only

6.15 When questioning a patient seeking advice for nausea and gastrointestinal upset, which of the following symptoms would indicate the need for direct referral to the general practitioner?

E. a. Feeling of impending vomiting
 b. Loss of appetite over the last 24 hours
 c. Dark coloured vomit

6.16 A common presentation of minor aphthous ulcers is

A. a. Pain
 b. Ulcers on the buccal mucosa and tongue
 c. Occur in crops of between one and five

6.17 Which symptoms in a patient presenting with constipation should be referred?

D a. Melaena
 b. Greater than 7 days duration
 c. Abdominal pain

Questions 6.18 to 6.20: these questions consist of a statement in the left-hand column followed by a statement in the right-hand column. You need to:

● decide whether the first statement is true or false
● decide whether the second statement is true or false

Then choose:

A. If both statements are true and the second statement is a correct explanation of the first statement
B. If both statements are true but the second statement is NOT a correct explanation of the first statement
C. If the first statement is true but the second statement is false
D. If the first statement is false but the second statement is true
E. If both statements are false

Directions summarised

	1st statement	2nd statement	
A	True	True	2nd statement is a correct explanation of the first
B	True	True	2nd statement is not a correct explanation of the first
C	True	False	
D	False	True	
E	False	False	

	First statement	*Second statement*
6.18	IBS is common in people under the age of 40	It is caused by stress C
6.19	Gingivitis is caused by plaque build-up	It is characterised by swollen and red gums B
6.20	Heartburn causes retrosternal pain	Sphincter incompetence is responsible for symptoms A

Case study

Mrs SJ, a 28-year-old women, asks to speak to the pharmacist because she wants something for stomach ache. You find out that the pain is located in the lower and upper left quadrant, but mainly the upper quadrant.

a. From which conditions might she be suffering?

Reflux, non-ulcer dyspepsia, gastritis, primary dysmenorrhoea, endometriosis, irritable bowel syndrome, pancreatitis, renal colic, MI and herpes zoster.

Further questioning reveals Mrs SJ to be suffering with pain she describes as 'an ache'.

b. Name the likely conditions that she could be suffering from?

The use of the word 'ache' means you can rule out those conditions that present with severe, stabbing, burning or gnawing pain:

- *pancreatitis, renal colic: severe*
- *reflux: burning*
- *herpes zoster: severe, lancing*

But it could still be any of: non-ulcer dyspepsia, gastritis, primary dysmenorrhoea, irritable bowel syndrome, endometriosis and MI. However, as the pain is primarily upper quadrant this makes primary dysmenorrhoea, endometriosis and irritable bowel syndrome less likely. This leaves non-ulcer dyspepsia, gastritis and MI as possibilities

c. Which questions would now allow you to differentiate between these conditions?

MI is the most unlikely of the three conditions and one would expect the patient to have more severe symptoms. Questions asking about radiation of pain, previous history of similar symptoms and precipitating/relieving factors should be asked.

You reach the differential diagnosis of non-ulcer dyspepsia but before you make any recommendations, you ask if she takes any medication from the GP, her response is as follows:

- Paracetamol prn: She has taken this for 6 months for knee pain
- Atorvastatin 40 mg od: She has taken this for the last 3 years for familial hyperlipidaemia
- Naproxen 500 mg bd prn: She has taken this for 6 months for knee pain.

d. Which of these medications, if any, do you consider are contributing to Mrs SJ's pain? Explain your rationale.

Of the three medicines that Mrs SJ is taking, the one most likely to cause GI irritation is Naproxen. However, she has been taking this for the last 6 months and you would expect that dyspepsia symptoms would have been experienced already if she was going to have a reaction to Naproxen. It is therefore unlikely that Naproxen has caused the problem, unless the dose has recently been changed. Atorvastatin can also cause GI side effects but has been taken for the last 3 years and is therefore almost certainly not the cause of the symptoms. Paracetamol is not known to cause GI irritation so can also be ruled out. In conclusion it is likely that none of the medicines have caused Mrs SJ's symptoms.

6

CASE STUDY 6.2

Mr LR, a male patient (approximately 50 to 60 years old), presents to the pharmacy at lunch time asking for something for diarrhoea. The following questions are asked, and responses received.

Information gathering	Data generated
Presenting complaint (possible questions)	
Describe symptoms	Going to the toilet three or four times a day. Normal habit is once or twice
Nature of movements	Very watery
Duration	4 or 5 days
Other symptoms/ provokes	Generally feels a bit rough. Headache and has a temperature. Been getting some cramping pains
Blood noticed	No
Eaten anything different in day or so before diarrhoea appeared	No
Additional questions	No foreign travel Doesn't seem to be worse at any time of day
Previous history of presenting complaint	Has had the odd bout of diarrhoea before but usually clears up after a couple of days
Past medical history	None
Drugs (OTC, Rx and compliance)	Ibuprofen 600 mg tds; aspirin 75 mg od; atenolol 25 mg od No change to medicines for last 6–9 months
Allergies	None known

Information gathering	Data generated
Social history	
Smoking	Alcohol mostly at weekends.
Alcohol	Does not smoke. Tries to
Drugs	exercise twice a week.
Employment	Married
Relationships	
Family history	No-one in family with similar symptoms
On examination	General appearance is of a healthy person. No obvious signs of dehydration. Pinch test normal

Epidemiology dictates that the most likely cause of diarrhoea seen in primary care is bacterial or viral infection. However, other conditions are possible and are noted below:

Probability	Cause
Most likely	Viral and bacterial infection
Likely	Medicine induced
Unlikely	Irritable bowel syndrome, giardiasis, faecal impaction
Very unlikely	Ulcerative colitis and Crohn's disease, colorectal cancer, malabsorption syndromes

Diagnostic pointers with regard to symptom presentation

The expected findings for questions when related to the different conditions that can be seen by community pharmacists are summarised on the following page.

Continued

CASE STUDY 6.2

	Age	Acute or chronic	Timing	Periodicity	Weight loss	Blood in stools
Infection	Any	Acute	Any	Acute	No	Unusual
Medicines	Any	Acute or chronic	Any	No	No	No
IBS	<45 years	Acute	Mornings?	Recurs	No	No
Giardiasis	Any	Acute	Any	Acute	No	No
Faecal impaction	Elderly	Chronic	Any	No	No	No
Ulcerative colitis	Young adults	Acute	AM and PM	Recurs	No	Yes
Crohn's disease	Young adults	Acute	AM and PM	Recurs	No	Yes
Coeliac disease	Infants or middle-aged	Chronic	Any	No	Yes	No
Carcinoma	>50 years	Chronic	Any	No	Yes	Unusual

When this information is applied to that gained from our patient (below) we see that from the questions asked the most likely cause of his symptoms is infection.

	Age	Acute or chronic	Timing	Periodicity	Weight loss (not asked)	Blood in stools
Infection	✓	✓	✓	✓	?	✓?
Medicines	✓	✓	✓	✗	?	✓
IBS	✗	✓	✗?	✓	?	✓
Giardiasis	✓	✓	✓	✓	?	✓
Faecal impaction	✗	✗	✓	✗	?	✓
Ulcerative colitis	✗	✓	✗	✓	?	✗
Crohn's disease	✗	✓	✗	✓	?	✗
Coeliac disease	✓	✗	✓	✗	?	✓
Carcinoma	✓	✗	✓	✗	?	✓?

CASE STUDY 6.2

Danger symptoms/signs (trigger points for referral)

As a final double check it might be worth making sure the person has none of the 'referral signs or symptoms'; this is the case with this patient.

Change in bowel (long term) habit in patients over 50	✗
Diarrhoea following recent travel to tropical or subtropical climate	✗
Duration longer than 2 to 3 days in children and elderly	N/A
Patients unable to drink fluids	?
Presence of blood or mucus in the stool	✗
Signs of dehydration	✗
Severe abdominal pain	✗
Steatorrhoea	✗
Suspected faecal impaction in the elderly	N/A

The question mark against 'unable to drink fluids' should be determined during advice and product selection, and so in this context is not applicable.

6

CASE STUDY 6.3

Mrs RH, an elderly patient (about 75 years old), picks her prescription up and at the same time says she wants something to help get rid of a funny patch on the inside of her cheek. The following questions are asked, and responses received.

Information gathering	Data generated
Presenting complaint (possible questions)	
Describe symptoms	White patch about the size of a 10 pence piece
How long have you had the symptoms	Had for a couple of weeks
Type/severity of pain	Not really painful
Other symptoms/ provokes	No other obvious symptoms
Additional questions	No systemic symptoms (e.g. fever, chills)
Previous history of presenting complaint	Had something similar a couple of years ago and the other chemist gave me some cream
Past medical history	RA, HT, stroke 2 years ago
Drugs (OTC, Rx and compliance)	Ibuprofen 600 mg tds; aspirin 75 mg od; dipyridamole 200 mg bd; atenolol 25 mg od
Allergies	None known

Information gathering	Data generated
Social history	
Smoking	Lives on her own and
Alcohol	watches TV most of the
Drugs	time. Loves quiz shows
Employment	
Relationships	
Family history	
On examination	Discrete white patch. No underlying redness

Epidemiology dictates that the most likely cause of white patches in the oral cavity seen in primary care is thrush. However, other conditions are possible and are noted below:

Probability	Cause
Most likely	Thrush
Likely	Minor aphthous ulcers, medicine induced, ill-fitting dentures
Unlikely	Underlying medical disorders, e.g. diabetes, xerostomia (dry mouth) and immunosuppression, major & herpetiform ulcers, herpes simplex
Very unlikely	Leukoplakia, squamous cell carcinoma

Diagnostic pointers with regard to symptom presentation

The expected findings for questions when related to the different conditions that can be seen by community pharmacists are summarised on the following page.

CASE STUDY 6.3

	Number	Location	Size and shape	Age	Pain
Thrush	'Single patch'	Anywhere	Irregular and variable size	Young and elderly	No
Minor ulcers	Up to five or so ulcers	Lips and inside cheeks	Less than 1 cm and round	10–40 years most common	Yes
Major ulcers	Numerous	Anywhere	Large (and variable shape)	All ages	Yes
Herpetiform	Very numerous	Back of the mouth	Pinpoint & round	All ages	Yes
Herpes simplex	Numerous	Anywhere	Small	Children	Yes
Lichen planus	Diffuse	Tongue, cheek, gums	'Spider's web'	Adults	No
Leukoplakia	Singular patch	Tongue or cheek	Irregular and variable size	Elderly	No
Carcinoma	Singular lesion	Tongue, mouth, lower lip	Irregular and variable size	Elderly	No, but latter stages yes

When this information is applied to that gained from our patient (below) we see that from the questions asked the diagnosis is either thrush, lichen planus or leukoplakia. Lichen planus can be ruled out because of the appearance of the white patch (plus lichen planus also commonly has a rash, but not always). This leaves a diagnosis between thrush and leukoplakia. Although the lady is not really complaining of pain, there is a possibility that this 'white patch' could be deemed potentially sinister, especially as she is of an age where leukoplakia is more likely. A positive smoking history would make leukoplakia even more of a possibility. This person must be referred.

	Number	Location	Size and shape	Age	Pain
Thrush	✓	✓	✓	✓	✗
Minor ulcers	✗	✓	✗	✗	✗
Major ulcers	✗	✓	✗	✗?	✗
Herpetiform	✗	✗	✗	✓	✗
Herpes simplex	✗	✓	✗	✗	✗
Lichen planus	✓?	✓	✓	✓	✓?
Leukoplakia	✓	✓	✓	✓	✓
Carcinoma	✗?	✓	✓	✓	✓?

Answers to multiple choice questions									
1 = c	2 = e	3 = b	4 = d	5 = c	6 = d	7 = d	8 = e	9 = e	10 = a
11 = a	12 = a	13 = b	14 = c	15 = e	16 = a	17 = d	18 = c	19 = b	20 = a.

Dermatology

Background

The skin is the largest organ of the body. It has a complex structure and performs many important functions. These include protecting underlying tissues from external injury and overexposure to ultraviolet light, barring entry to microorganisms and harmful chemicals, acting as a sensory organ for pressure, touch, temperature, pain and vibration and maintaining the homeostatic balance of body temperature.

It has been reported that dermatological disorders account for up to 15% of the workload of UK GPs, with similar findings reported from community pharmacies. It is therefore important that community pharmacists are able to differentiate between common dermatological conditions that can be managed appropriately without referral to the GP and those that require further investigation or treatment with a prescription-only medicine.

General overview of skin anatomy

Principally the skin consists of two parts, the outer and thinner layer called the epidermis and an inner, thicker layer named the dermis. Beneath the dermis lies a subcutaneous layer, known as the hypodermis (Fig. 7.1).

The epidermis

The epidermis is the major protective layer of the skin and has four distinct layers when viewed under the microscope. The basal layer actively undergoes cell division, forcing new cells to move up through the epidermis and form the outer keratinised horny layer. This process is continual and takes approximately 35 days. Pathological changes in the epidermis produces a rash or a lesion with abnormal scale, loss of surface integrity or changes to pigmentation.

The dermis

The dermis is the layer below the epidermis. The majority of the dermis is made of connective tissue; collagen for strength and elastic fibres to allow stretch. It provides support to the epidermis as well as its blood and nerve supply. Also located in the dermis are the hair follicle, sebaceous and sweat glands and arrector pili muscle. Under cold conditions the arrector pili muscle contracts, pulling the hair into a vertical position and causing 'goosebumps'. Conditions of the dermis usually result in changes in the elevation of the skin, e.g. papules and nodules.

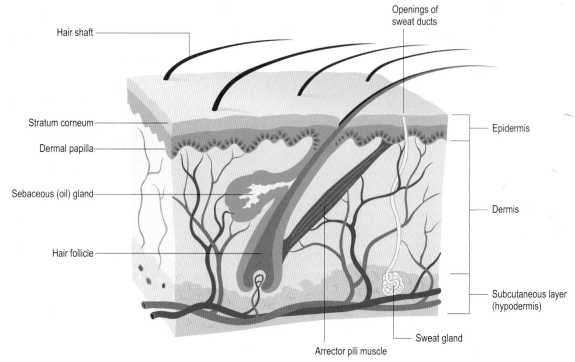

Fig. 7.1   The epidermis, dermis and associated structures

The hair

The primary function of hair is one of protection. Each hair consists of a shaft, the visible part of the hair, and a root. Surrounding the root is the hair follicle, the base of which is enlarged into a bulb structure. A sebaceous gland secretes sebum into each hair follicle that lubricates the hair and protects it from damage.

Sebaceous glands

Sebaceous glands are found in large numbers on the face, chest and upper back. During puberty these glands become large and active due to hormonal changes.

Sweat glands

These are the most numerous of the skin glands and are classed as apocrine or eccrine. Eccrine glands are located all over the body and play a role in elimination of waste products and maintaining a constant core temperature. Apocrine sweat glands are mainly located in the axilla and begin to function at puberty.

History taking

Unlike internal medicine, the majority of dermatological complaints presenting in community pharmacy can be seen. This affords the community pharmacist an excellent

opportunity to base his or her differential diagnosis not only on questioning but also on physical examination. General questions that should be considered when dealing with dermatological conditions are listed in Table 7.1. Terminology describing skin lesions can be confusing and the more common terms used are shown in Table 7.2.

Physical examination

A more accurate differential diagnosis will be made if the pharmacist actually sees the person's athlete's foot or 'rash' on the back. Providing adequate privacy can be obtained there is no reason why the majority of skin complaints cannot be seen. Pharmacies with specific private areas or consultation rooms should be able to perform such exams relatively easy. It is worth remembering that many patients will be embarrassed by skin conditions and might be ashamed of their appearance. When performing an examination of the skin, a number of things should be looked for (Table 7.3).

Hyperproliferative disorders

Background

Hyperproliferative disorders are characterised by a combination of increased cell turnover rate and a shortening

Table 7.1
Questions to consider when taking a dermatological history

Question	Relevance
Where did the problem first appear?	• Certain skin problems start in one particular location before spreading to other parts of the body, e.g. impetigo* usually starts on the face before spreading to the limbs • Patients might need prompting to tell you where the problem started as they are likely to want help for the most obvious or large skin lesion but neglect to tell you about smaller lesions that appeared first
Are there any other symptoms?	• These are generally itch and/or pain • Mild itch is associated with many skin conditions including psoriasis and medicine eruptions • Severe itch is associated with conditions such as scabies, atopic and contact dermatitis
Occupational history (relevant to adults only)	• This is particularly pertinent for contact dermatitis, e.g. do symptoms improve when away from work?
General medical history	• Many skin signs can be the first marker of internal disease, e.g. diabetes can manifest with pruritus; fungal or bacterial infection and thyroid disease can present with hair loss and pruritus — ITCHING
Travel	• More people are taking long-haul holidays and therefore expose themselves to tropical diseases that can manifest as skin lesions
Family and household contact history	• Infections such as scabies can infect relatives and others with whom the patient is in close contact
The patient's thoughts on the cause of the problem	• Ask for the patient's opinion. This might help with the diagnosis or alternatively shed light on anxieties and theories as to the cause of the condition

*impetigo — a contagious skin disease especially of children, usually caused by streptococcal bacteria, marked by a superficial pustular eruption, particularly on the face.

[handwritten margin note: atopy: an allergy, involving an inherited immunoglobulin of the IgE type, that predisposes a person to certain allergic responses, as atopic dermatitis]

of the time it takes for cells to migrate from the basal layer to the outer horny layer. Typically, cell turnover rate is ten times faster than normal and cell migration takes 3 or 4 days rather than 35 days.

Psoriasis

Background

Psoriasis is a chronic relapsing inflammatory disorder characterised by a variety of morphological lesions that present in a number of forms. The commonest form of psoriasis is plaque psoriasis and will be the form most familiar to pharmacists. Depending on the extent and severity of lesions, psoriasis can have a profound effect on the person's work and social life.

Prevalence and epidemiology

Psoriasis is a common skin disorder with an estimated worldwide prevalence between 1 and 3%. In the UK it has been reported to affect 1 to 2% of the population. However, this is probably an underestimate, as many patients with mild psoriasis do not present to their GP.

Psoriasis can present at any time in life, although it appears to be more prevalent in the second and fifth decade. It is rare in infants and uncommon in children. The sexes are equally affected but it is more common in Caucasians.

Aetiology — the study of the causes of disease.

The exact aetiology of psoriasis still remains unclear but it is known that inherited factors are important. For example, if the patient has one parent with psoriasis then they have a 25 to 30% chance of developing psoriasis and if both parents suffer from psoriasis then the figure rises to 50 to 60%. However, studies in twins also suggest that environmental factors might be needed for clinical expression of the disease because only 70% of genetically identical twins both develop the condition. Psoriasis lesions often develop at sites of skin trauma, such as sunburn and cuts (known as the Koebner phenomenon), following streptococcal throat infection and during periods of stress. *[handwritten: → type of bacteria (pathogenic to humans)]*

Arriving at a differential diagnosis

Psoriasis can be located on various parts of the body (Fig. 7.2) and presents in a variety of different forms.

—itis → inflammation.

Table 7.2
Common terms used to describe skin lesions

Term	Description
Macule	A flat lesion that is less than 1 cm in diameter
Patch	A flat lesion that is greater than 1 cm in diameter
Papule	A raised solid lesion less than 1 cm in diameter
Nodule	A raised solid lesion greater than 1 cm in diameter
Vesicle	A clear fluid-filled lesion lasting a few days that is less than 1 cm in diameter
Bulla	A clear fluid-filled lesion lasting a few days that is greater than 1 cm in diameter
Pustule	A pus-filled lesion lasting a few days that is less than 1 cm in diameter
Comedone	A papule that is 'plugged' with keratin and sebum
Erythema	Redness due to dilated blood vessels that blanche when pressed
Excoriation	Localised damage to the skin due to scratching
Lichenification	Thickening of the epidermis with increased skin markings due to scratching

acne – inflammatory disease of the sebaceous glands, characterized by comedones and pimples, especially on the face, back and chest, and in sever cases, by cysts and nodules resulting in scarring. Acne – Vulgaris.

Table 7.3
Things to consider when performing a dermatological examination

Lesions	Relevance
Temperature	Use the backs of your fingers to make the assessment. This should enable you to identify generalised warmth or coolness of the skin and note the temperature of any red areas, e.g. generalised warmth can indicate fever whereas local warmth might indicate inflammation or cellulitis *inflammation of cellular tissue.*
Lesions	Distribution Many skin diseases have a 'typical' or 'classic' distribution: • Symmetrical. e.g. acne and psoriasis • Asymmetrical, e.g. contact dermatitis • Unilateral, e.g. shingles *inflammation of the skin* • Localised, e.g. nappy rash Arrangement • Discrete (with healthy skin in between), e.g. psoriasis *common chronic inflammat—scaly patches* • Coalescing (merging together), e.g. eczema • Grouped, e.g. insect bites Feel of lesions Remember that very few skin conditions are infectious, so do not be afraid to touch the patient's skin: • Smooth, e.g. urticaria • Rough, e.g. solar keratosis
Recent trauma	Is there any sign that individual lesions have developed on a site of trauma or injury such as a scratch? This is seen in a number of conditions such as psoriasis and viral warts

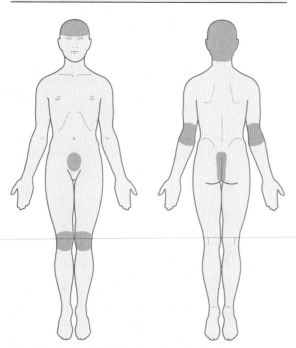

Fig. 7.2 Typical distribution of psoriatic plaques

As plaque and scalp psoriasis are the only forms of the condition that can be managed by the community pharmacist, it is necessary that other forms of psoriasis, and conditions that look like psoriasis, can be distinguished. Asking symptom-specific questions will help the pharmacist to determine if referral is needed (Table 7.4).

Clinical features of plaque psoriasis

Plaque psoriasis classically presents with characteristic salmon-pink lesions with slivery-white scales and

Table 7.4
Specific questions to ask the patient: Psoriasis

Question	Relevance
Onset	• Psoriasis can develop in patients of any age, although it first occurs most commonly in early adult life. However, in young and elderly patients the lesions tend to be atypical, which can complicate the diagnosis
Distribution of rash	• Psoriasis often presents in a symmetrical distribution and most commonly involves the scalp, extensor aspects of the elbows and knees. However, the gluteal cleft and umbilicus can also be affected (see Fig. 7.2) • Conditions such as lichen planus (often inside of the wrists) and pityriasis rosea (thighs and trunk) have a different distribution to psoriasis
Other symptoms	• Itch is not normally the predominant feature of psoriasis, unlike other conditions such as dermatitis and fungal infections *ONYCHOLYSIS.* • Nail involvement in the form of pitting and <u>onycholysis</u> (separation of the nail plate from the nail bed) is often seen and can involve one or more of the nails. However, this is normally observed in patients with long-standing psoriasis and is therefore of little value in patients presenting with rash of recent onset
Look of rash	• Scalp and plaque psoriasis usually show scaling as a predominant feature. This is not seen with other common skin conditions (e.g. dermatitis) or other forms of psoriasis • When scalp involvement is mild, psoriasis can be impossible to distinguish from seborrhoeic dermatitis
Previous history of lesions	• Psoriasis is a chronic relapsing and remitting disease and it is likely that the patient will have had lesions in the past. Other skin diseases, such as fungal infections, are acute and patients do not normally have a history of the problem

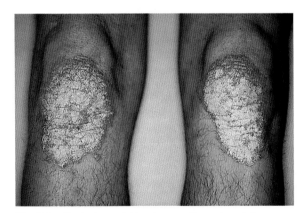

Fig. 7.3 Typical psoriatic plaques. Reproduced from *Dermatology: An Illustrated Colour Text* by D J Gawkrodger, 2008, Churchill Livingstone, with permission

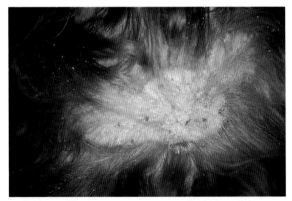

Fig. 7.4 Scaly plaques of psoriasis in the scalp, with localised hair loss. Reproduced from *Dermatology: An Illustrated Colour Text* by D J Gawkrodger, 2008, Churchill Livingstone, with permission

well-defined boundaries (Fig. 7.3). Lesions can be single or multiple and vary in size from pinpoint to covering extensive areas. If the scales on the surface of the plaque are gently removed and the lesion is then rubbed, it reveals pinpoint bleeding from the superficial dilated capillaries. This is known as the <u>Auspitz</u> sign and is diagnostic.

Clinical features of scalp psoriasis

Scalp psoriasis can be mild, exhibiting slight redness of the scalp through to severe cases with marked inflammation and thick scaling (Fig. 7.4). The redness often extends beyond the hair margin and is commonly seen behind the ears.

Conditions to eliminate for plaque psoriasis

Pustular psoriasis

In this rare form of psoriasis sterile pustules are an obvious clinical feature. The pustules tend to be located on the advancing edge of the lesions and typically occur on the palms of the hands and soles of the feet (Fig. 7.5).

Seborrhoeic psoriasis (also known as flexural psoriasis)

Seborrhoeic psoriasis refers to classic lesions that affect the scalp but with less typical lesions (lack scaling) in the body folds, especially the groin and axillae. Often, in mild cases the scalp might be the only part of the body involved. Itch can be prominent. *noticeable*

Guttate psoriasis (also known as rain drop psoriasis)

Guttate psoriasis is characterised by crops of scattered small lesions (less than 1 cm) covered with light flaky scales that often affect the trunk and proximal part of the limbs (Fig. 7.6). This form of psoriasis usually occurs in adolescents and often follows a streptococcal throat infection, in persons genetically predisposed to psoriasis. The condition is usually self-limiting.

Erythrodermic psoriasis

Erythrodermic psoriasis presents as an extensive erythema and shows very few classical lesions. It is therefore difficult to diagnose. The condition is serious and even life-threatening. Systemic symptoms can be severe and include fever, joint pain and diarrhoea. Patients are extremely unlikely to present at a community pharmacy with such symptoms.

Tinea corporis

Tinea corporis can superficially look like plaque psoriasis. For further information on tinea infection see page 199.

Lichen planus

Lichen planus is an uncommon condition and is reported to only account for 0.2 to 0.8% of dermatological outpatient consultations. The lesions are similar in appearance to plaque psoriasis but are itchy and are normally located on the inner surfaces of the wrists and on the shins, an atypical distribution for psoriasis. Additionally, oral mucous membranes are normally affected with white, slightly raised lesions that look a little like a spider's web. The person will not have a family history of psoriasis.

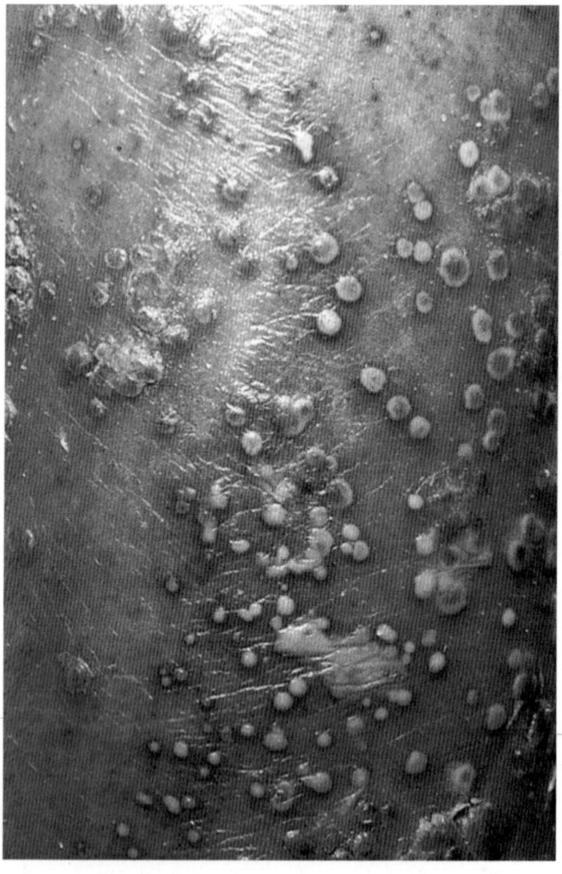

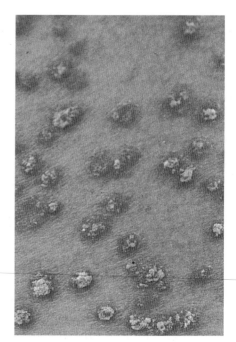

Fig. 7.5 Pustular psoriasis. Reproduced from *Dermatology in Focus* by J Wilkinson et al, 2005, Churchill Livingstone, with permission

Fig. 7.6 Guttate psoriasis. Reproduced from *Dermatology in Focus* by John Wilkinson et al, 2005, Churchill Livingstone, with permission

Pityriasis rosea

The condition is characterised by erythematous scaling mainly on the trunk, but also on the thighs and upper arms. The colour of the rash tends to be a lighter pink colour than psoriasis and can be mildly itchy. A 'target' disc lesion, often misdiagnosed as ringworm, is followed 1 week later by an extensive rash. It most commonly affects young adults. The condition usually remits spontaneously after 4 to 8 weeks. An accurate history will normally eliminate pityriasis rosea from psoriasis, as the condition is acute in onset and the patient can often identify the initial 'target' lesion.

Medication that can trigger or aggravate psoriasis

A number of medicines can cause rashes that look like psoriasis or aggravate existing psoriasis. These include ACE inhibitors, alcohol, beta-blockers, chloroquine, lithium, NSAIDs, terbinafine and steroid withdrawal.

Conditions to eliminate for scalp psoriasis

Seborrhoeic dermatitis

Mild scalp psoriasis can be very difficult to distinguish from seborrhoeic dermatitis. However, in practice this is rarely a problem as treatment for both conditions is often the same. For further information on seborrhoeic dermatitis see page 195.

Tinea capitis (fungal infection of the scalp)

Tinea capitis is an uncommon infection but if the patient has scaling skin, broken hairs and a patch of alopecia then a tinea infection should be considered. For further information on fungal infections see pages 198–203.

Figure 7.7 will aid in the differentiation of plaque psoriasis.

> **❗ TRIGGER POINTS indicative of referral: Psoriasis**
>
> - Lesions that are extensive, follow recent infection or cause moderate to severe itching
> - Patients with psoriatic-type lesions but who have no family history or past personal history of psoriasis
> - Pustular psoriatic lesions

Evidence base for over-the-counter medication

Before any treatment is offered to the patient it is first worth noting that simple OTC remedies should be limited to mild to moderate plaque psoriasis and scalp psoriasis, as these are most likely to respond to such measures. A patient who presents with severe plaque psoriasis or another form of psoriasis should be referred.

Any treatment recommended should also be in conjunction with patient education. Reassurance should be given about its benign, non-contagious nature but it should be emphasised that the condition is chronic and long term and the probable benefit the patient can expect from treatment should be made clear.

Treatment OTC is limited to the use of emollients, keratolytics, coal tar or dithranol, although there is limited published literature supporting efficacy of these treatments. Other topical treatments and systemic agents available on prescription have evidence of efficacy if OTC options are ineffective. A future candidate for deregulation to pharmacy status is calcipotriol (Dovonex) as it has proven efficacy for mild to moderate plaque psoriasis and has few side effects.

Emollients

No published literature appears to have addressed either emollient efficacy or whether one emollient is superior

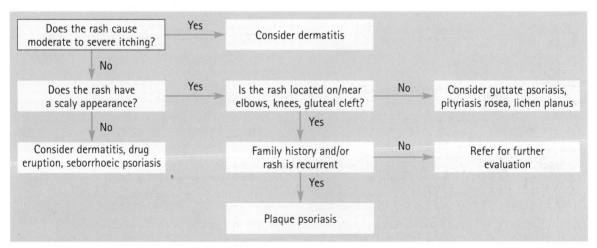

Fig. 7.7 Primer for differential diagnosis of plaque psoriasis

to another in treating psoriasis. Subjective evidence over a long period of time has shown that emollients are useful and are an important aspect of psoriasis treatment. Emollients are frequently prescribed and used to help soften scaling and soothe the skin so reducing irritation, cracking and dryness. On current evidence there is no way of knowing if one emollient is superior to another. Patients might have to try several emollients before finding one that is most effective for their skin.

Keratolytics

Keratolytics, such as salicylic acid and lactic acid, have been incorporated into emollients to aid clearing scale and are often used for scalp psoriasis where very thick scaling can occur. Although there appears to be no published evidence for their efficacy in clearing scale, clinical practice suggests that they should be used first when significant scaling is present before using other treatments.

Coal tar

Goeckerman demonstrated the effectiveness of coal tar as early as 1925. This remained the mainstay of treatment until the introduction of dithranol, corticosteroids and, more recently, vitamin D analogues. A number of clinical studies have confirmed the beneficial effect coal tar has on psoriasis, although a major drawback in assessing the effectiveness of coal tar preparations is the variability in their composition making meaningful comparisons between studies difficult. Comparisons between coal tar and other treatment regimens have been conducted. Tham et al (1994) compared the effectiveness of calcipotriol 50 µg twice daily versus 15% coal tar solution each day. Both treatments were shown to be effective, although calcipotriol was significantly better than the coal tar solution. Harrington (1989) compared two pharmacy-only products, Psorin and Alphosyl. Findings showed that both helped in the treatment of psoriasis but Psorin (which includes 0.11% dithranol) was significantly more effective. Testament to coal tar's effectiveness is that it still features in the current *British National Formulary* (edition 55).

Dithranol

Dithranol was first used in the 1950s and has become an established treatment option as clinical trials have established its efficacy. A systematic review in 2002 identified three placebo-controlled trials with dithranol, all demonstrating a statistically significant improvement over placebo (Mason et al 2002). There appears to be no definitive answer as to which strength is most appropriate; however, current practice dictates starting on the lowest possible concentration and gradually increasing the concentration until improvement is noticed. In addition, short contact regimens are advocated. However, one

review of published studies (Naldi et al 1992) involving short-contact dithranol therapy concluded that due to methodological flaws in many of the trials it is impossible to objectively determine the efficacy of this regimen.

Practical prescribing and product selection

Prescribing information relating to the medicines used to treat psoriasis discussed in the section 'Evidence base for over-the-counter medication' is summarised in Table 7.5; useful tips relating to patients presenting with psoriasis are given in Hints and Tips Box 7.1.

Emollients

There are a large number of emollient products. All emollients should be regularly and liberally applied with no upper limit on how often they can be used. All are chemically inert and can therefore be safely used from birth onwards by all patients. They do not have any interactions with other medicines. For a summary of marketed emollient products see Table 7.32 on page 231.

Tar-based products

Most non-emollient OTC products are coal tar-based but some are combinations of coal tar with salicylic acid or dithranol. All patient groups, including pregnant and breast-feeding women, can use the majority of products on either the skin or scalp. They have no drug interactions but can cause local skin or scalp irritation and stain skin and clothes. There has been recent concern over coal tar's association with an increased risk of skin cancer, although there is at present no firm epidemiological evidence, and the 2006 British Association of Dermatologists' guidelines (http://www.bad.org.uk/healthcare/guidelines/psoriasis.asp) still advocate the use of topical tar products.

Dithranol (Dithrocream)

Dithranol preparations are pharmacy-only medicines so long as the strength does not exceed a maximum of 1.0%.

Short-contact therapy is often advocated for dithranol because prolonged exposure can lead to irritation and burning skin. This involves using the lowest strength available (0.1%) for 15 to 30 minutes, which is then washed off. The concentration of dithranol is increased gradually to 1%. If psoriasis fails to respond with 1% treatment then referral to the GP is needed for higher strength treatment or an alternative product.

The patient might experience burning, even at low concentrations, and if this becomes apparent therapy should either be discontinued or the concentration and/or the contact time reduced. Dithranol will stain skin a

Table 7.5
Practical prescribing: Summary of tar-based products

	Scalp, skin or both	Salicylic acid	Sulphur	Other ingredients	Children	Application
Alphosyl 2 in 1 Shampoo	Scalp	No	No	No	All ages	Every 2 to 3 days
Capasal	Scalp	Yes	No	No	All ages	Daily
Carbo-Dome	Skin	No	No	No	All ages	Two or three times a day
Clinitar	Skin	No	No	No	All ages	Once or twice daily
Cocois	Scalp	Yes	Yes	No	>6 years	Weekly
Exorex	Scalp	No	No	No	>2 years	Two to three times a day
Pentrax shampoo	Scalp	No	No	No	All ages	Twice weekly
Pinetarsol	Skin	No	No	No	All ages	Use as a soap substitute
Polytar & Polytar Plus	Scalp	No	No	No	All ages	Once or twice weekly
Polytar AF	Scalp	No	No	Zinc pyrithione 1%	All ages	Once or twice weekly
Psoriderm	Both	No	No	No	All ages	Once or twice a day
SebCo	Scalp	Yes	Yes	No	>6 years	Daily when needed
T/Gel	Scalp	No	No	No	All ages	When needed

HINTS AND TIPS BOX 7.1: PSORIASIS

Problems with tar and dithranol products	Coal tar and dithranol share common problems of patient compliance. Both are messy to use, have an unpleasant odour and can stain skin and clothing
UV light	90% of patients with psoriasis improve when exposed to sunlight and most patients notice an improvement when they go on holiday
Emollient use	Remind patients that these should be used regularly and liberally
Emollient bath additives	Some bath additives, for example oilatum, will make the bath slippery and patients should be warned to exercise care when getting out of the bath

purple-brown colour but does clear in time. It should not be used on the face. It has been used safely in pregnancy and breast-feeding but should be limited to small areas for as short a period as possible.

Further reading

Clark C. Psoriasis: first-line treatments. Pharm J 2004;274:623–6.

Dodd WA. Tars. Their role in the treatment of psoriasis. Dermatol Clin 1993;11:131–5.

Downs A. Scale of the problem. Chemist and Druggist 22 April, 2006:19–22.

Gelfand JM, Weinstein R, Porter SB, et al. Prevalence and treatment of psoriasis in the United Kingdom: a population-based study. Arch Dermatol 2005;141:1537–41.

Harrington Cl. Low concentration dithranol and coal tar (Psorin) in psoriasis: a comparison with alcoholic coal tar extract and allantoin (Alphosyl). Br J Clin Pract 1989;43:27–9.

Henseler T. Genetics of psoriasis. Arch Dermatol Res 1998;290:463–76.

Leary MR, Rapp SR, Herbst KC, et al. Interpersonal concerns and psychological difficulties of psoriasis patients: effects of disease severity and fear of negative evaluation. Health Psychol 1998;17:530–6.

Mason J, Mason AR, Cork MJ. Topical preparations for the treatment of psoriasis: a systematic review. Br J Dermatol 2002;146:351–64.

MacKie RM. Clinical dermatology. Hong Kong: Oxford University Press; 1999.

Naldi L, Carrel CF, Parazzini F, et al. Development of anthralin short-contact therapy in psoriasis: survey of published clinical trials. Int J Dermatol 1992;31:126–30.

Scon P, Henning-Boehncke W. Psoriasis. N Eng J Med 2005;352:1899–912.

Tham SN, Lun KC, Cheong WK. A comparative study of calcipotriol ointment and tar in chronic plaque psoriasis. Br J Dermatol 1994;131:673–7.

Tristani-Firouzi P, Kruegger CG. Efficacy and safety of treatment modalities for psoriasis. Cutis 1998;61:11–21.

Swanbeck G, Inerot A, Martinsson T, et al. Age at onset and different types of psoriasis. Br J Dermatol 1995;133: 768–73.

Web sites

The Psoriasis Association: http://www.psoriasis-association. org.uk/

Psoriatic Arthropathy Alliance: http://www.paalliance.org/

Australian Psoriasis Association: http://www.psoriasis.org.au/

Markham T. Current approaches to the treatment of psoriasis (2005 article in The Prescriber): http://www.escriber.com/ Prescriber/Features.asp?ID=945&GroupID=6&Action=View

Dandruff (pityriasis capitis)

Background

Dandruff is a chronic relapsing non-inflammatory hyper-proliferative skin condition that is often seen as socially unsightly and a source of embarrassment. Consequently, there are many products marketed to help with the problem.

Prevalence and epidemiology

Dandruff is very common and affects both sexes and all age groups, although it is unusual in prepubescent children. It has been estimated that 50 to 80% of Caucasians will experience dandruff at some time.

Aetiology

Increased cell turnover rate is responsible for dandruff but the reason why cell turnover increases is unknown. Increasingly, research has focused on the role that micro-organisms have on the pathogenesis of dandruff, and in particular the yeast *Malassezia* (previously known as *Pityrosporum*) *ovale*, although the evidence is inconclusive as to whether M. *ovale* is the primary cause of dandruff or is a contributory factor. It has been shown that M. *ovale* makes up more of the scalp flora of dandruff sufferers and might explain why dandruff improves in the summer months (fungal organisms thrive in warm and moist environments that exist on the scalp due to wearing of hats and caps). Further evidence to support a role of M. *ovale* in the aetiology of dandruff is the positive effect that antifungal therapy has on the resolution of dandruff.

Arriving at a differential diagnosis

Most patients will diagnose and treat dandruff without seeking medical help. However, for those patients that do ask for help and advice it is important to differentiate dandruff from other scalp conditions. Asking symptom-specific questions will help the pharmacist to determine if referral is needed (Table 7.6).

Clinical features of dandruff

The scalp will be dry, itchy and flaky. Flakes of dead skin are usually visible in the hair close to the scalp and are visible on the shoulders and collars of clothing.

Conditions to eliminate

Seborrhoeic dermatitis

Typically, seborrhoeic dermatitis will affect areas other than the scalp. In adults, the trunk is commonly involved, as are the eyebrows, eyelashes and external ear. If only scalp involvement is present then the patient might

Table 7.6
Specific questions to ask the patient: Dandruff

Question	Relevance
Presence of erythema	• Dandruff is not associated with scalp redness unless the person has been scratching. Redness is characteristic of psoriasis and is common in adult seborrhoeic dermatitis
Itch	• Dandruff tends to cause itching of the scalp unlike psoriasis and seborrhoeic dermatitis
Presence of other skin lesions	• An adult with scalp involvement only is likely to have dandruff, especially in the absence of erythema • Many patients who have scalp psoriasis also have plaque psoriasis affecting arms, legs and the back

complain of severe and persistent dandruff and the skin of the scalp will be red. For further information on seborrhoeic dermatitis see page 195.

Contact dermatitis

Enquiry should be made to the use of new hair products such as dyes and perms. These can cause irritation and scaling. Avoidance of the irritant should see an improvement in the condition. If improvement is not observed after avoidance of 1 to 2 weeks then a re-assessment of the condition is needed.

Tinea capitis

If the problem is persistent and associated with hair loss then fungal infection of the scalp should be considered. For further information see page 207.

Figure 7.8 will aid the differentiation of dandruff from other scalp disorders.

TRIGGER POINTS indicative of referral: Dandruff

- OTC treatment failure with a 'medicated shampoo'
- Suspected fungal infection

Evidence base for over-the-counter medication

The use of a hypoallergenic shampoo on a daily basis will usually control mild symptoms. In more persistent and severe cases a 'medicated' shampoo can be used to control the symptoms. Treatment options include coal tar, selenium sulphide, zinc pyrithione and ketoconazole.

Coal tar

The mechanism of action for crude coal tar in the management of dandruff is unclear, although it appears that tars affect DNA synthesis and have an antimitotic effect. There are virtually no published studies in the literature to assess the efficacy of coal tars in the treatment of dandruff. One study compared the efficacy between a tar and a non-tar shampoo (containing salicylic acid) but found no statistical difference between the two shampoos. Despite the lack of evidence, tar derivatives are found in a plethora of OTC medicated shampoos and have been granted FDA approval in America as an antidandruff agent.

Selenium sulphide

Selenium is thought to work by its antifungal action. It is accepted that selenium is effective as an antidandruff agent and studies have shown it be significantly better than placebo and non-medicated shampoos.

Zinc pyrithione

Zinc pyrithione, like selenium, exhibits antifungal properties but also reduces cell turnover rates. It is believed that one or both of these properties confers its effectiveness in treating dandruff. Few trials have been conducted with zinc pyrithione although trials have shown significant improvement in dandruff severity scores.

Ketoconazole

Ketoconazole, an azole antifungal, inhibits *M. ovale* replication by interfering with cell membrane formation. It helps in controlling the itching and flaking associated with dandruff. Studies have shown it to be an effective treatment. It has been demonstrated that ketoconazole is significantly better than zinc pyrithione and has similar efficacy to selenium, although it is better tolerated than selenium. Ketoconazole has also been shown to act as a prophylactic agent in preventing relapse.

In addition to the ingredients listed, salicylic acid is an ingredient in some combined products (e.g. Capasal and Meted) included for its keratolytic properties, although trials are lacking to substantiate its effect.

Practical prescribing and product selection

Prescribing information relating to the specific products used to treat dandruff and discussed in the section 'Evidence base for over-the-counter medication' is discussed and summarised in Table 7.7; useful tips relating to dandruff shampoo are given in Hints and Tips Box 7.2.

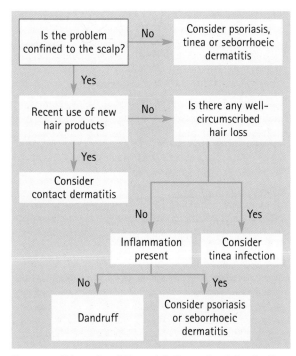

Fig. 7.8 Primer for differential diagnosis of dandruff

Table 7.7
Practical prescribing: Summary of medicines for dandruff

Name of medicine	Use in children	Likely side effects	Drug interactions of note	Patients in whom care should be exercised	Pregnancy and breast-feeding
Coal tar products	All ages	Local irritation and dermatitis reported but rare	None	None	OK
Selenium	>5 years				Manufacturers state to avoid in first trimester but safety data show it to be OK when used on small areas over a limited time
Zinc pyrithione	No lower age limit				OK
Ketoconazole	All ages				

HINTS AND TIPS BOX 7.2: DANDRUFF

Selsun Shampoo	Gold, silver and other metallic jewellery should be removed prior to use, because they can discolour. It also has an unpleasant odour

All antidandruff shampoos can cause local scalp irritation. If this is severe the product should be discontinued. Any patient group can use them, although some manufacturers state products should be avoided during the first 3 months of pregnancy. However, there appear to be no data to substantiate this precaution during pregnancy. They have no drug interactions.

Coal tar products

Products containing coal tar are discussed under practical prescribing for psoriasis. For further information on coal tar products see page 190.

Selenium sulphide (e.g. Selsun)

Adults and children over the age of 5 should use the product twice a week for the first 2 weeks and then once a week for the next 2 weeks. The hair should be thoroughly wet before applying the shampoo, which should be left in contact with the scalp for 2 to 3 minutes before rinsing out. Selenium should be avoided if the patient has inflamed or broken skin because irritation can occur. Selenium can also cause discoloration of the hair and alter the colour of hair dyes.

Zinc pyrithione (e.g. Head and Shoulders)

Zinc-based products can be used by all patients and at any age. It should be used on a daily basis until dandruff clears. Dermatitis has been reported with zinc pyrithione and should be borne in mind when treating patients with pre-existing dermatitis.

Ketoconazole (Nizoral Dandruff and Nizoral Anti-Dandruff Shampoo)

Nizoral can either be used to treat acute flare-ups of dandruff or as prophylaxis. To treat acute cases adults and children should wash the hair thoroughly, leaving the shampoo on for 3 to 5 minutes before rinsing it off. This should be repeated every 3 or 4 days (twice a week) for between 2 and 4 weeks. If used for prophylaxis, the shampoo should be used once every 1 to 2 weeks. It can cause local itching or a burning sensation on application and may rarely discolour hair.

Further reading

Arrese JE, Pierard-Franchimont C, De-Doncker P, et al. Effect of ketoconazole-medicated shampoos on squamometry and *Malassezia ovalis* load in pityriasis capitis. Cutis 1996;58:235–7.

Danby FW, Maddin WS, Margesson LJ, et al. A randomized double-blind controlled trial of ketoconazole 2% shampoo versus selenium sulfide 2.5% shampoo in the treatment of moderate to severe dandruff. J Am Acad Dermatol 1993;29:1008–12.

Nigam PK, Tyagi S, Saxena AK, et al. Dermatitis from zinc pyrithione. Contact Dermat 1988;19:219.

Orentreich N. Comparative study of two antidandruff preparations. J Pharm Sci 1969;58:1279–84.

Pereira F, Fernandes C, Dias M, et al. Allergic contact dermatitis from zinc pyrithione. Contact Dermat 1995;33:131.

Peter RU, Richarz-Barthauer U. Successful treatment and prophylaxis of scalp seborrheic dermatitis and dandruff with 2% ketoconazole shampoo: results of a multicentre, double blind, placebo-controlled trial. Br J Dermatol 1995;132:441–5.

Pierard-Franchimont C, Goffin V, Decroix J, Pierard GE. A multicenter randomized trial of ketoconazole 2% and zinc pyrithione 1% shampoos in severe dandruff and seborrhoeic dermatitis. Skin Pharmacol Appl Skin Physiol 2002;15:434–41.

Rigoni C, Toffolo P, Cantu A, et al. 1% econazole hair shampoo in the treatment of pityriasis capitis; a comparative study versus zinc pyrithione shampoo. G Ital Dermatol Venereol 1989;124:67–70.

Van Custem J, Van Gerven F, Fransen J, et al. The in vitro antifungal activity of ketoconazole, zinc pyrithione and selenium sulfide against Pityrosporum and their efficacy as a shampoo in the treatment of experimental pityrosporosis in guinea pigs. J Am Acad Dermatol 1990;22:993–8.

Seborrhoeic dermatitis

Background

There are two distinct types of seborrhoeic dermatitis – an infantile form, often referred to as cradle cap, and an adult form. Seborrhoeic dermatitis can present with varying degrees of severity, ranging from mild dandruff to a severe and explosive form in AIDS patients.

Prevalence and epidemiology

Estimates of its prevalence range from 1 to 5% of the population, although cradle cap is reported to be more prevalent than the adult form. Cradle cap usually starts in infancy, before the age of 6 months, and is usually self-limiting; the adult form tends to be chronic and persistent. In addition men are six times more likely to suffer from the adult form than women and it is also more common in people with underlying neurological illness, for example, Parkinson's disease.

Aetiology

Despite its name, there appear to be no changes in sebum secretion. Like psoriasis and dandruff, seborrhoeic dermatitis is characterised by an increased cell turnover rate. The precise cause of seborrhoeic dermatitis remains unknown and several theories have been put forward,

ranging from immunological, hormonal and nutritional mechanisms. Like dandruff, *Malassezia ovale* plays an important role in the development of seborrhoeic dermatitis; however, it has not yet been established whether it has a primary or secondary role in the clinical presentation of seborrhoeic dermatitis.

Arriving at a differential diagnosis

Infantile seborrhoeic dermatitis is relatively easy to recognise but can sometimes be confused with atopic dermatitis. Arriving at a differential diagnosis of the adult form is more problematic as the condition can affect different areas and present with different degrees of severity. In mild cases it needs to be differentiated from dandruff and in more severe forms from allergic contact dermatitis, psoriasis and pityriasis versicolor. Asking symptom-specific questions will help the pharmacist to determine if referral is needed (Table 7.8).

Clinical features of seborrhoeic dermatitis

Cradle cap appears as large yellow, greasy scales and crusts on the scalp. This can become thick and cover the whole scalp (Fig 7.9). Other areas can be involved such as the face and nappy area.

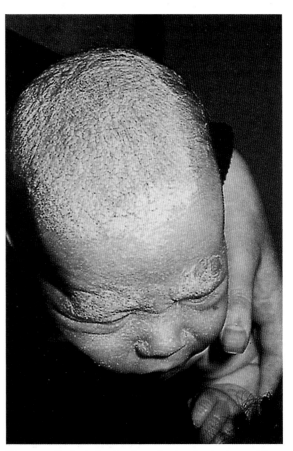

Fig. 7.9 Typical distribution of seborrhoeic dermatitis

Table 7.8
Specific questions to ask the patient: Seborrhoeic dermatitis

Question	Relevance
Itching	• In cradle cap the rash does not itch. This is useful in differentiating cradle cap from atopic dermatitis as there is often overlap in the age at which they present
Location	• Infantile and adult forms of seborrhoeic dermatitis do present in different locations (see Fig. 7.10). Additionally, the distribution in the adult form varies from other similar skin conditions (e.g. psoriasis typically involves knees, elbows and sacral area)
Positive family history	• Patients tend not to have a family history in seborrhoeic dermatitis. This is in contrast to patients with psoriasis and those patients suffering from atopic dermatitis
Other symptoms	• Ear and eyelid problems are associated with seborrhoeic dermatitis. It is useful to rule out contact dermatitis when the ear is involved and atopic dermatitis when the eyelids are involved • The general health of a child with seborrhoeic dermatitis will be unaffected. In contrast a child who is fractious and miserable is more likely to have atopic dermatitis • Seborrhoeic dermatitis usually has yellow greasy scale, unlike psoriasis, which has a silvery scale
Physical signs	• If you run your fingers through the hair of someone with seborrhoeic dermatitis little is felt. In psoriasis, accumulation of scales give the scalp an uneven, lumpy feel

The adult form of seborrhoeic dermatitis is characterised by a history of intermittent skin problems. The distribution of rash is synonymous with skin areas with high numbers of sebaceous glands, typically the central part of the face, scalp, eyebrows, eyelids, ears, nasolabial folds and mid chest (Figs 7.10 and 7.11) The rash is red with greasy looking scales and is mildly itchy. Blepharitis and otitis externa are also common secondary complications.

Conditions to eliminate

Atopic dermatitis

In infants, atopic dermatitis usually presents as itchy lesions on the face and trunk. Scalp involvement is less common and the nappy area is usually spared. A positive family history of the atopic triad of dermatitis, asthma or hay fever is common. For further information on differentiating atopic dermatitis see Chapter 9, pages 275–277.

Psoriasis

Adults with scalp psoriasis can be confused with those patients who present with severe and persistent dandruff caused by seborrhoeic dermatitis. However, in scalp psoriasis the plaques tend to be crusty and extend away from the hairline whereas seborrhoeic dermatitis causes scaling with underlying redness. It also affects the eyebrows and eyelids, unlike psoriasis.

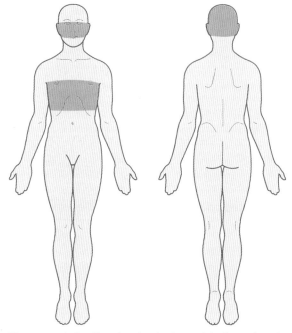

Fig. 7.10 Infantile seborrhoeic dermatitis. Reproduced from *Dermatology in Focus* by J Wilkinson et al, 2005, Churchill Livingstone, with permission

Pityriasis versicolor (meaning bran-like scaly rash of various colour)

Pityriasis versicolor, a yeast infection, can be mistaken for adult seborrhoeic dermatitis because the lesions exhibit fine superficial scale and are located on the upper

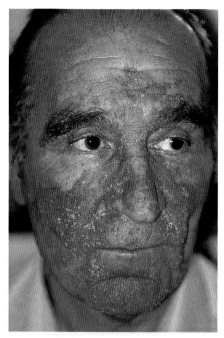

Fig. 7.11 Seborrhoeic dermatitis affecting the face. Reproduced from *Dermatology: An Illustrated Colour Text* by D J Gawkrodger, 2008, Churchill Livingstone, with permission

trunk. The lesions are usually small (less than 1 cm) but can join together to form larger plaques. The condition is associated with warm climates and most people will have picked the infection up when on holiday. The rash does not itch significantly and the face is usually spared. It can be treated with antifungal lotions and shampoos (see 'Dandruff' page 192) or if there is a small number of lesions with imidazole creams (see 'Fungal skin infections' page 198). Antifungal shampoos such as ketoconazole and selenium sulphide (2.5%) are applied for 10 minutes and then washed off, and this is repeated daily for 10 days. Imidazole creams are applied daily for 10 days.

Medication that can trigger or aggravate seborrhoeic dermatitis

A number of medicines are associated with triggering or aggravating existing seborrhoeic dermatitis. These include buspirone, cimetidine, gold, griseofulvin, haloperidol, interferon alfa, lithium, methyldopa and phenothiazines.

 TRIGGER POINTS indicative of referral: Seborrhoeic dermatitis

- Treatment failure with OTC medicines
- Lesions that appear after holiday to warm climates

Evidence base for over-the-counter medication

Treatment options for seborrhoeic dermatitis are the same as dandruff. Unfortunately, seborrhoeic dermatitis tends to be more resistant to therapy and often recurs whatever treatment is chosen.

For infants with cradle cap simple measures are usually only required in most cases. Daily use of a baby shampoo followed by gentle brushing will improve the condition. If this fails, the scales can be removed by applying olive oil to the scalp overnight followed by using a baby shampoo the next morning. If symptoms persist a medicated shampoo containing a keratolytic (e.g. Meted) or keratolyic-tar combination (e.g. Capasal) could be tried. If this fails the child should be referred to the GP.

In adults, OTC preparations should only be used on mild to moderate seborrhoeic dermatitis involving the scalp. In mild cases of scalp involvement zinc pyrithione can be tried, reserving selenium and ketoconazole for resistant or more moderate disease. For involvement on the face and torso antifungals and corticosteroids are effective but OTC product licences preclude their use.

Practical prescribing and product selection

Prescribing information relating to specific products used to treat seborrhoeic dermatitis is discussed under 'Dandruff' on pages 193–194. In addition, at least one product is marketed specifically for cradle cap and is discussed and summarised in Table 7.9.

Dentinox Cradle Cap Shampoo

This contains sodium lauryl ether sulpho-succinate 6% and sodium lauryl ether sulphate 2.7%. The shampoo should be applied twice during each bath time until the scalp clears, after which it can be used when needed.

Table 7.9 Practical prescribing: Summary of medicines for cradle cap					
Name of medicine	Use in children	Likely side effects	Drug interactions of note	Patients in whom care should be exercised	Pregnancy and breast-feeding
Dentinox Cradle Cap Shampoo	Birth onwards	None reported	None	None	Not applicable

Further reading

Bergbrant IM, Faergemann J. The role of *Pityrosporum ovale* in seborrheic dermatitis. Semin Dermatol 1990;9:262–8.

Danby FW, Maddin WS, Margesson LJ, et al. A randomized double-blind controlled trial of ketoconazole 2% shampoo versus selenium sulfide 2.5% shampoo in the treatment of moderate to severe dandruff. J Am Acad Dermatol 1993;29:1008–12.

Go IH, Wientjens DP, Koster M. A double-blind trial of 1% ketoconazole shampoo versus placebo in the treatment of dandruff. Mycoses 1992;35:103–5.

Gupta AK, Bluhm R. Seborrhoeic dermatitis. J Eur Acad Dermatol Venereol 2004;18:13–26

Johnson BA, Nunley JR. Treatment of seborrheic dermatitis. Am Fam Physician 2000;61:2703–10.

McGrath J, Murphy GM. The control of seborrhoeic dermatitis and dandruff by antipityrosporal drugs. Drugs 1991;41:178–84.

Fungal skin infections

Background

Two main groups of fungi infect man, *Candida* yeasts and the dermatophytes; however, in this section only dermatophyte infections are considered. Fungal infections are commonly referred to as ringworm (although this is inaccurate, as a worm does not cause the infection and most variants are not observed as a ring). This terminology only serves to cause confusion and should be avoided. Dermatophyte skin infections are classed by anatomical location, for example: athlete's foot (tinea pedis); groin infection (tinea cruris or 'jock itch'); ringworm of the skin (tinea corporis); and scalp ringworm (tinea capitis).

Prevalence and epidemiology

Globally, dermatophytic fungi are more prevalent in tropical and subtropical areas because fungal organisms prefer high temperatures and high humidity. Having said this, dermatophyte infections are commonly met in more temperate Western countries. Tinea pedis (athlete's foot) is the most common fungal infection, although prevalence rates vary depending on the population studied and whether diagnosis is made by clinical symptoms or culture confirmation. Despite these discrepancies, athlete's foot is said to affect about 15% of the UK population and is common in people of all ages.

Other tinea infections such as tinea corporis and tinea cruris might present in the community pharmacy but are uncommon. Tinea unguium (nail infection) is covered separately on pages 203–205. Tinea capitis is the commonest infection in children worldwide but in Western nations is rare (for further information on fungal scalp infection see page 207).

Aetiology

Dermatophyte infections are contagious and transmitted directly from one host to another. They invade the stratum corneum of the skin, hair and nails but do not generally infiltrate living tissues. The fungus then begins to grow and proliferate in the non-living cornified layer of keratinised tissue of the epidermis. Transmission of athlete's foot is thought to be commonly acquired from communal rooms (e.g. changing rooms) whereas infection of the groin can be acquired from contaminated towels and bed sheets, or by autoinoculation from an existing foot infection.

Arriving at a differential diagnosis

Dependent on the area affected the infection will manifest itself in a variety of clinical presentations (Fig. 7.12). Recognition of symptoms for each site affected will facilitate recognition and accurate diagnosis.

All forms of tinea infection should be relatively easy to recognise, perhaps with the exception of isolated lesions on the body.

Patients with athlete's foot will often accurately self-diagnose the condition. However, the pharmacist should still confirm this self-diagnosis through a combination of questions (Table 7.10) and inspection of the feet. This is important as it also provides an opportunity to check for fungal nail involvement.

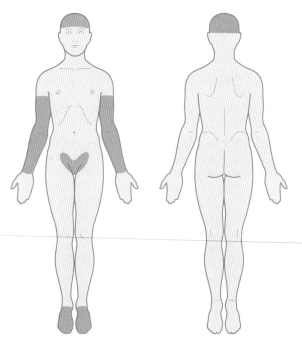

Fig. 7.12 Distribution of fungal infections

Table 7.10
Specific questions to ask the patient: Fungal infections

Question	Relevance
Age and sex of patient	• Athlete's foot is most prevalent in adolescents and young adults, especially men • Nail involvement usually occurs in older adults • Infection in the groin is much more common in men than women
Presence of itch	• Fungal infections usually cause itch, irritation or burning sensations. This usually eliminates conditions such as psoriasis but not dermatitis/eczema
Associated symptoms	• Fungal lesions tend to be dry and scaly (except athlete's foot) and have a sharp margin between infected and non-infected skin
Previous and family history	• Fungal infections are usually acute in onset with no previous episodes, although athlete's foot may become recurrent • For lesions that do not show a classic textbook description, a positive family history of dermatitis or psoriasis might influence your differential diagnosis

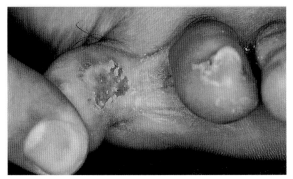

Fig. 7.13 Athlete's foot. Reproduced from *20 Common Problems* by A. Fleischel, 2000, McGraw-Hill.

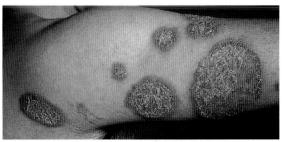

Fig. 7.14 Tinea corporis. Reproduced from *Dermatology: An Illustrated Colour Text* by D J Gawkrodger, 2008, Churchill Livingstone, with permission

Clinical features of tinea infections

Athlete's foot

Athlete's foot is characterised by itching, flaking and fissuring of the skin and will appear white and 'soggy' due to maceration of the skin (Fig. 7.13). The feet often smell. The usual site of infection is in the toe webs, especially the fourth web space (web space next to the little toe).

Once acquired the infection can spread to other sites including the sole and in-step of the foot. Over time this can infect the nails (see pages 203–205 for fungal nail infection). Cases of tinea infection where the plantar surface has become involved may be persistent and difficult to treat.

Tinea corporis

Tinea corporis is defined as an infection of the major skin surfaces that do not involve the face, hands, feet, groin or scalp. The usual clinical presentation is of itchy pink or red scaly slightly raised patches with a well-defined inflamed border (Fig. 7.14). Over time the lesions often show 'central clearing' as the central area is relatively resistant to colonisation. This appearance led to the term ringworm. Lesions can occur singly, be numerous or overlap to produce a single large lesion and appear poly-cyclic (several overlapping circular lesions).

Tinea cruris

The rash is usually isolated to the groin and inner thighs, but can spread to the buttocks. It is often bilateral and is normally intensely itchy, reddish brown and has a well-defined edge.

Conditions to eliminate

Tinea faciei

Fungal infections on the face are rare and are consequently often mistaken for other facial skin conditions. The lesions are similar in appearance to tinea corporis in that they will normally have a sharp well-defined border, show scaling and be itchy. Conditions such as acne, rosacea and lupus need to be considered in its differential diagnosis.

Tinea manuum

Tinea manuum is often misdiagnosed as eczema or psoriasis due to its atypical tinea appearance. The patient usually suffers from chronic diffuse scaling of one palm. Often, athlete's foot will be present, as the infection has spread to the hands from the feet due to the patient scratching their feet. The condition is not common and if no foot involvement is implicated then the diagnosis strongly points to dermatitis.

Psoriasis

Isolated fungal body lesions can be difficult to distinguish from plaque psoriasis. However, if the patient has psoriasis there will normally be a family history of psoriasis and the lesions tend not to itch, exhibit more scaling and do not show central clearing.

Dermatitis – allergic and contact forms

Both fungal infections and dermatitis exhibit red itchy lesions and therefore can be difficult to distinguish from one another. Patients with dermatitis will often have a family and personal history of dermatitis or be able to describe an event that triggered the onset of the rash. Misdiagnosis of a fungal infection for dermatitis and subsequent treatment with a steroid-based cream will diminish the itch, redness and scaling but the infecting organism will proliferate. On withdrawal of the steroid cream the visible signs of the infection will return and be worse than before, often in a papular form (tinea incognito). Discoid eczema also needs to be considered. This presents as round, raised, coin-shaped lesions that particularly affect the arms and legs. It can itch and show superficial scale. It occurs mainly in middle-aged people.

> **TRIGGER POINTS indicative of referral: Tinea infections**
>
> - Involvement of large areas of the trunk (possible oral treatment needed)
> - OTC treatment failure
> - Suspected facial or scalp involvement

Evidence base for over-the-counter medication

Superficial dermatophyte infections can be treated effectively with topical OTC preparations. Six classes of medicines have proven efficacy in their treatment.

Allylamines

Terbinafine has been exempt from POM control in the UK since 2000. It inhibits the biosynthesis of ergosterol – an essential component of fungal cell membranes. Reviews have shown terbinafine to have high cure rates.

Benzoic acid

Benzoic acid acts by lowering intracellular pH of dermatophytes and is combined with salicylic acid (Whitfield's ointment). Although Whitfield's ointment has been on the market for nearly a century it still has a role to play as an effective antifungal but newer products – with higher cure rates, quicker resolution and more cosmetically acceptable formulations – have replaced its widespread use in Western society. However, it remains one of the essential medicines on the World Health Organization's model list.

Imidazoles

Imidazoles, like allylamines, act by inhibiting ergosterol production but at a later stage in the ergosterol biosynthesis pathway. They have largely replaced benzoic acid, undecenoates and tolnaftate, because they have greater efficacy and an excellent safety record. There appear to be no clinically significant differences in cure rates between the different imidazoles.

Griseofulvin

Griseofulvin (as a 1% spray) was exempt from POM control in the UK in 2003; it works by inhibiting cellular mitosis. It has proven effectiveness when taken orally but has only limited trial data as a topical formulation. One trial reported an 80% mycological cure rate after 4 weeks with once-daily application (Aly et al 1994).

Tolnaftate

Tolnaftate is thought to work by distorting fungal hyphae. It appears to have the least amount of trial data supporting its efficacy. Low patient numbers involved in the studies further compounds the difficulty in assessing its efficacy.

Undecenoates

The exact mechanism of action of undecenoates is not understood. They have been used to treat athlete's foot for over 30 years and feature in the most recent United States Pharmacopoeia.

Summary

On current evidence, an imidazole derivative or terbinafine would be first-line treatment for superficial fungal infection. Both have similar mycological and symptom cure rates, although terbinafine might be preferred because it clears symptoms in a shorter space of time, although it is more expensive. Treatment choice will therefore probably be driven by patient acceptability and cost.

Practical prescribing and product selection

Prescribing information relating to specific products used to treat fungal infections and discussed in the section 'Evidence base for over-the-counter medication' is summarised in Tables 7.11 and 7.12; useful tips relating to patients presenting with fungal infections are given in Hints and Tips Box 7.3.

Imidazoles

All topical imidazoles have excellent safety records and can be used by all patient groups, including pregnant and breast-feeding women. They do not have any drug interactions and the major side effect associated with their use is irritation on application. To prevent reinfection,

imidazoles should be used after the lesions have cleared, although the length of time varies from product to product.

Clotrimazole (e.g. Canesten range)

Clotrimazole-containing products can be used for all dermatophyte and candida infections. Canesten and Canesten AF cream should be applied two or three times a day, whereas Canesten Hydrocortisone can only be used twice a day.

Ketoconazole (Daktarin Gold)

Ketoconazole has a licence for athlete's foot, groin infection and candidal intertrigo. For athlete's foot the cream should be applied twice a day for 1 week. For groin infections and candidal intertrigo, the cream should be applied once or twice daily. If no improvement in symptoms is experienced after 4 weeks' treatment then the patient should be referred to a GP. For all conditions treatment should be continued for 2 to 3 days after all signs of infection have disappeared to prevent relapse.

Table 7.11
Practical prescribing: Summary of medicines for tinea infections

Name of medicine	Use in children	Likely side effects	Drug interactions of note	Patients in whom care should be exercised	Pregnancy and breast-feeding
Imidazoles Clotrimazole	All ages	Mild burning or itching	None	None	OK
Miconazole					
Ketoconazole					
Imidazole/steroid combination	>10 years				
Tolnaftate Mycil	No lower age stated	None reported	None	None	OK
Tinaderm					
Undecenoates Mycota	No lower age stated	None reported	None	None	OK
Monphytol	>12 years	Stinging			OK, but manufacturer states avoid
Benzoic acid Whitfield's ointment	No lower age stated	None reported	None	None	OK
Terbinafine Lamisil AT	>16 years	Redness, itching	None	None	OK
Lamisil Once	>18 years				
Griseofulvin (Grisol AF)	No lower age stated	Stinging	None	None	OK

Table 7.12
Summary of antifungal products and formulations

Active ingredient	Brand	Formulations
Clotrimazole 1%	Canesten AF	Cream, spray, powder
	Canesten	Cream, spray, powder, solution
Clotrimazole 1% & hydrocortisone 1%	Canesten hydrocortisone	Cream
Miconazole 2%	Daktarin Activ	Cream, spray, powder
	Daktarin	Cream and powder
Miconazole 2% & hydrocortisone 1%	Daktacort HC	Cream
Ketoconazole	Daktarin Gold	Cream
Terbinafine	Lamisil AT	Spray, cream, gel
	Lamisil Once	Solution
Tolnaftate	Mycil	Ointment, spray, powder
	Scholl Athlete's Foot	Cream, spray, powder
	Tinaderm	Cream
Undecenoic acid	Mycota	Cream, spray, powder
	Monphytol	Paint

HINTS AND TIPS BOX 7.3: FUNGAL INFECTION

Reinfection and transmission	It is not known if improving foot hygiene or changing footwear can help to cure athlete's foot but measures to reduce transmission include: 1. Dry the skin thoroughly after showering or having a bath. Keep a personal towel and do not share it to prevent the infection spreading from person to person 2. Wear cotton socks and change at least once a day 3. Avoid the use of occlusive non-breathable shoes 4. Dust shoes and socks with antifungal powder 5. Avoid scratching infected skin 6. Use flip-flops (or equivalent) when using communal changing rooms
Steroid-containing products	The licences state that the maximum period of treatment is 7 days. This limits their usefulness, as many fungal infections will take longer to clear than 7 days, especially if the product needs to be used after the lesions have cleared for a number of days. The pharmacist has to either break the law or recommend the use of an imidazole-only product after the initial 7 days' treatment with the product containing a steroid

---

Miconazole (e.g. Daktarin range, Daktacort HC)

Products containing miconazole only are suitable for patients of all ages and should be used twice a day. Treatment should continue for 10 days after all lesions have disappeared to prevent relapse. Daktacort HC is suitable for children aged over 10 and is licensed for sweat rash and athlete's foot.

Tolnaftate (e.g. Mycil, Tinaderm)

Products containing tolnaftate have no interactions or side effects and can be used by all patients. They can be used for athlete's foot and infections of the groin and should be used twice a day with treatment continuing for at least 1 week after the infection has cleared up.

Undecenoates (e.g. Mycota, Monphytol)

Products containing undecenoates have no interactions and can be used by all patients. They are licensed for athlete's foot and should be used twice a day and treatment continued for at least 1 week after the infection has cleared up. Local irritation has been reported.

Benzoic acid (e.g. Whitfield's ointment)

Benzoic acid (in combination with salicylic acid) is now rarely used. However, it is a safe medicine and can be used by all patients.

Terbinafine (Lamisil AT and Lamisil Once)

Terbinafine can be used to treat athlete's foot, groin infection and tinea corporis. The cream should be applied once or twice a day whereas the spray should be used only once daily. It has no interactions, has few reported side effects and can be used by all patients. Lamisil AT products are licensed for people over 16 compared to Lamisil Once, which is for patients over 18 years of age.

Griseofulvin (Grisol AF spray)

Licensed for athlete's foot, Grisol should be applied to the area once daily. Each spray delivers 400 µg of griseofulvin with a maximum of three sprays in 24 hours for more extensive or severe infection. The spray should be used for 10 days after the lesions clear to prevent reinfection. It has no interactions, has few reported side effects and can be used by all patients.

Further reading

Aly R, Bayles CI, Oakes RA, et al. Topical griseofulvin in the treatment of dermatophytoses. Clin Exp Dermatol 1994;19:43–6.

Crawford F, Hart R, Bell-Syer S, et al. Topical treatments for fungal infections of the skin and nails of the foot. The Cochrane Database of Systematic Reviews 1999, issue 3.

Drake LA, Dinehart SM, Farmer ER, et al. Guidelines of care for superficial mycotic infections of the skin: tinea corporis, tinea cruris, tinea faciei, tinea manuum, and tinea pedis. Guidelines/Outcomes Committee. American Academy of Dermatology. J Am Acad Dermatol 1996;34:282–6.

Elewski B. Tinea capitis. Dermatol Clin 1996;14:23–31.

Pierard GE, Arrese JE, Pierard-Franchimont C. Treatment and prophylaxis of tinea infections. Drugs 1996;52:209–24.

Web sites

Bandolier issue 107: http://www.jr2.ox.ac.uk/bandolier/band107/b107-3.html#Heading2

Prodigy guidance: http://cks.library.nhs.uk/fungal_skin_infections

General site on tinea infection: http://www.nlm.nih.gov/medlineplus/ency/article/001439.htm

Fungal nail infection (onychomycosis)

7

Background

The deregulation of amorolfine in the UK and other Western countries (e.g. Australia) now makes it possible for community pharmacists to treat infection affecting the toenails. Onychomycosis is defined as a chronic fungal infection of the fingernails or toenails, although only infection of the toenail is covered in the text. The infection is common but is probably under-reported because of patient embarrassment or ignorance that they have an infection. If left untreated it can lead to pain and discomfort, which can make wearing shoes difficult. Nails, over time, will disfigure and crumble away.

Prevalence and epidemiology

It is estimated that 3 to 8% of the general population suffer from onychomycosis. The incidence of infection increases with increasing age and is particularly common in peopled aged over 60 years of age (e.g. estimated at between 14 and 28%).

Aetiology

Over 90% of cases are caused by dermatophytes (*Trichophyton rubrum* and *T. interdigitale*), with the remainder caused by yeasts and moulds. In most cases predisposing factors can be determined in the development of nail infection, for example, an initial skin infection (tinea pedis), immunocompromisation or poor peripheral circulation and neuropathies (e.g. diabetes).

Arriving at a differential diagnosis

There are a number of different types of onychomycosis and it is important to be able to differentiate between them because amorolfine is only licensed for the treatment of distal lateral subungual onychomycosis. Taking a history of the presenting symptom will be helpful but a visual inspection of the toenails is strongly advocated.

Clinical features of distal lateral subungual onychomycosis (DLSO)

DLSO is usually asymptomatic and people often seek medical help because of concerns about the appearance of the nail. The nail takes on a dull opaque and yellow appearance. Over time the nail thickens and distorts and as infection spreads and worsens the nail becomes brittle and crumbles away or falls off (Fig. 7.15). The key clinical symptoms that differentiate DLSO from other types of onychomycosis are summarised in Table 7.13.

Table 7.13
Main types of onychomycosis

Type	Key characteristics	Spread of infection
Distal lateral subungual onychomycosis (DLSO)	Mainly big toe	Note yellowing starts at distal part of toe or side of nail
Proximal subungual onychomycosis (PCO)	Immunocompromised patients	Yellow spots appear at the base of the nail (i.e. in the half-moon area of the nail)
Superficial white onychomycosis	Often occurs in previously damaged nails Chalky-white in appearance and can be scraped off the nail surface	Located on the surface of the nail

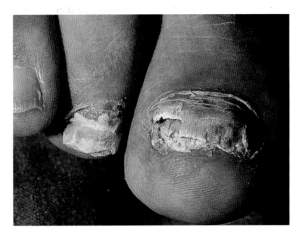

Fig. 7.15 Tinea unguium. Reproduced from *Dermatology: An Illustrated Colour Text* by D J Gawkrodger, 2008, Churchill Livingstone, with permission

(For more images of fungal nail infection visit http://www.dermnetnz.org/fungal/onychomycosis.html)

Other conditions to eliminate

Psoriasis, eczema and trauma can affect the nail and need to be considered; in psoriasis, nail pitting is visible; for trauma there should be an identifiable event that affected the nail; and in eczema and psoriasis the skin should be affected, either near and around the feet (eczema) or remotely (psoriasis plaques on areas such as knees and elbows).

> ❗ **TRIGGER POINTS indicative of referral: DLSO**
>
> - OTC treatment failure
> - Suspected poor compliance

Evidence base for over-the-counter medication

Amorolfine is a broad-spectrum antifungal agent that works by inhibiting ergosterol synthesis. An open-labelled, non-randomised trial has shown it to be effective, producing clinical cure in 37% of toenail infections (Zaug 1992). However, the study suffered from large drop out rates (nearly 30%), and there were no comparisons with other available topical antifungal treatments. A further trial comparing once versus twice weekly application of amorolfine reported similar cure rates (46%) with weekly application (Reinel 1992). Prodigy guidance (July 2008) advocates topical treatment only in DLSO confined to the distal edge of the nail, or when systemic treatment is contraindicated.

Practical prescribing and product selection

Prescribing information relating to amorolfine is summarised in Table 7.14; useful tips relating to patients presenting with fungal nail infection are given in Hints and Tips Box 7.4.

Amorolfine (Curanail)

Amorolfine is available as a 5% nail lacquer. It is used weekly and treatment lasts until the affected nail(s) have regrown and are clear of infection. This takes 9 to 12 months. Each pack of Curanail gives 3 months' treatment, which affords the pharmacist an opportunity to review treatment before further medication is given. The product licence restricts use to no more than two nails in people aged 18 or over who have no underlying medical conditions that predispose them to fungal infection (e.g. immunocompromised and diabetic patients). It cannot be used in pregnant or breast-feeding women. To apply amorolfine the nail must be first filed and cleaned. Files and cleaning pads are provided in the treatment pack and are not reusable. The lacquer should then be evenly applied and left to dry. Amorolfine is unlikely to cause side effects, but skin irritation has been reported.

Table 7.14
Practical prescribing: Summary of medicines for fungal nail infections

Name of medicine	Use in children	Likely side effects	Drug interactions of note	Patients in whom care should be exercised	Pregnancy and breast-feeding
Amorolfine (Curanail)	>18 years	Skin irritation (rare)	None	None	Avoid

HINTS AND TIPS BOX 7.4: CURANAIL

Why only two nails?	This is in line with Prodigy guidance as more severe infections require systemic treatment (e.g. terbinafine)
Hygiene measures	Keep the area clean Change socks regularly Avoid trauma to the nails Avoid sharing towels

Further reading

Baran R, Kaoukhov A. Topical antifungal drugs for the treatment of onychomycosis: an overview of current strategies for monotherapy and combination therapy. J Eur Acad Dermatol Venereol 2005;19:21–9.

Crawford F, Hart R, Bell-Syer S, et al. Topical treatments for fungal infections of the skin and nails of the foot. Cochrane Database of Systematic Reviews 1999, issue 3.

Finch JJ, Warshaw EM. Toenail onychomycosis: current and future treatment options. Dermatol Ther 2007;20:31–46.

Reinel D. Topical treatment of onychomycosis with amorolfine 5 per cent nail lacquer: comparative efficacy and tolerability of once and twice weekly use. Dermatology 1992;184(Suppl):21–4.

Seebacher C, Brasch J, Abeck D, et al. Onychomycosis. JDDG 2007;1:61–6.

Zaug M, Bergstraesser M. Amorolfine in the treatment of onychomycosis and dermatomycoses (an overview). Clin Exp Dermatol 1992;17(Suppl 1):61–70.

Web sites

Prodigy guidance: http://cks.library.nhs.uk/fungal_candidal_nail_infection

Hair loss

Background

Each hair consists of a shaft, made up of dead keratinized cells, and a root (see Fig 7.1). Hair is found on most skin surfaces (hands, feet and lips being notable exceptions). Each hair follicle goes through a growth cycle, which consists of a long growing phase (anagen) followed by a short resting phase (telogen). At the end of resting phase, the hair falls out (catagen) and a new hair starts growing in the follicle, beginning the cycle again. The hair cycle occurs randomly for each follicle so that normal hair loss from the adult scalp is approximately 100 hairs per day; where the rate is greater than this then the clinical signs of hair loss can be observed. Hair loss affects both men and women and is associated with strong emotional and psychological consequences. People have been socialised to link a full head of hair with youth and vitality, whereas baldness portrays a feeling of unattractiveness and loss of youth. Hair loss can be due to a number of aetiologies; however, this section concentrates on androgenetic alopecia (male pattern baldness) because it is the most common cause of hair loss.

Prevalence and epidemiology

Men are more susceptible than women to androgenetic alopecia and usually experience more severe hair loss. Men tend to be affected from the second decade onwards (30% of 30-year-old men will be affected to some degree) and the prevalence of male pattern baldness in Caucasians who reach old age approaches 100%. In women the condition becomes more pronounced after menopause.

Patients usually have a positive family history. The nature and extent of hair loss will follow identical patterns to those seen in the patient's immediate parents and grandparents, which can be used as a predictor to the patient's potential hair-loss pattern.

Aetiology

Hair is classed as either terminal or vellus hair. Terminal hair is longer and thicker and found on the scalp and eyebrows. Vellus hair covers the remainder of the body and is shorter and downy. In androgenetic alopecia terminal hair follicles transform into more vellus-like hair follicles as a result of preferential binding by dihydrotestosterone (produced from the conversion of androgen by 5-alpha-reductase) to hair follicle receptors. Eventually the follicle ceases activity completely with resulting hair loss. It appears that there is a genetic component determining the age of onset and the severity of the problem.

Arriving at a differential diagnosis

Hair loss is obviously easy to detect. Empathy and understanding towards the patient needs to be exercised. Although androgenetic alopecia is the most common form of hair loss, other causes need to be eliminated (Fig. 7.16). Asking symptom-specific questions will help the pharmacist to determine if referral is needed (Table 7.15).

Clinical features of androgenetic alopecia

Men initially notice a thinning of the hair and a frontal receding hairline that might or might not be accompanied with hair loss at the crown. In women the frontal hairline is maintained with diffuse hair loss that is somewhat accentuated at the crown.

Conditions to eliminate

Telogen effluvium

Telogen effluvium represents a shift of more hairs into the resting phase (telogen) of the hair cycle, which results in shedding of hair. This can be caused by a number of factors:

Postpartum
During pregnancy, circulating levels of oestrogen increase, with a resulting rise in the number of follicles in anagen (growth phase); the hair therefore thickens. However, after delivery the hair follicles return to the

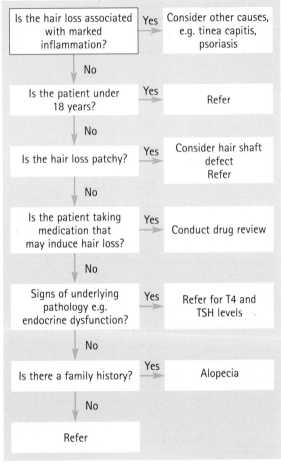

Fig. 7.16 Primer for differential diagnosis of hair loss

Table 7.15 **Specific questions to ask the patient: Hair loss**	
Question	**Relevance**
Hair loss accompanied by other symptoms	• Androgenetic alopecia is not associated with other symptoms. Itch and/or erythema are indicators that another cause, e.g. fungal scalp infection, psoriasis or seborrhoeic dermatitis, might be responsible for the hair loss
Pattern of hair loss	• In men, hair loss begins at the front of the head and recedes backwards or at the crown. In women, hair loss tends to be generalised and diffuse. Presentations that differ from this or are sudden in onset suggest another cause of hair loss
Deficiency states	• There is now strong evidence that iron deficiency in women can cause hair loss
Underlying pathology	• A number of endocrine conditions can cause hair loss, most notably thyroid disorders
Medicine-induced hair loss	• A number of medicines can cause hair loss (see Table 7.16)
Hair loss triggered by a specific event	• Hair loss can be caused by a stressful event or following surgery or after childbirth

resting phase and the hair is shed. Women might believe that they are experiencing hair loss when in reality the hair is returning to the normal prepregnancy state. Reassurance should be given that this is a temporary and self-limiting problem.

Stress

Stress is known to induce hair loss. The reason behind this is poorly understood. Enquiry to ascertain lifestyle factors that might have caused recent stress and anxiety to the patient should be explored.

Nutritional factors

Iron deficiency is associated with female hair loss. If iron deficiency is the cause, a 2-month course of iron supplementation should result in thickening of the hair. If the patient fails to respond to treatment then the patient should be reassessed.

Underlying endocrine disorder

Diabetes mellitus, hypopituitarism and hypothyroidism can result in poor hair growth. In hypothyroidism the hair is thin and brittle and the patient might be lethargic and have a history of recent weight gain. If the patient is currently taking levothyroxine then T4 measurements should be performed to ensure the condition is not being treated subtherapeutically.

Fungal scalp infection (tinea capitis)

The first signs of infection are the appearance of a well-circumscribed round patch of alopecia that is associated with itch and scaling. Common areas of involvement include the occipital, parietal and crown region. Inspection of the area might reveal erythema and 'black dots' on the scalp as a result of infected hairs.

Alopecia areata

This refers to hair loss of unknown origin, although there is often an association with atopy and autoimmune disease and a positive family history is found in up to 25% of patients. It is relatively uncommon affecting 0.1 to 0.2% of the UK population. Unlike androgenetic alopecia the hair loss is sudden and mainly affects children and adolescents (60% will have had their first episode before the age of 20). It most commonly involves only small patches of hair loss although the whole scalp can be affected. The condition is usually self-limiting and regrowth of hair is often observed but repeated episodes are not unusual.

Traction alopecia

Most commonly seen in women, traction alopecia refers to hair loss due to excess and sustained tension on the hair, usually as a result of styling hair with rollers or a

Table 7.16 Medicines known to cause hair loss

Medicine or medicine class	Incidence of hair loss
Antineoplastics	Almost 100% (to varying degrees)
Anticoagulants	Telogen effluvium in approximately 50%
Lithium carbonate	Telogen effluvium in approximately 10%
Interferons	Telogen effluvium in 20 to 30%
Oral contraceptives	Seen 2 to 3 months after stopping
Retinoids	Approximately 20% of patients
Colchicine, carbimazole	Rare

particular type of hairstyle. It is reversible if the tension on the hair is removed.

Medicine-induced causes

Many medicines can interfere with the hair cycle and cause transient hair loss, cytotoxic medicines being one of the most obvious examples. However, many medicines have been associated with hair loss. Table 7.16 lists some of the more commonly implicated medicines. If medicines other than cytotoxics are suspected of causing hair loss, the prescriber should be contacted to discuss other possible treatment options.

Trichotillomania

Trichotillomania is a psychiatric disorder, which refers to patients who have an impulsive desire to twist and pull scalp hair but often deny it. Hair loss is asymmetrical and an unusual shape. It would be very unusual for such patients to present to a community pharmacy.

TRIGGER POINTS indicative of referral: Hair loss

- Fungal infection of the scalp
- Patients under 18
- Possible endocrine cause
- Sudden onset
- Suspected iron deficiency for blood test
- Trichotillomania

Evidence base for over-the-counter medication

Currently, minoxidil is the only product marketed for androgenetic alopecia. It is available as either a 2 or 5% solution.

A number of clinical trials have investigated the efficacy and safety of minoxidil at 2 and 5% concentrations. The majority of these have been conducted on precisely the population that would respond the best to treatment; men aged between 18 and 50, with mild to moderate thinning of the hair at the vertex. Despite this, trial results are not totally convincing. Minoxidil is superior to placebo (although placebo does invoke a large initial response) and promotes a small increase in regrowth of vellus hair and increases the diameter of the hair shaft. However, longitudinal studies show that less than half of patients treated experience moderate to marked hair growth. Hair counts appear to be greatest after 12 months of treatment but, by 30 months, hair counts have decreased (albeit still above baseline) and the bald area increases in size to its initial diameter.

Minoxidil therefore appears to delay and slow down hair loss in less than half of its target patient population. Furthermore, if treatment is stopped any hair growth achieved is lost within 6 to 8 weeks on discontinuation of therapy and baldness returns to pretreatment levels.

The situation in women is not too dissimilar, although the 5% solution offers no advantage over the 2% solution and has therefore not been granted a product licence at that strength.

Summary

Minoxidil will not significantly help the majority of balding individuals. It will promote hair growth in approximately 50% of minimally balding young men but, over time, the effect tails off. After 30 months the effect is still greater than baseline but, on the whole, will not achieve cosmetically acceptable hair growth. In other words the use of minoxidil is useful for specific patients who want to 'buy' themselves time from the inevitable balding process.

Oral finasteride (1 mg per day) is used to treat androgenetic alopecia in men because it has been shown to promote hair growth and prevent further loss in a significant proportion of men with male pattern baldness; up to a third of men will have marked regrowth and a further third moderate regrowth. If treatment with minoxidil is unsatisfactory then the patient could be referred for evaluation by the GP and potentially be given finasteride.

Practical prescribing and product selection

Prescribing information relating to minoxidil is discussed and summarised in Table 7.17; useful tips relating to the treatment of patients with monoxidil are given in Hints and Tips Box 7.5.

Minoxidil (e.g. Regaine Regular (2%) and Extra (5%) Strength and Gel)

The dose for minoxidil solution or gel is 1 mL applied to dry hair to the total affected areas of the scalp twice daily. If fingertips are used to facilitate drug application, hands should be washed afterwards. Although minoxidil is applied topically, absorption into the systemic circulation can occur and result in chest pain, rapid heart beat, faintness or dizziness. If these occur the patient should stop using the product immediately. Other less important

Table 7.17
Practical prescribing: Summary of medicines for hair loss

Name of medicine	Use in children	Likely side effects	Drug interactions of note	Patients in whom care should be exercised	Pregnancy and breast-feeding
Minoxidil (Regaine)	Not applicable	Skin irritation	None	Avoid in hypertensive patients	Avoid

HINTS AND TIPS BOX 7.5: HAIR LOSS

Changes to hair colour and texture	Some patients have experienced changes in hair colour and/or texture with Regaine use. The patient should be warned of this possible problem before using Regaine
How long should the patient use Regaine?	It can take 4 months or more before evidence of hair growth can be expected. Users should discontinue treatment if there is no improvement after 1 year

adverse effects associated with topical minoxidil are local irritation, redness and itching but these appear to be related to the vehicle – propylene glycol – rather than minoxidil. Changes in blood pressure should not occur because the serum level of minoxidil after topical application is below that needed to cause changes to blood pressure; however, as a precaution minoxidil should be avoided in hypertensive patients if possible. Some patients also report a temporary increase in hair shedding 2 to 6 weeks after beginning treatment. This subsides and is most likely due to the action of minoxidil, shifting hairs from the resting telogen phase to the growing anagen phase.

Further reading

Burke KE. Hair loss. What causes it and what can be done about it. Postgrad Med 1989;85:52–8, 67–73, 77.

Hong D, Hart LL. Topical minoxidil for hair loss in women. DICP 1990;24:1062–3.

Katz HI, Hien NT, Prawer SE, et al. Long-term efficacy of topical minoxidil in male pattern baldness. J Am Acad Dermatol 1987;16:711–8.

Koperaki JA, Orenberg EK, Wilkinson DL. Topical minoxidil therapy for androgenetic alopecia: a 30 month study. Arch Dermatol 1987;123:1483–7.

Price VH. Treatment of hair loss. N Engl J Med 1999;341:964–73.

Price VH, Menefee E, Strauss PC. Changes in hair weight and hair count in men with androgenetic alopecia, after application of 5% and 2% topical minoxidil, placebo, or no treatment. J Am Acad Dermatol 1999;41:717–21.

Rietschel RL, Duncan SH. Safety and efficacy of topical minoxidil in the management of androgenetic alopecia. J Am Acad Dermatol 1987;16:677–85.

Roberts JL. Androgenetic alopecia in men and women: an overview of cause and treatment. Dermatol Nurs 1997;9:379–88.

Tosti A, Misciali C, Piraccini BM, et al. Drug-induced hair loss and hair growth: incidence, management and avoidance. Drug Safety 1994;10:310–17.

Web sites

General medical site containing information on hair loss: http://www.nlm.nih.gov/medlineplus/ency/article/003246.htm

Prodigy guidance on alopecia areata: http://cks.library.nhs.uk/alopecia

Hair loss article in The Prescriber (Oct 2001): http://www.escriber.com/Prescriber/Features.asp?ID=319&GroupID=8&Action=View

Warts and verrucas

Background

Warts and verrucas are benign growths of the skin caused by the human papilloma virus (HPV). Certain types of HPV have an affinity for certain body locations, for example hands, face, anogenital region and feet. Spontaneous resolution is seen in 30% of people within 6 months and two-thirds of cases within 2 years. Despite their self-limiting nature they are cosmetically unacceptable to many patients and with nearly 60% of people trying an OTC treatment before visiting a GP the pharmacist has a major role to play in their management.

Prevalence and epidemiology

The prevalence of warts has not been accurately documented and published prevalence data vary widely. However, it is clear children are most affected, having been reported to affect between 2 and 20% of schoolchildren, with a peak incidence in children aged between 12 and 16 years. Warts are uncommon in infants and the elderly and caution should be exercised if an elderly patient presents to the pharmacy with a self-diagnosed wart. One UK study involving 1000 children reported that warts were three times more common than verrucas.

Aetiology

HPV gain entry to the host by epithelial defects in the epidermis. It is transmitted by direct skin-to-skin contact, although contact with an infected person's shed skin can also transmit the virus. Infection via the environment is more likely to occur if the skin is macerated and in contact with roughened surfaces, for example, in swimming pools and communal washing areas. Once established in the epithelial cells, the virus stimulates basal cell division to produce the characteristic lesion.

Patients, especially children, should be warned not to pick, bite or scratch warts as this can allow viral particle shedding to penetrate skin breaks. This process is known as autoinoculation and is responsible for multiple lesions becoming established and transferred to other parts of the body.

Arriving at a differential diagnosis

Warts and verrucas are not difficult to diagnose. However, pharmacists must be able to recognise other similar conditions that superficially look like warts and verrucas. Asking symptom-specific questions will help the pharmacist to determine if referral is needed (Table 7.18). It is worth noting that HPV infections involving the anogenital area are outside the remit of community pharmacists and must be referred.

Clinical features of warts and verrucas

Warts

Warts most often occur on the backs of the hands, fingers and knees, either singly or in crops. When examined the

7

Table 7.18
Specific questions to ask the patient: Human papilloma virus

Question	Relevance
Age of patient	• Warts are unusual in very young children, e.g. infants. Young children and adolescents are most likely to get warts but this is also the age group in which molluscum contagiosum is most prevalent • The likelihood that nodular lesions are caused by seborrhoeic warts or carcinoma increases with increasing age
Location	• Warts are common on the hands and knees; verrucas are usually on the weight-bearing parts of the sole • Warts can occur on the face but so too can plane warts and carcinoma. Referral is always needed as all OTC treatment can cause scarring
Associated symptoms	• Itching and bleeding is not associated with warts and verrucas and must be viewed with suspicion especially in older patients • Pain on walking is often associated with verrucas
Colour/appearance	• Typically warts have a 'cauliflower' appearance and are raised and pale • Warts with a reddish hue or change colour should be referred • Lesions that are raised, smooth and have a central 'dimple' suggests molluscum contagiosum

wart appears as a raised, hyperkeratotic papule with thrombosed, black vessels visible as black dots within the wart. They tend to be rough textured, skin-coloured and are usually less than 1 cm in diameter (Fig. 7.17).

Verrucas

Verrucas are found on the sole of the foot, usually in weight-bearing areas, for example on the metatarsal heads or heel. Owing to constant pressure imparted on the sole of the foot the normal outward expansion of the wart is thwarted and instead grows inward. Pressure on nerves can then cause considerable pain and patients often complain of pain when walking. Inspection of the lesion will normally reveal tiny black dots (thrombosed capillaries) on the surface (Fig. 7.18). Owing to keratin build-up this characteristic sign might not be visible unless the hardened skin is first shaved away. Verrucas, like warts, are rarely larger than 1 cm in diameter and can occur singly or in crops. A number of closely located plantar warts can coalesce to form a large single plaque and this is termed a mosaic wart.

Conditions to eliminate

Plane warts (flat warts or verruca plana)

These most frequently occur in groups on the face and the back of the hands. They are small in size (1 to 5 mm in diameter), slightly raised and can take on the skin colour of the patient (Fig. 7.19). As drug treatment is destructive in nature, plane warts located on the face should be referred to avoid the risk of scarring.

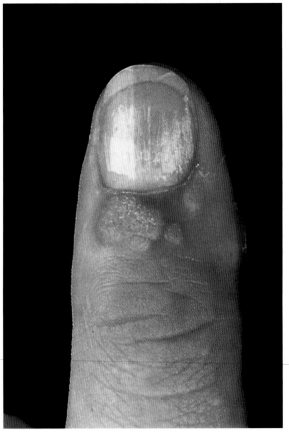

Fig. 7.17 Common wart. Reproduced from *Dermatology in Focus* by J Wilkinson et al, 2005, Churchill Livingstone, with permission

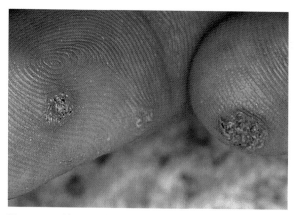

Fig. 7.18 Verruca. Reproduced from *Dermatology: An Illustrated Colour Text* by D J Gawrodger, 2008, Churchill Livingstone, with permission

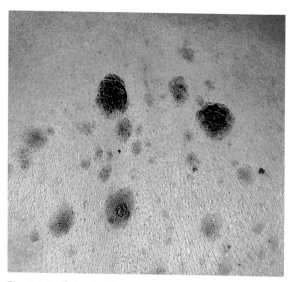

Fig. 7.20 Seborrhoeic wart. Reproduced from *Dermatology: An Illustrated Colour Text* by D J Gawrodger, 2008, Churchill Livingstone, with permission

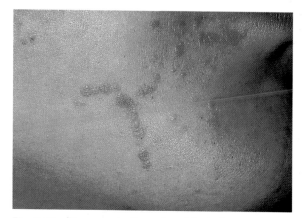

Fig. 7.19 Plane warts. Reproduced from *Dermatology: An Illustrated Colour Text* by D J Gawrodger, 2008, Churchill Livingstone, with permission

Molluscum contagiosum

Molluscum contagiosum primarily affects children under 5 years old. It is not particularly common and a GP with a list size of 2000 will probably see 5 new cases per year. It is caused by a pox virus and patients present with multiple lesions usually on the face and neck, although the trunk can be involved. The lesions resemble common warts but each raised papule tends to be smooth and have a central dimple, the latter is a useful diagnostic point (see Fig. 9.6, page 284). Lesions tend to be between 1 and 5 mm in diameter. The condition is self-limiting and will resolve without medical intervention. Patients should be told this, but if they believe treatment is necessary, referral to the GP is advisable. Cryotherapy or imiquimod might be considered.

Corns

Corns and plantar warts can be confused. The reader is referred to page 214 on corns and calluses for information on differentiating corns from verrucas.

Basal cell papilloma (seborrhoeic wart)

Basal cell papillomas are benign growths that are increasingly common with increasing age. They usually occur on the trunk and present as raised, often multiple lesions that have a superficial 'stuck on' or waxy appearance (Fig. 7.20). Lesion colour can range from pink to black but they are often brown.

Basal cell carcinoma

Basal cell carcinoma is the commonest form of skin cancer and its incidence is related to sunlight exposure. It typically occurs in older age groups and there is a history of prolonged sun exposure. Men are twice as likely to be affected. The usual site where lesions develop is the face. Any wart-like lesion that is itchy, has an irregular outline, is prone to bleeding and exhibits colour change should be referred to eliminate serious pathology. For more information on skin cancers see page 232.

> **❗ TRIGGER POINTS indicative of referral: Warts and verrucas**
>
> - Anogenital warts
> - Diabetic patients
> - Lesions on the face
> - Multiple and widespread warts
> - Patients aged over 50 presenting with a first-time wart
> - Warts that itch or bleed without provocation
> - Warts that have grown and changed colour

Evidence base for over-the-counter medication

A number of ingredients can be used to treat warts and verrucas; however, salicylic acid is the most commonly used agent and can be found in many OTC treatments both alone and combined with lactic acid or podophyllum. The concentration of salicylic acid in proprietary preparations varies widely from 11 to 50%.

A recent Cochrane review (Gibbs et al 2006) investigated topical treatments for the cure of warts. This review identified 60 trials that met their inclusion criteria. Overall, the quality of the trials was low due to poor methodology and reporting. However, placebo was found to have a substantial effect although salicylic acid in comparison was significantly more effective. Cure rates for salicylic acid (from pooled data) showed 73% cure rates compared to control cure rates of 48% over a 6- to 12-week period. However, there appears to be no evidence to suggest which concentration of salicylic acid is most effective.

In addition, there is some evidence to show that common warts are more responsive to keratolytic therapy than plantar warts and resolution might be enhanced by soaking the wart or verruca prior to application and/or occlusion of the site (by use of plasters or collodion-like vehicle) to aid penetration.

Compliance with treatment has been identified as a limiting factor in the cure rate for warts and verrucas. One study that investigated Occlusal reported an 80% cure rate after only 2 weeks of therapy. This might be an alternative option for patients whose compliance could be questioned. However, the study suffered from poor design and had only a small number of patients and the results must be viewed with caution.

Salicylic acid is often combined with other ingredients, in particular lactic acid. However, there is no evidence to support additional efficacy when lactic acid is added. Monochloroacetic acid has also been combined with salicylic acid. Cure rates for this combination are comparable to cure rates of salicylic acid alone or when monochloroacetic acid is used singly. It therefore appears that the combination has no additional benefit to when active ingredients are used as monotherapy. As far as the author is aware, no commercially available preparation contains monochloroacetic acid.

Other agents commercially available include formaldehyde, gluteraldehyde, podophyllum resin and silver nitrate pencils. Information regarding their effectiveness stems from either small-scale or poorly designed studies, and their use should therefore be relegated to second-line choices. However, it should be noted that cure rates reported with these agents were equal if not better than those reported with salicylic acid.

Until recently, cryotherapy was a treatment option that was only available via the GP. However, there is now a commercially available product OTC (Wartner).

Evidence suggests cryotherapy is effective but not clinically superior to salicylic acid.

Summary

Any salicylic acid-based product should have modest success rates in clearing warts and verrucas after a 12-week treatment period, providing patient compliance is good. If treatment has been unsuccessful with salicylic acid then a second-line medicine such as glutaraldehyde, formaldehyde or podophyllum could be tried. Cryotherapy is probably still best left to the GP to perform rather than the patient.

Practical prescribing and product selection

Prescribing information relating to specific products used to treat warts and verrucas in the section 'Evidence base for over-the-counter medication' is summarised in Table 7.19; useful tips relating to patients presenting with warts and verrucas are given in Hints and Tips Box 7.6.

As the majority of warts and verrucas will spontaneously resolve after 2 years, treatment is not necessarily needed. Pharmacists should determine from the patient how much the wart or verruca affects day-to-day life and also what social impact the lesions have on the patient. It is also worth assessing patient motivation to comply with medication regimes because treatment is over a period of months not days or weeks.

Salicylic acid products (e.g. Compound W (17%), Bazuka Extra Strength (26%), Occlusal (26%), Verrugon (50%), Wartex (50%)) and salicylic acid/lactic acid combinations (Bazuka, Cuplex, Duofilm, Salactol, Salactac)

There is a wide choice of salicylic acid-based products for the removal of warts, verrucas (and corns). Prior to using a salicylic acid-based product the affected area should be soaked in warm water and towelled dry. The surface of the wart or verruca should be rubbed with a pumice stone or emery board to remove any hard skin. This should be done at least once per week. A few drops of the product should be applied to the lesion, taking care to localise the application to the affected area. The procedure should be repeated daily. Salicylic acid can be recommended to most patients, although those with diabetes are a notable exception. Salicylic acid does not interact with any medicines. It can cause local skin irritation and because of its destructive action should be kept away from unaffected skin.

Glutaraldehyde (Glutarol)

Application of glutaraldehyde is the same as salicylic acid but it should be used twice a day. It can cause skin irritation and stains the outer layer of the skin brown.

Table 7.19
Practical prescribing: Summary of medicines for warts and verrucas

7

Name of medicine	Use in children	Likely side effects	Drug interactions of note	Patients in whom care should be exercised	Pregnancy and breast-feeding
Salicylic acid					
Compound W	>6 years	Local skin irritation	None	Avoid in diabetic patients	OK
Bazuka Extra Strength	No lower age stated				
Occlusal					
Verrugon					
Wartex					
Salicylic acid and lactic acid					
Bazuka	No lower age stated	Local skin irritation	None	Avoid in diabetic patients	OK
Cuplex					
Duofilm	>2 years				
Salactol	No lower age stated				
Salatac					
Glutaraldehyde					
Glutarol	No lower age stated	Local skin irritation. Skin will be stained brown	None	Avoid in diabetic patients	OK
Formaldehyde					
Veracur	No lower age stated	No local effects reported	None	Avoid in diabetic patients	Manufacturer advises avoidance, although there are no reports of teratogenicity
Posalfilin	No lower age stated	Local skin irritation	None	Avoid in diabetic patients	Avoid
Silver nitrate (Avoca)	No lower age stated	Local skin irritation	None	Avoid in diabetic patients	OK

HINTS AND TIPS BOX 7.6: VERRUCAS AND WARTS

Is it a verruca or a corn?	If diagnosis is uncertain then removal of the top layer of skin from the lesion can be performed. If black spots are not visible this implies the lesion is a corn and not a verruca
Length of treatment	Patients should be told that it is a slow process. Treatment commonly lasts 3 months. If OTC medication has been unsuccessful after this time then the patient could be referred to the GP
Salatac gel	The gel forms an elastic film after application. This has to be removed each time before the gel can be reapplied
Bazuka and Bazuka Extra Strength	Don't be fooled into thinking the extra strength has better cure rates. It has a higher concentration of salicylic acid (26% as opposed to 12%) but this does not necessarily equate to a more efficacious product

Formaldehyde (Veracur)

Veracur is marketed particularly for verrucas and, like glutaraldehyde, is applied twice a day. In all other respects it has the same side effects and precautions for use as salicylic acid.

Posalfilin (Podophyllum Resin BP and 25% salicylic acid)

Posalfilin is licensed for verrucas only. As with all other products containing salicylic acid, it must not be used in diabetic patients; however, it is also contraindicated in pregnancy and breast-feeding because podophyllum is cytotoxic and possesses teratogenic properties. To apply the ointment, a corn ring should be placed around the verruca and a minimal amount of ointment applied onto the verruca. The verruca and corn ring should be covered with a plaster and the treatment repeated daily.

Silver nitrate (e.g Avoca)

To use silver nitrate pencils the tip must be first moistened and then applied to the wart or verruca for 1 to 2 minutes. This should be repeated after 24 hours. It is recommended that three applications are used for warts and six applications for verrucas. Like other treatments the process is destructive and the surrounding skin should be protected.

Further reading

Ahmed I. Management of viral warts in primary care. The Prescriber 5 May 2001:43–54.

Bunney MH, Nolan MW, Williams DA. An assessment of methods of treating viral warts by comparative treatment trials based on a standard design. Br J Dermatol 1976;94:667–79.

Cobb MW. Human papillomavirus infection. J Am Acad Dermatol 1990;22:547–66.

Gibbs S, Harvey I. Topical treatments for cutaneous warts. Cochrane Database of Systematic Reviews 2006, issue 3.

Hirose R, Hori M, Shukuwa T et al. Topical treatment of resistant warts with glutaraldehyde. J Dermatol 1994;21:248–53.

Johnson LW. Communal showers and the risk of plantar warts. J Fam Pract 1995;40:136–8.

Steele K, Irwin WG. Liquid nitrogen and salicylic/lactic acid paint in the treatment of cutaneous warts in general practice. J R Coll Gen Pract 1988;38:256–8.

Steele K, Shirodaria P, O'Hare M et al. Monochloroacetic acid and 60% salicylic acid as a treatment for simple plantar warts: effectiveness and mode of action. Br J Dermatol 1988;118:537–43.

Yazar S, Basaran E. Efficacy of silver nitrate pencils in the treatment of common warts. J Dermatol 1994;21:329–33.

Web sites

British Association of Dermatologists – information on seborrhoeic warts: http://www.bad.org.uk/patients/skin_disorders/seborrhoeic/index.htm

Prodigy guidance on warts and verrucas: http://cks.library.nhs.uk/warts_including_verrucas

Effectiveness and cost-effectiveness of salicylic acid and cryotherapy for cutaneous warts. An economic decision model – A Health Technology Assessment Monograph: http://www.nelm.nhs.uk/Record%20Viewing/viewRecord.aspx?id=567931 and http://www.nelm.nhs.uk/Record%20Viewing/viewRecord.aspx?id=567931

Corns and calluses

Background

In general, people do not tend to give their feet the care they deserve. It is estimated that on average a person walks the equivalent of 1000 miles a year. It is therefore hardly surprising that people experience foot problems. Foot disorders can be broadly subdivided into either those that result from opportunistic infection or those resulting from incorrect distribution of pressure. This section discusses the latter.

Prevalence and epidemiology

The exact prevalence of corns and calluses is not known. Surveys have indictated that up to 18% of working people complain of corns and calluses (Springett et al 2003). Corns and calluses tend to be seen more often in older patients.

Aetiology

Corns form due to a combination of friction and intermittent pressure against one of the bony prominences of the feet (e.g. heel and metatarsal heads). Inappropriate footwear is frequently the cause. Continued pressure and friction results in hyperkeratoses (excessive skin growth of the keratinised layer) leaving even less space between the shoe and the foot and therefore the corn is pressed even more firmly against the underlying soft tissues and bone.

Callus formation is also caused by constant friction and pressure. Calluses can be beneficial, providing a natural barrier to objects and protecting underlying tissues; however, when such a thickened mass of skin occurs in abnormal places (e.g. border of the big toe) pain is experienced.

Arriving at a differential diagnosis

Diagnosis of corns and calluses is best done by appearance. Pharmacists should therefore ask to inspect the person's feet because trying to take a description of what the problem looks like can be difficult. This might be met with resistance from patients, although use of consultation rooms should make examination easier.

Differential diagnosis should be straightforward and is usually between corns, calluses and verrucas. Most patients will accurately self-diagnose and seek advice and help to remedy the situation. The pharmacist's role will be to confirm the self-diagnosis and give advice and/or treatment where appropriate. Asking symptom-specific questions will help the pharmacist to determine the best course of action (Table 7.20).

Clinical features of corns

Corns (helomas) have been classified into a number of types, although only soft and hard corns are commonly met in practice. Hard corns (heloma durum) are generally located on the top of the toes. Corns exhibit a central core of hard grey skin surrounded by a painful, raised, yellow ring of inflammatory skin. Any of the toes can be affected but it is commonest on the second toe. Soft corns (heloma molle) form between the toes rather than on the tops of toes and are due to pressure exerted by one toe against another. They have a whitened appearance and remain soft due to moisture being always present between the toes, which causes maceration of the corn. Soft corns are most common in the fourth web space.

Clinical features of calluses

Calluses, depending on the cause and site involved, can range in size from a few millimetres to centimetres. They appear as flattened, yellow-white and thickened skin. In women, the balls of the feet are a common site as a result of prolonged wearing of ill-fitting high-heeled shoes. Other sites that can be affected are the heel and lower border of the big toe. Patients frequently complain of a burning sensation resulting from fissuring of the callus.

Conditions to eliminate

Verrucas

Verrucas can be mistaken for a corn or callus, although verrucas tend to have a spongy texture with the central area showing tiny black spots. They are also rarely located on or between the toes and are more common in younger patients than corns and calluses. For further information see page 210.

Bunions

Bunions are 10 times more common in women than men and are directly related to wearing tight shoes. Initially, irritation of skin by ill-fitting shoes causes bursitis of the big toe. Over time the inflamed area begins to harden and subsequently bursal fluid solidifies into a gelatinous mass. The result will be a bunion joint (the first metatarsal phalangeal joint). Patients often complain of pain, have difficulty in wearing normal shoes and walking. Referral to a podiatrist is recommended.

 TRIGGER POINTS indicative of referral: Corns and calluses

Initially a patient should be referred to a podiatrist if:

- Discomfort/pain is causing difficulty in walking
- Impaired peripheral circulation, e.g. diabetes
- Soft corns
- Treatment failure

Evidence base for over-the-counter medication

Corns and calluses are due to friction and pressure. Removal of the precipitating factors will result in

 Table 7.20
Specific questions to ask the patient: Corn/callus

Question	Relevance
Location	• Lesions on the tops or between the toes suggest a corn compared with verrucas, which are on the plantar surface of the foot
Aggravating or relieving factors	• Pain experienced with corns is a result of pressure between footwear and the toes. If footwear is taken off the pain is relieved • Pain associated with verrucas will be felt irrespective of whether footwear is worn
Appearance	• Corns and calluses appear as white or yellow hyperkeratinised areas of skin unlike verrucas, which show black thrombosed capillaries seen as black dots on the surface of the verruca
Previous history	• Patients will often have a previous history of foot problems. The cause is usually due to poorly fitting shoes, such as high heels. Prolonged wear of such footwear can lead to calluses and permanent deformity of bunions

resolution of the problem. Therefore, preventative measures should form the mainstay of treatment. Correctly fitting shoes are essential to help prevent corn and callus formation. If pressure and friction still persist when correctly fitted shoes are worn then patients can obtain relief by shielding or padding. Moleskin or thin podiatry felt placed around the corn allows pressure to be transferred from the corn to the padding. Specific proprietary products are available for such purposes. In callus formation a 'shock absorbing' insert such as a metatarsal pad is useful to relieve weight off the callus and so reduce stress on the plantar skin.

Treatment should be avoided if possible, but if deemed appropriate keratolytics can be used although there is no evidence to suggest that they are effective.

Practical prescribing and product selection

Products used to treat corns and calluses are exactly the same as those used for warts and verrucas. Prescribing information relating to specific products used to treat corns and calluses is therefore discussed in the section 'Evidence base for over-the-counter medication' for warts and verrucas on page 212. See also Hints and Tips Box 7.7. However, a number of proprietary products are marketed for sufferers with corns and calluses, for example, products in the Carnation and Scholl ranges. These products contain high concentrations of salicylic acid that are surrounded by a non-medicated self-adhesive ring

Further reading
Robbins JM. Recognizing, treating and preventing common foot problems. Cleve Clin J Med 2000;67:45–56.
Silfverskiold JP. Common foot problems. Relieving the pain of bunions, keratoses, corns and calluses. Postgrad Med. 1991;89:183–8.
Springett K, Whiting M, Marriott C. Epidemiology of plantar forefoot corns and callus, and the influence of dominant side. The Foot 2003;13:5–9.

Scabies

Background

Scabies can be defined as a pruritic skin condition caused by the mite *Sarcoptes scabiei*. It is easily missed or misdiagnosed as dermatitis. The diagnostic burrows are small and difficult to locate because they are often obscured by the effects of scratching.

Prevalence and epidemiology

Scabies is not gender- or age-specific. Infants to the elderly can acquire the infestation, although it is more common in the elderly. Outbreaks in schools and care homes are not uncommon. The incidence of scabies in the UK is low but epidemics can occur on a cyclical basis approximately every 15 years. In temperate climates (e.g. the UK), it appears to be more prevalent in urban areas and in the winter months.

Aetiology

The mite is usually transmitted by direct physical contact (e.g. holding hands, hugging or sexual contact). Rarely, it can be caught from bed linen because the mite can survive away from human skin for 24 to 36 hours at room temperature. The female mite burrows into the stratum corneum to lay eggs. The faecal pellets she leaves in the burrow cause a local hypersensitivity reaction and this is assumed to cause the release of inflammatory mediators that trigger an allergic reaction invoking intense itching. This normally takes 15 to 20 days in a primary infestation but can take up to 6 weeks to develop. In subsequent infestations this hypersensitivity reaction develops much more quickly. During the asymptomatic period the mite can be passed onto others unknowingly. The eggs hatch and mature in 14 days, after which the cycle can begin again.

Arriving at a differential diagnosis

The diagnosis of scabies is confirmed by extraction of the mite from its burrow, although in primary care this is rarely performed and a differential diagnosis is made on clinical appearance, patient history and symptoms reported by close family. Confusion can arise from mistaking scabies for other pruritic skin disorders such as allergic contact dermatitis or dermatitis herpetiformis, especially when the condition is extensive. Asking symptom-specific questions will help the pharmacist to determine the best course of action (Table 7.21).

Clinical features of scabies

Severe pruritus, especially at night, is the hallmark symptom of scabies. Besides classic location of lesions, in men the penile and scrotal skin and in women beneath the breasts and nipples can be affected. Infants who are not yet walking may have marked sole involvement. The rash is usually made up of small red papules that over time can change into vesicles.

7

Table 7.21
Specific questions to ask the patient: Scabies

Question	Relevance
Visible signs of the mite	• Burrows, which are up to 1 cm long and blue-grey in colour, might be visible although in practice this characteristic is often not present. For the pharmacist, who will only see a limited number of cases, it is best to concentrate on other clinical signs rather than attempt to look for signs of burrows
Location of rash	• Scabies classically affects the finger webs, the sides of the fingers and wrists. Hand involvement is rare in dermatitis herpetiformis
History of presenting complaint	• If contact dermatitis is suspected then questioning should reveal a past history of similar skin lesions • Often people with scabies will be care workers looking after institutionalised people • A positive history in other family members increases the likelihood that the patient has scabies

Conditions to eliminate

Insect bites

A host of insects, fleas and mites can inflict a bite or sting. This usually results in an itchy papule that can become firm and last several days. Occasionally, the rash can become blistered, normally as a result of scratching, and secondary bacterial infection can occur. Bites often tend to be in groups and are asymmetrical. See Chapter 10, pages 306–307 for further information.

Allergic contact dermatitis

The condition presents as an area of inflamed, itchy skin with either papules or vesicles being present. However, enquiry into the patient's history should reveal a past history of similar lesions in allergic contact dermatitis. For further information on dermatitis see page 226.

Dishydrotic eczema (Pompholyx)

Pompholyx simply means bubble and refers to the presence of intensely itchy vesicles or blisters on the palms of the hands and occasionally on the soles of the feet. Stress is known to precipitate the condition.

Dermatitis herpetiformis

Dermatitis herpetiformis is a condition characterised by intense itchy clusters of papules and vesicles. It is more often seen in middle-aged people, especially men. It commonly involves the buttocks, elbows, knees and sacral region. The lesions usually exhibit a symmetrical distribution and hand involvement is rare. On investigation up to 90% of patients are found to have a gluten enteropathy.

 TRIGGER POINTS indicative of referral: Scabies

• Severe and extensive symptoms
• Suspected dermatitis herpetiformis

Evidence base for over-the-counter medication

The efficacy and safety of scabicidal agents is difficult to determine due to limited trial data. Benzyl benzoate, crotamiton, permethrin and malathion have all been used. A Cochrane review (Walker et al 2000) and a subsequent study by Usha et al (2000) found permethrin to have cure rates of 90% or higher. The Cochrane review also compared permethrin with other scabicidal agents and concluded that it was superior to crotamiton in relieving itching and parasite clearance. When compared to gamma benzene hexachloride (also known as lindane – this was withdrawn from the UK market in 1995 because of concerns about possible adverse effects) in two small trials it appeared to have a better clinical cure rate, although a larger trial found no difference.

The efficacy of malathion is questionable as no random controlled trials appear to have been conducted. However, case reports have suggested malathion is effective in curing scabies with a cure rate of approximately 80%.

Benzyl benzoate has been used to treat scabies for many years. However, its efficacy has not been demonstrated in randomised controlled trials. In uncontrolled trials benzyl benzoate has been shown to provide cure rates of approximately 50%. Unfortunately, up to 25% of patients experience side effects such as burning, irritation and itching on application.

Summary

On current evidence, permethrin (Lyclear dermal cream) is the medicine of choice as it has the highest cure rate, resistance appears rare and is associated with minimal side effects. Malathion 0.5% aqueous liquid should be reserved as a second-line treatment. Benzyl benzoate and crotamiton should be avoided where possible. However, crotamiton can be used to relieve the itch caused by scabies.

Practical prescribing and product selection

Prescribing information relating to specific products used to treat scabies in the section 'Evidence base for over-the-counter medication' is discussed and summarised in Table 7.22; useful tips relating to patients presenting with scabies are given in Hints and Tips Box 7.8.

It is important that all people in the same household and close contacts are treated at the same time to prevent re-infection even though they might be asymptomatic (latent period before itch develops) and treatment should be repeated after 7 days. Current recommendations are that the head and neck should be treated. (This is at odds with some manufacturers' advice who recommend application to the body but to exclude the head and neck.)

All products for scabies can be used by all patient groups and have no drug interactions.

Permethrin (Lyclear Dermal Cream)

Permethrin is suitable for use by adults and children over 2 months of age, although the summary of product characteristics (SPC) states that for children under the age of 2 years medical supervision is required. Interpretation of what constitutes medical supervision is unclear and the manufacturer was unable to give the author a definitive response. General guidance for application of Lyclear is that adults and children over 12 should use up to a full tube as a single application. Some adults might need to use more than one tube to ensure total body coverage, but a maximum of two tubes (60 g in total) is recommended for a single application. For children under 12 the manufacturers suggest the following: 2 months to 1 year should use up to $\frac{1}{8}$ of a tube, children aged between 1 and 5 years, up to $\frac{1}{4}$ of a tube and for those aged between 6 and 12 years, $\frac{1}{2}$ a tube. The whole body should be washed thoroughly 8 to 12 hours after treatment.

Malathion (Derbac M and Quellada M liquid)

Of the malathion products marketed, only Derbac M and Quellada M have a licensed indication for the treatment of scabies.

The liquid can be used on adults and children over 6 months old and is left on for 24 hours. If hands, or any other parts of the body must be washed during this period, the treatment must be reapplied to those areas immediately.

Benzyl benzoate (e.g. Ascabiol)

Benzyl benzoate can be used by adults and children, although recommendations (*British National Formulary*

Table 7.22
Practical prescribing: Summary of medicines for scabies

Name of medicine	Use in children	Likely side effects	Drug interactions of note	Patients in whom care should be exercised	Pregnancy and breast-feeding
Permethrin	>2 months	Burning, stinging or tingling	None	None	OK
Benzyl benzoate	>12 years	Burning, irritation			
Crotamiton	>3 years	Skin irritation reported			
Malathion Derbac M Quellada M	>6 months	Skin irritation but rare			

HINTS AND TIPS BOX 7.8: SCABIES

Itching after treatment	Pruritus can persist for 2 to 3 weeks after treatment and the patient might benefit from crotamiton. Antihistamines appear to have a limited role in relieving itch but their sedative effect (e.g. chlorphenamine) might be useful for temporary help in aiding sleep
Hygiene measures	Clothes, towels and bed linen should be machine-washed (at 50°C or above) after the first application of treatment, to prevent reinfestation and transmission to others
Bathing	Treatment should not be applied after a hot bath because this increases systemic absorption and removes the drug from its treatment site

edition 55) state it should be avoided in children. This is because dilution is advocated in children to lessen irritation but it also reduces its efficacy. If the application is thorough, one treatment should suffice, but the possibility of failure is lessened if a second application is made within 5 days of the first. Alternatively, benzyl benzoate can be applied to the whole body, on three occasions, at 12-hourly intervals.

There are no reports of teratogenicity, although the manufacturers of Ascabiol recommend it should be avoided wherever practicable and breast-feeding suspended until after the treatment is complete. The main drawback with benzyl benzoate is its side effects. It causes skin irritation and a transient burning sensation. This is usually mild but can occasionally be severe in sensitive individuals. In the event of a severe skin reaction the preparation should be washed off using soap and warm water. Ascabiol is also irritating to the eyes, which should be protected if it is applied to the scalp.

Crotamiton (Eurax)

Eurax should be rubbed into the entire body surface once a day for between three and five consecutive days for adults and children over the age of 3. It can cause irritation on application.

Further reading

Angarano DW, Parish LC. Comparative dermatology: parasitic disorders. Clin Dermatol 1994;12:543–50.

Buffet M, Dupin N. Current treatments for scabies. Fundam Clin Pharmacol 2003;17:217–25.

Burgess I, Robinson R, Robinson J, et al. Aqueous malathion 0.5% as a scabicide: clinical trial. Br Med J 1986;292:1172.

Chosidow O. Clinical practices. Scabies. New Engl J Med 2006;354:1718–27.

Glaziou P, Cartel JL, Alzieu P, et al. Comparison of ivermectin and benzyl benzoate for treatment of scabies. Trop Med Parasitol 1993;44:331–2.

Hanna NF, Clay JC, Harris JR. *Sarcoptes scabiei* infestation treated with malathion liquid. Br J Vener Dis 1978;54:354.

Johnston G, Sladden M. Scabies: diagnosis and treatment. Br Med J 2005;331:619–22.

Usha V, Gopalakrishnan Nair TV. A comparative study of oral ivermectin and topical permethrin cream in the treatment of scabies. J Am Acad Dermatol 2000;42;236–40.

Walker GJA, Johnstone PW. Interventions for treating scabies. Cochrane Database of Systematic Reviews 2000, issue 3.

Web sites

Prodigy guidance: http://www.cks.library.nhs.uk/scabies

New York State Department of Health and Communicable Disease Fact Sheet: http://www.health.state.ny.us/nysdoh/consumer/scabies.htm

For images of scabies visit: http://www.dermis.net/index_e.html

Acne vulgaris

Background

Acne can be defined as an inflammatory disease of the pilosebaceous follicles causing comedones, papules and pustules on the face (99% of cases), chest (60%) and upper back (15%). It affects virtually all adolescents, to varying degrees of severity, and usually appears at the time of puberty. Diagnosis is usually straightforward and most patients presenting in the community pharmacy will generally be seeking appropriate advice on correct product selection rather than wanting someone to put a name to their rash. The majority of cases seen in the pharmacy setting will be mild and can be managed appropriately without referral to the GP. However, more persistent and severe cases need referral for more potent topical or systemic treatment. Acne often causes significant psychological impact such as lack of confidence, low self-esteem and depression.

Prevalence and epidemiology

Acne lesions develop at the onset of puberty. Girls therefore tend to develop acne at an earlier age than boys. The peak incidence for girls is between the ages of 14 and 17 compared with 15 to 19 years of age for boys. Although acne is closely associated with adolescence up to 5% of women and 1% of men aged 25 to 40 either continue to get acne or develop acne (late-onset acne) after adolescence. There might be a familial tendency to acne and it is slightly more common in boys, who also experience more severe involvement. In addition, white patients are more likely to experience moderate to severe acne than black patients, although black skin is prone to worse scarring.

Aetiology

At the onset of puberty a cascade of events takes place resulting in the formation of non-inflammatory and inflammatory lesions. In response to increased testosterone levels, the pilosebaceous gland begins to produce sebum (if the sebaceous glands become oversensitive to testosterone they produce excess oil and the skin becomes greasy; a hallmark of acne). At the same time epithelial cells lining the follicle undergo change. Prior to puberty dead cells are shed smoothly out of the ductal opening but at puberty this process is disrupted and in patients with acne these cells develop abnormal cohesion and partially block the opening and effectively reduce sebum outflow. Over time the opening of the duct becomes blocked trapping oil in the hair follicle. Bacteria, particularly *Propionibacterium acnes*, proliferate in the stagnant oil stimulating cytokine production, which in turn produces local inflammation leading to the appearance

Question	Relevance
Severity	• Mild acne – consists mainly of non-inflammatory comedones • Moderate acne – can be described as having many inflammatory spots that are not confined to the face. Lesions are often painful and there is a real possibility of scarring • Severe acne – has all the characteristics of moderate acne plus the development of nodules and cysts. Lesions are often widespread involving the upper back and chest. Scarring will usually result
Age of onset	• Patients presenting with acne-type lesions who fall outside the normal age range should be closely questioned. Adverse drug reactions and rosacea should be considered
Occupation	• Certain jobs can predispose patients to acne-like lesions and acne is commonly associated with long-term contact with oils

Table 7.23
Specific questions to ask the patient: Acne vulgaris

of a spot. In response to the proliferation of bacteria white blood cells infiltrate the area to kill the bacteria and in turn die leading to pus formation. The pustule eventually bursts on the skin surface, carrying the plug away. The whole process then starts again.

Arriving at a differential diagnosis

Up to 60% of affected people seek treatment for acne with a substantial proportion self-medicating rather than consulting their GP. Differential diagnosis of acne is routine and should not be difficult. The pharmacist will, however, need to assess the severity of the acne. Several rating scales have been developed with the aim of trying to grade the severity of an individual's condition. None have gained universal acceptance although most dermatology texts simply grade the severity of acne into mild, moderate or severe. Asking symptom-specific questions will help the pharmacist to determine if referral is needed (Table 7.23).

Clinical features of mild acne vulgaris

Patients suffering from mild acne characteristically have predominate open and closed comedones with a small number of active lesions normally confined to the face.

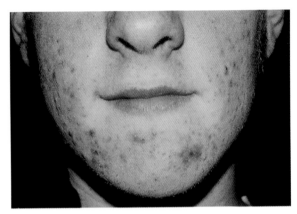

Fig. 7.21 Mild acne. Reproduced from *20 Common Problems in Dermatology* by A Fleischer et al, 2000, with permission of the McGraw-Hill Companies

Mild acne will not cause permanent scarring (Fig. 7.21). Acne can sometimes consist predominately of blackheads and whiteheads with very few inflammatory lesions. This is termed comedonal acne and occurs most commonly in Asian and Afro-Caribbean patients.

Conditions to eliminate

Rosacea

Rosacea is an inflammatory disease of the skin follicles. It is uncertain what causes rosacea although successful treatment with antibiotics suggests that bacterial pathogens play a significant role in the disease. It is normally seen in patients over 40 years of age and is classically characterised by recurrent flushing and blushing of the central face especially the nose and medial cheeks. Crops of inflammatory papules and pustules are also a common feature, although comedones are not present (Fig. 7.22). Eye irritation and blepharitis is present in about 20% of rosacea patients.

Medicines causing acne-like skin eruptions

A number of medicines can produce acne-like lesions and include lithium, oral contraceptives (especially those with high progestogen levels), phenytoin, azathioprine, rifampicin and steroids.

Perioral dermatitis

Perioral dermatitis tends to affect young women aged between 25 and 40 and exhibits an acne-like rash generally around the mouth and nasolabial folds (Fig. 7.23). Itching and burning can also be present and the rash can take on a dermatitis-like quality.

Polycystic ovary syndrome

A clinical manifestation of this condition can be acne vulgaris. Any patient that also exhibits hirsuitism, is

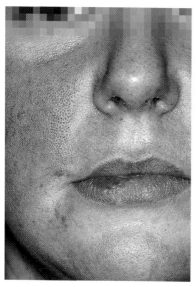

Fig. 7.22   Rosacea. Reproduced from *Dermatology in Focus* by J Wilkinson et al, 2005, Churchill Livingstone, with permission

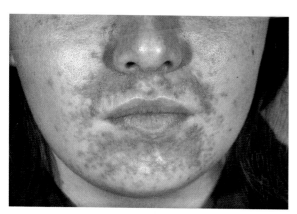

Fig. 7.23   Perioral dermatitis. Reproduced from *Dermatology in Focus* by J Wilkinson et al, 2005, Churchill Livingstone, with permission

overweight and has menstrual irregularity must be referred for further investigation.

 TRIGGER POINTS indicative of referral: Acne

- Moderate or severe acne
- Occupational acne
- OTC treatment failure
- Patients over 25 presenting for the first time
- Rosacea

Evidence base for over-the-counter medication

The aim of treatment must be to clear the lesions and prevent scarring. Mild acne can be managed OTC but it

is important to show understanding and empathy when advising patients. Acne is predominantly a condition that affects adolescents, a time when appearance is all-important. It is worth taking a few minutes to counsel patients about their condition, ally fears and make sure their expectations of treatment are realistic.

OTC acne treatments contain either benzoyl peroxide, salicylic acid, sulphur, nicotinamide or an antibacterial.

Benzoyl peroxide

Benzoyl peroxide exerts its main effect by reducing the concentration of *Propionibacterium acnes*. Additionally, it has slight anti-inflammatory and mild anticomedogenic effects. Many studies have investigated the efficacy of benzoyl peroxide. It has been proven to be effective, especially in mild to moderate acne. However, there is no evidence to suggest that 10% benzoyl peroxide is more effective than lower strengths. Therefore, because of its potential to cause erythema and irritation, concentrations of 10% should probably be avoided.

A variety of other agents have been compared against or in combination with benzoyl peroxide. None of these products has been shown to be significantly better than benzoyl peroxide alone. For example, the addition of miconazole 2% (Acnidazil) was shown to be no more effective than benzoyl peroxide alone despite manufacturer claims to the contrary. Likewise, when Quinoderm was compared to Quinoderm HC (benzoyl peroxide and hydrocortisone) no significant differences in efficacy were observed.

Evidence of efficacy for salicylic acid and sulphur is poor. Both agents have been used for many years on the basis of their keratolytic action but on current evidence they are best avoided. Nicontinamide (Nicam) is a more recent addition to the products available OTC. Trial data for nicotinamide suggest it is as effective as clindamycin 1% gel but because of the paucity of trial data, UK guidance (e.g. Prodigy) currently do not recommend its use.

CAM treatments

Evidence is lacking to support the use of CAM. Reviews of CAM to treat acne report studies that were small in size and of poor quality. In one trial, the herb *Ocimum gratissimum* was compared with benzoyl peroxide and placebo. However, because various concentrations were investigated, the number of patients in each group was too small to allow any firm conclusions. A further trial that compared tea tree oil with benzoyl peroxide lacked a placebo group and was underpowered, yet benzoyl peroxide was more effective than tea tree oil. Another study, which compared gluconolactone versus benzoyl peroxide, found gluconolactone to be better than placebo but not significantly different from benzoyl peroxide.

HINTS AND TIPS BOX 7.9: ACNE

Myths surrounding acne	Sunshine helps reduce acne – there is no convincing evidence that this is the case Poor hygiene causes acne – there is no evidence that improved cleaning of the skin improves acne Chocolate causes spots. There is no proof that any food causes acne Stress causes acne. Stress cannot cause acne although it can make it worse
Applying benzoyl peroxide	Benzoyl peroxide has a potent bleaching effect. It has the ability to permanently bleach clothing and bed linen. Patients should be advised to always wash their hands after applying the product
Formulation	Choice should take into account patient preference but: • Gels and solutions might be useful in patients with oily skin because they have a drying effect • Creams might suit those with dry skin • Lotions are useful if large areas of skin need to be covered

Table 7.24
Practical prescribing: Summary of medicines for acne

Name of medicine	Use in children	Likely side effects	Drug interactions of note	Patients in whom care should be exercised	Pregnancy and breast-feeding
Benzoyl peroxide	Not appropriate	Skin irritation, burning or peeling	None	None	OK

Summary

First-line treatment of acne should be benzoyl peroxide 2.5 or 5%. Patients should see an improvement in their symptoms after 6 weeks. If the patient's symptoms fail to improve in this time then referral to the GP would be appropriate. However, if beneficial, treatment should be continued for at least 4 to 6 months.

Practical prescribing and product selection

Prescribing information relating to benzoyl peroxide is discussed and summarised in Tables 7.24 and 7.25; useful tips relating to patients presenting with acne are given in Hints and Tips Box 7.9.

Benzoyl peroxide

Benzoyl peroxide is licensed for use in adults and children (for products see Table 7.25). However, acne is very uncommon in children under 12 and should not be given to this age group. Benzoyl peroxide is usually applied once or twice daily depending on patient response, although once-daily application is often sufficient. It should be applied to all areas of the skin where acne occurs and not just to the active lesions. It can cause drying, burning and peeling on initial application. If this occurs the patient should be told to stop using the product for a day or two before starting again. Patients should

Table 7.25
Products available in the UK containing benzoyl peroxide

Name	Form	Strength	Other ingredients
Acnecide	Gel	5%	
Brevoxyl	Cream	4%	
PanOxyl	Aquagel	2.5%, 5%, 10%	
	Cream	5%	
	Gel	5%	
	Wash	10%	
Quinoderm	Cream	5%, 10%	Antimicrobial hydroxyquinoline sulphate 0.5%
Oxy 10	Lotion	10%	

therefore start on the lowest strength commercially available, especially if the patient suffers from sensitive or fair skin. Occasionally, patients will experience contact dermatitis, although it has been reported to affect only 1 to 2% of patients. Apart from local adverse effects benzoyl peroxide is safe and can be used by all patient groups, including pregnant and breast-feeding women. It has no drug interactions, although it does bleach clothing.

Further reading

Bassett IB, Pannowitz DL, Barnetson RS. A comparative study of tea-tree oil versus benzoyl peroxide in the treatment of acne. Med J Aust 1990;153:455–8.

Burke B, Eady EA, Cunliffe WJ. Benzoyl peroxide versus topical erythromycin in the treatment of acne vulgaris. Br J Dermatol 1983;108:199–204.

Cunliffe B. Rosacea. Pharm J 2001;267:782–3.

Fluckiger R, Furrer HJ, Rufli T. Efficacy and tolerance of a miconazole-benzoyl peroxide cream combination versus a benzoyl peroxide gel in the topical treatment of acne vulgaris. Dermatologica 1988;177:109–14.

Haider A, Shaw JC. Treatment of acne vulgaris. JAMA 2004;292:726–35.

Hunt MJ, Barnetson RS. A comparative study of gluconolactone versus benzoyl peroxide in the treatment of acne. Australas J Dermatol 1992;33:131–4.

Johnson BA, Nunley JR. Topical therapy for acne vulgaris. How do you choose the best drug for each patient? Postgrad Med 2000;107:69–70, 73–6, 79–80.

Kligman AM. Acne vulgaris: tricks and treatments. Part II: The benzoyl peroxide saga. Cutis 1995;56:260–1.

Magin P, Pond D, Smith W, Watson A. A systematic review of the evidence for 'myths and misconceptions' in acne management: diet, face washing and sunlight. Fam Pract 2005;22:62–70.

Purdy S, de Berker D. Clinical review: acne. Br Med J 2006;333:949–53.

Shalita AR, Smith JG, Parish LC, et al. Topical nicotinamide compared with clindamycin gel in the treatment of inflammatory acne vulgaris. Int J Dermatol 1995;34:434–7.

Web sites

Prodigy guidance: http://www.cks.library.nhs.uk/acne_vulgaris
Acne Support Groups: http://www.m2w3.com/acne/, http://www.stopspots.org/ and http://www.talkacne.com/

Cold sores

Background

A cold sore is an infection caused by the herpes simplex virus (HSV). There are two main subtypes of the virus: HSV1 and HSV2. Cold sores are caused by HSV1, whereas HSV2 is most commonly implicated in genital lesions.

Prevalence and epidemiology

Herpes simplex virus infection is one of the most commonly encountered human viral infections. It is estimated that more than 50% of adults in the Western world show serological evidence of having been infected by HSV1, although this might not manifest as symptoms. When first contracted, the virus is known as the primary infection. This is often asymptomatic, and is most commonly contracted by preschool children. It is reported that 20 to 40% of people have experienced cold sores at some time.

Aetiology

Infection is spread by viral shedding into saliva and results from direct mucous membrane (e.g. kissing) contact at sites of abraded skin between an infected individual and an uninfected individual. The virus then infects epidermal and dermal cells, causing skin vesicles. At the same time, nerve endings are also infected with the virus, which travels to the sensory ganglia where it lies dormant in the dorsal root ganglia of the trigeminal nerve until reactivation. The virus remains dormant until triggered by a stimulus. During reactivation the virus actively replicates, leading to lesions in the distribution of the affected nerve. Once contracted the infection lasts the lifetime of the host.

Arriving at a differential diagnosis

Cold sores should not be too difficult to diagnose, although conditions such as impetigo can look similar to cold sores. Asking symptom-specific questions will help the pharmacist to determine if referral is needed (Table 7.26).

Clinical features of cold sores

Patients with cold sores typically experience prodromal symptoms of itching, burning, pain or tingling symptoms prior to vesicle eruption. These symptoms might be noticed from a few hours to a couple of days before the lesions develop. The lesions appear as blisters and vesicles with associated redness (Fig. 7.24). These crust over – usually within 24 hours – and tend to itch and be painful. The lesions spontaneously resolve in 7 to 10 days, therefore most outbreaks last 14 days from the recognition of prodromal symptoms to the resolution of lesions.

Many patients can identify a cause of their cold sore, with sunlight (UV light) reported to induce cold sores in 20% of sufferers. Recurrence is common and lesions tend to occur in the same location. Patients will often experience two or three episodes each year. Immunocompromised patients or patients taking immunosuppressive medication can experience severe symptoms and should be referred.

Table 7.26
Specific questions to ask the patient: Cold sores

Question	Relevance
Appearance	• Patients with cold sores will often have symptoms prior to the skin eruption whereas no warning symptoms are present with impetigo
Location	• Cold sores typically occur around the mouth and for this reason are known as herpes simplex libialis. They can also occur around and inside the nose, but this is less common • Impetigo also occurs in the same areas but is much more likely to spread to other areas of the face or move to other parts of the body, for example the arms • Angular cheilitis occurs at the corners of the mouth and can be mistaken for cold sores due to their similar locations
Trigger factors	• Stress, ill health, sunlight, viral infection (e.g. the common cold) and menstruation are all implicated in triggering cold sore attacks. These triggers are not seen with other similar conditions and the patient should be asked if they can identify what brought on the lesions if possible

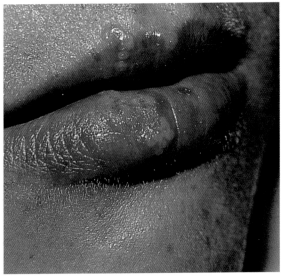

Fig. 7.24   Cold sore. Reproduced from *Color Atlas of Dermatology* by G White, 2004, Churchill Livingstone, with permission

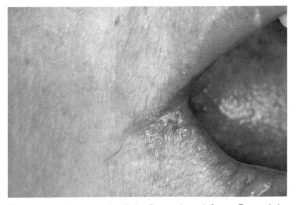

Fig. 7.25   Angular cheilitis. Reproduced from *Essentials of Oral Pathology and Oral Medicine* by R Cawson et al, 2002, Churchill Livingstone, with permission

Angular cheilitis

Angular cheilitis can occur at any age but is more common in patients who wear dentures. The corners of the mouth become cracked, fissured and red. The lesions can become boggy and macerated and are slow to heal because movement of the mouth hinders healing of the lesions (Fig. 7.25). It is painful but generally does not itch or crust over as is typical with cold sores.

Conditions to eliminate

Impetigo

Impetigo usually starts as a small, red, itchy patch of inflamed skin that quickly develops into vesicles that rupture and weep. The exudate dries to a brown, yellow sticky crust. Currently, referral is needed for either topical (e.g. fusidic acid) or systemic (flucloxacillin) therapy. However, patient group directions for supply of topical antibiotics by community pharmacists are in use in certain areas of the UK. It is likely that deregulation from POM to P will occur in the future for topical antibiotics to treat impetigo.

TRIGGER POINTS indicative of referral: Cold sores

- Duration of longer than 14 days
- Lesions that are located within the mouth
- Lesions that spread rapidly over the face
- Patients who are immunocompromised or take immunosuppressive medicines
- Severe and widespread lesions
- Systemic symptoms such as fever and malaise

Evidence base for over-the-counter medication

A number of products are marketed for the relief and treatment of cold sores. None have shown conclusively to be effective in both prevention and treatment. Products containing ammonia, zinc and povidone-iodine appear to have no evidence of efficacy. However, they might be useful in drying lesions and preventing secondary bacterial infections. Local anaesthetics (e.g. lidocaine) and choline salicylate might also be useful for mildly painful lesions. For information on these products see Chapter 6, page 128.

Only the antivirals aciclovir and penciclovir, which work by inhibiting the herpes virus DNA polymerase, have demonstrated clinical effectiveness against the herpes virus. Orally, antivirals such as aciclovir are highly effective but the evidence for topical administration is less conclusive. Trial data for both found weak evidence that they reduce the duration of pain compared with placebo. Pain and healing is reduced by about half a day if they are applied at the first symptom or sign of recurrence, whether this is prodromal or a later stage.

Summary

Aciclovir and penciclovir are first-line therapy for the treatment and prevention of cold sores. However, they should be used as soon as the patient experiences symptoms for them to have an effect.

Practical prescribing and product selection

Prescribing information relating to aciclovir is discussed and summarised in Table 7.27. For completeness the table also contains some of the other commonly used cold sore products; useful tips relating to patients presenting with cold sores are given in Hints and Tips Box 7.10.

Aciclovir (e.g. Lypsyl aciclovir cold sore cream, Soothelip, Virasorb, Zovirax)

Aciclovir can be used topically by all patient groups, including pregnant and breast-feeding women, although the manufacturers advise caution because of limited data regarding the exposure of pregnant women to aciclovir. It has no drug interactions and causes only transient stinging after first application in the minority of patients. Aciclovir should be applied five times daily at approximately 4-hourly intervals and treatment should be continued for 5 days.

Penciclovir (Fenistil cold sore cream)

Penciclovir, like aciclovir, has the same side effect profile, cautions and contraindications although the

Table 7.27
Practical prescribing: Summary of medicines for cold sores

Name of medicine	Use in children	Likely side effects	Drug interactions of note	Patients in whom care should be exercised	Pregnancy and breast-feeding
Aciclovir Lypsyl aciclovir cold sore cream Soothelip Virasorb Zovirax	All (except Lypsyl product) state can be used in children but no lower age limit stated	Stinging	None	OK	OK
Penciclovir (Fenistil)	>12 years	None	None	None	Manufacturers recommend avoidance
Ammonia Blisteze, Blistex	Yes, but no lower age stated	None	None	None	OK
Povidone iodine Brush Off	>2 years	None	None	None	OK
Zinc & Lidocaine Lypsyl cold sore gel	>12 years	Stinging	None	None	OK
Urea Cymex	Yes, but no lower age stated	None	None	None	OK

> ## HINTS AND TIPS BOX 7.10: COLD SORES
>
> | | |
> |---|---|
> | Sun-induced cold sores | For those patients in whom the sun triggers cold sores, a sun block would be the most effective prophylactic measure |
> | Applying products | Patients should be encouraged to use a separate towel and wash their hands after applying products because viral particles are shed from the cold sore and can be transferred to others |
> | Decrease transmission | Risk of transmission is highest during the first 1 to 4 days of symptoms and people should be advised not to kiss others |

manufacturers advise avoidance in pregnancy and breast-feeding, presumably on lack of safety data. For people aged over 12 years it should be applied every 2 hours and treatment continued for 4 days.

Further reading
Emmert DH. Treatment of common cutaneous herpes simplex virus infections. Am Fam Physician 2000;61:1697–704.

Raborn QW, McGaw WT, Grace M et al. Treatment of herpes labialis with acyclovir. Am J Med 1988;85:39–42.

Scully C, Gorsky M, Lozada-Nur F. The diagnosis and management of recurrent aphthous stomatitis: a consensus approach. J Am Dental Assoc 2003;134:200–7.

Spruance SL, Nett R, Marbury T, et al. Acyclovir cream for treatment of herpes simplex labialis: results of two randomized, double-blind, vehicle-controlled, multicenter clinical trials. Antimicrob Agents Chemother 2002;46:2238–43.

Whitley RJ, Kimberlin DW, Roizman B. Herpes simplex viruses. Clin Infect Dis 1998;26:541–55.

Web sites
Mayo Foundation for Medical Education and Research: http://www.mayoclinic.com/invoke.cfm?id=DS00358

Eczema and dermatitis

Background

The terms 'eczema' and 'dermatitis' are often used interchangeably. Dermatitis simply means inflammation of the skin whereas eczema has no universally agreed definition but in some countries indicates a more acute condition. Many authorities subdivide eczema and dermatitis into either exogenous (due to an obvious external cause) or endogenous (assumed to be of a genetic cause); however, the distinction is not clear. The condition is also referred to as either acute (a single exposure to an irritant) or chronic (repeated exposure). In this section, for consistency, the term dermatitis will be used.

Dermatitis is characterised by sore, red, itching skin. In primary care, the two commonest forms of dermatitis are irritant and allergic dermatitis.

Prevalence and epidemiology

The exact prevalence and incidence of irritant and allergic contact dermatitis (ICD and ACD) is unclear, although ICD is much more common than ACD and has been reported to account for 80% of all occupational skin disorders. ACD is said to affect 1 to 2% of the population with certain patient groups, such as patients with leg ulcers, at higher risk of developing ACD.

Aetiology

Different physiological mechanisms are responsible for ICD and ACD. In ICD an agent must penetrate the outer layer of skin – the stratum corneum – to invoke a physiological response. The type of irritant, the concentration, quantity involved and length of exposure will affect the severity of reaction. This can occur with a single exposure or, more commonly, with frequent exposures when the irritant accumulates in the statum corneum. For example, strong acids and alkaline substances can produce ulceration on a single exposure, whereas other agents (e.g. zinc oxide tape) potentially require multiple exposure and tend to invoke a weaker reaction and cause a prickly heat type of dermatitis.

ACD first requires sensitisation to occur. This leads to specific cell-mediated sensitisation. Once the skin has become sensitised to an allergen, re-exposure to the allergen triggers memory T cells to initiate an inflammatory response 24 to 48 hours after re-exposure. Because these T cells are distributed throughout the body the reaction is not limited to the site of exposure and explains why lesions are seen away from the site of exposure. The risk of sensitisation can depend on the individual's susceptibility as well as the particular allergen's concentration and quantity. Re-exposure can occur days and sometimes years after initial exposure. A list of common irritants and allergens is shown in Table 7.28.

Arriving at a differential diagnosis

Many patients will present in the pharmacy with an itchy red rash. Gaining an accurate diagnosis can be difficult as identification of the cause is difficult and clinical features are similar. Generally speaking, treatment is the

Table 7.28 Irritants and allergens known to precipitate dermatitis*	
Irritants that can precipitate ICD	Allergens that can precipitate ACD
Detergents and soaps	Nickel (especially jewellery in women) Chromate in cement
Solvents and abrasives	Topical corticosteroids (5% of patients)
Oils	Cosmetics – particularly fragrances, hair dyes, preservatives and nail varnish resin
Acids and alkalis, including cement	Rubber, including latex
Reducing agents and oxidizing agents	Dyes, formaldehyde and epoxy resins

*Many causes of dermatitis are occupationally related. Questions about exposure to irritants and allergens at work can often identify the cause of symptoms

Table 7.29 Specific questions to ask the patient: Dermatitis	
Question	Relevance
Location	The distribution of rash for contact dermatitis is closely associated with clothing and jewellery (see Fig. 7.26)
Exposure	A history of when the rash occurs gives a useful indication as to the cause, e.g. a construction worker might complain of sore hands while at work but when on holiday the condition improves only for it to worsen when they go back to work
Patch testing	If the rash persists despite avoiding likely irritants and allergens then patch testing could be tried

same for both forms of dermatitis so making a definitive diagnosis is less important. However, asking symptom-specific questions will help the pharmacist to determine if referral is needed (Table 7.29).

Figure 7.26 shows the distribution of contact dermatitis.

Clinical features of ACD and ICD

In both cases rash develops at the site of exposure. In the acute phase, lesions appear rapidly – within 6 to 12 hours – of contact. The skin appears red, itchy, inflamed and might show papules and vesicles. In chronic exposure the skin becomes dry, scaly and can crack and fissure (Fig. 7.27). Itching is a prominent feature and often causes the patient to scratch, which results in broken skin with subsequent weeping. The rash in ICD tends to be well demarcated. In ACD the rash tends to be less well defined; milder involvement away from the site of exposure is seen on repeated exposure and can reactivate at previously exposed sites.

Conditions to eliminate

Psoriasis

Isolated lesions of psoriasis can be superficially similar to dermatitis; they appear red and scaly, although a key

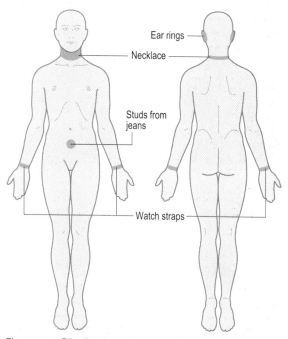

Fig. 7.26 Distribution of contact dermatitis

difference is the general lack of itch in psoriasis. The distribution of lesions is also usually different, and psoriasis is not precipitated by exposure to certain irritants or allergens. For further information on psoriasis see page 185.

Fungal infections

Fungal infections exhibit the classical dermatitis-type symptoms of itchy red rash and can therefore be easily confused. Very clear lesion demarcation along with differing location and central clearing all point towards fungal infection. For further information on fungal infections see page 198.

Discoid dermatitis

Discoid eczema differs from other forms of eczema as the lesions have clearly demarcated edges and are circular or oval. Lesions tend to affect the arms and legs and are often distributed symmetrically. It is more common in middle-aged people.

Dishydrotic eczema (Pompholyx)

Pompholyx simply means 'bubble' and refers to the presence of intensely itchy vesicles or blisters on the palms of the hands and occasionally on the soles of the feet. Stress and heat are known to precipitate the condition.

Urticaria

Urticarial rashes can result from many causes, most notably due to food allergies, food additives (Table 7.30) and medicines. Like dermatitis, the rash is itchy and red but resembles the rash seen when stung by a stinging nettle (Fig. 7.28). In addition, the skin can be oedematous and blanches when pressed. Urticarial reactions often respond well to systemic antihistamines.

Figure 7.29 will aid the differentiation of dermatitis.

TRIGGER POINTS indicative of referral: Eczema and dermatitis

- Children under 10 in need of corticosteroids
- Lesions on the face unresponsive to emollients
- OTC treatment failure
- Widespread or severe dermatitis

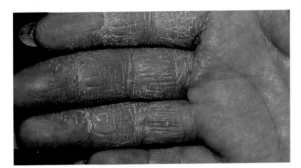

Fig. 7.27 Irritant dermatitis. Reproduced from *Color Atlas of Dermatology* by G White, 2004, Churchill Livingstone, with permission

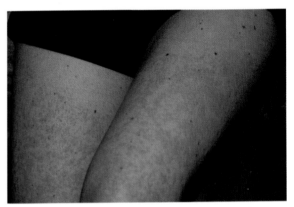

Fig. 7.28 Urticarial reaction to grass

Table 7.30 **Food additives known to cause allergic reaction**	
Sulphites (E220–E227)	Sulphites are used to preserve smoked and processed meats, dried fruit (apricots) and salads. They are commonly found in liquid form in cold drinks, fruit juice concentrates and wine, and are sprayed onto foods to keep them fresh and prevent discolouration or browning
Benzoic acid and parabens (E 210–E 219)	Benzoates and parabens have antibacterial and antifungal properties for prevention of food spoilage. These agents are added to pharmaceutical and food products and occur naturally in prunes, cinnamon, tea and berries
Antioxidants (E320–321)	Fat and oils in food turn rancid when exposed to air. Synthetic phenolic antioxidants butylated hydroxyanisole and butylated hydroxytoluene prevent this spoilage from happening but can trigger asthma, rhinitis and urticaria
Flavour enhancers (E620–E635)	These are used to enhance food palatability, most notably aspartame, which can trigger urticaria and swelling and monosodium glutamate (E620), which can trigger the 'Chinese restaurant syndrome' of headache and burning plus tightness in the chest, neck and face
Colourings (E100–E180)	Colourings are used to make food visually more attractive; the azo dyes (tartrazine, E102, Sunset Yellow, E110) and non-azo dyes (erythrocine) have been associated with triggering urticaria, asthma and generalised allergic reactions

Evidence base for over-the-counter medication

All forms of dermatitis cause redness, drying of the skin and irritation/pruritus to varying degrees. Treatment should include three steps: managing the itch, avoiding irritants and maintaining skin integrity.

Non-pharmacological interventions include avoidance of the causative agent; however, determining the cause is often difficult and avoidance is sometimes impractical.

Sweating intensifies the itching so strategies to keep the person cool will help; cotton and loose-fitting clothing can be worn.

Pharmacological treatment of dermatitis should be managed with a combination of emollients and steroid-based products.

Emollients

Emollients should be used on a regular basis to keep the condition under control and flare-ups can then be treated with corticosteroids. Choosing the most efficacious emollient for an individual is difficult due to the lack of comparative trial data between products and the variable nature of patient response. In general, patients respond to a thicker emollient rather than an elegant cosmetic brand because these allow greater retention of water, for example 50% liquid paraffin and 50% white soft paraffin. However, patient acceptability of such products needs to be considered. Cream formulations rather than ointments tend to be more readily accepted by patients, as they are easier and less messy to use. In general, skin that is moderately dry to very dry will respond best to an ointment and skin that is mildly dry, a cream. If the skin is broken or weeping then a water-soluble cream can be useful. To avoid the drying effects of soap, a soap substitute should be used.

Steroids

In the UK, two steroids are available OTC: hydrocortisone and clobetasone. Both have proven efficacy in treating dermatitis and should be considered first-line treatment for acute dermatitis. Once symptoms are controlled then the patient should be instructed to revert back to emollient therapy.

Practical prescribing and product selection

Prescribing information relating to specific products used to treat dermatitis discussed in the section 'Evidence base for over-the-counter medication' is summarised in Table 7.31; useful tips relating to using products to treat dermatitis are given in Hints and Tips Box 7.11.

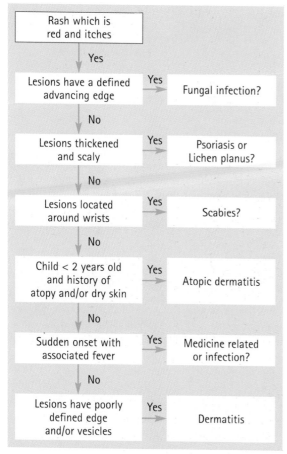

Fig. 7.29 Primer for differential diagnosis of dermatitis

Table 7.31
Practical prescribing: Summary of medicines for dermatitis

Name of medicine	Use in children	Likely side effects	Drug interactions of note	Patients in whom care should be exercised	Pregnancy and breast-feeding
Emollients	From birth onwards	None	None	None	OK
Corticosteroids Hydrocortisone	>10 years	None	None	None	OK
Clobetasone	>12 years				

HINTS AND TIPS BOX 7.11: DERMATITIS

How much to apply?	Patients should be instructed to use a fingertip unit. This is the distance from the tip of the adult index finger to the first crease. One unit is sufficient to cover an area twice the size of an adult flat hand
Quantity required?	The BNF gives the following guidance for a week's use: • Both hands – 15 to 30 g • Both arms – 30 to 60 g • Both legs or trunk – 100 g
When to apply emollients and corticosteroids?	After using a corticosteroid an emollient can be applied to the same area 30 minutes later

Emollients

There are a large number of emollients on the market. They come in a range of formulations to suit all skin types and patient preference (Table 7.32). Patients should be instructed to apply emollients both liberally and whenever needed. They are pharmacologically inactive and so can be used by all patients regardless of age or medical status. A number of ingredients incorporated into emollients do have the potential to sensitise skin and patients should be advised to patch test the product on the back of the hand before starting to routinely use it.

Corticosteroids

Although corticosteroids can be sold to patients OTC, there are a number of restrictions to their sale. In the UK these are:

- the patient must be over 10 for hydrocortisone (over 2 in Australia) and 12 for clobetasone
- duration of treatment is limited to a maximum of 1 week
- a maximum of 15 g can be sold at any one time
- they cannot be used on facial skin, the anogenital region, broken or infected skin

In the opinion of the author, these restrictions limit their usefulness and mean that many patients, who could be otherwise treated successfully if the product licences were not so prohibitive, must be referred to a GP. For example, 1% hydrocortisone cream, if used short term, is an ideal steroid to use on the face with no adverse events; also, 15 g of product is often insufficient for surface areas such as limbs and the body even if used only for a week.

Despite these restrictions, corticosteroids can be used by many patients and, when used short term, have been shown to have minimal side effects, no drug interactions and can be used by all patient groups.

Hydrocortisone

Hydrocortisone can either be bought alone (e.g. Dermacort, Hc45, Lanacort, Zenoxone) or in combination with other ingredients (e.g. Eurax HC, Canesten Hydrocortisone). It is prudent to use products solely containing hydrocortisone for dermatitis, applying them twice a day for a maximum of 7 days. If secondary infection is suspected, for example with a fungal infection, then products such as Canesten Hydrocortisone should be used.

Clobetasone (Eumovate eczema and dermatitis cream)

Clobetasone is classed as moderately potent, whereas hydrocortisone is classed as mild. This affords the pharmacist choice in tailoring treatment to the severity of the condition. It would seem reasonable to reserve clobetasone for more severe flare-ups of dermatitis, or those patients in whom hydrocortisone has in the past failed to control symptoms. Like hydrocortisone, clobetasone should be applied twice a day.

Further reading
Bellingham C. Proper use of topical corticosteroids. Pharm J 2001;267:377.
Clark C, Hoare C. Making the most of emollients. Pharm J 2001;266:277–9.
Cunliffe B. Eczema. Pharm J 2001;267:855–6.

Web sites
Prodigy guidance on contact dermatitis: http://www.cks. library.nhs.uk/dermatitis_contact
National Eczema Society: http://www.eczema.org/
National Eczema Association: http://www.nationaleczema. org/

Table 7.32
Summary of proprietary emollient products

Product name	Formulation	Combination product	Contains potential sensitising agents
Alha Keri	Bath oil		Yes
Aveeno	Bath oil, cream and lotion		Yes
Aquadrate	Cream	Urea	No
Balneum	Bath oil		Yes
Balneum Plus	Bath oil, cream	Urea (cream)	Yes
Calmurid	Cream	Urea, lactic acid	No
Cetraben	Cream, bath oil		Yes
Decubal	Cream		Yes
Dermamist	Spray		No
Dermalo	Bath oil		No
Dermol	Lotion, shower and bath emollient	Antimicrobials	Yes
Diprobase	Cream, ointment		Yes (cream)
Diprobath	Bath oil		No
Doublebase	Gel		No
E45	Cream, lotion, bath oil, emollient wash cream		Yes (cream and lotion only)
E45 Itch Relief	Cream	Urea	Yes
Emulsiderm	Bath emulsion	Antimicrobials	Yes
Epaderm	Ointment		Yes
Eucerin	Cream, lotion	Urea	Yes
Hewletts	Cream		Yes
Hydromol	Cream, ointment, bath oil		Yes (cream and ointment)
Imuderm	Bath oil		Yes
Keri	Lotion		Yes
Linola Gamma	Cream		Yes
Lipobase	Cream		Yes
Neutrogena	Cream		Yes
Nutraplus	Cream	Urea	Yes
Oilatum	Cream, Junior, shower emollient, bath oil		Yes
Oilatum Plus	Bath oil	Antimicrobials	Yes
QV	Cream, lotion, wash, bath oil		Yes
Ultrabase	Cream		Yes
Unguentum M	Cream		Yes
Vaseline Dermacare	Cream, lotion		Yes
Zerobase	Cream		Yes

Sun exposure and melanoma risk

Background

The ultraviolet spectrum is subdivided into three regions: UVA (320 to 400 nm); UVB (290 to 320 nm); and UVC (200 to 290 nm). Light from the UVA spectrum causes skin tanning and UVB light sunburn, whereas UVC light is effectively filtered out by the ozone layer. It is now well recognised that excessive or prolonged exposure to the sun's rays and inadequate skin protection can result in precancerous and cancerous neoplasms. There are many types of skin cancer, but three types are associated with sun exposure – squamous cell carcinoma (SCC), basal cell carcinoma (BCC) and malignant melanoma (MM) – and are responsible for more than 95% of all skin cancers. SCC and BCC result from chronic long-term exposure to sunlight, whereas MM is associated with acute, intense and intermittent blistering sunburns. BCC and SCC are often grouped together as non-melanoma skin cancer (NMSC).

Prevalence and epidemiology

The incidence of cancers related to skin damage has dramatically increased since the 1980s, and is greatest in white-skinned people living in equatorial regions. For example, in Australia there are over 8000 new cases of MM reported each year, and over 1000 deaths. In the UK it is estimated that there are 60 000 new cases of all types of skin cancer each year, although this is believed to be a significant underestimate. MM accounts for just 10% of all cases but has a much higher mortality rate than NMSC. MMs are more common in women, although the incidence in both sexes has been steadily increasing. Affluent women appear to be at highest risk of developing MM, whereas men from lower socioeconomic groups are at greatest risk of developing NMSC.

Aetiology

The body's response to the effects of UVA and UVB light is protective. On exposure to ultraviolet light melanocytes increase production of melanin, thus causing a darkening of the skin, the all-important suntan! Melanin absorbs both UVA and UVB and effectively protects the skin from damage. Unfortunately, melanin synthesis is slow and skin damage might occur manifesting as sunburn. Sunburn is an inflammatory response to excessive exposure to ultraviolet light whereby an increase in inflammatory mediators results in capillary vasodilatation and increased capillary permeability. In addition to melanin production, epidermal hyperplasia occurs, causing the skin to thicken; this provides further protection against the sun.

Arriving at a differential diagnosis

Pharmacists have a major role to play in dealing with patients who have been exposed to excessive amounts of sunlight. They can promote sun safety messages, both passively and actively (when dealing with requests for sunburn), and make appropriate referrals with regard to suspicious lesions. Pharmacists must be able to recognise suspicious lesions, especially those resembling MM because it has the highest mortality of skin cancers, but if treated early is curable.

Clinical features of malignant melanoma

MM is one of the few cancers that is associated with young adults. It can appear on all body sites but the distribution in men and women differs (Fig. 7.30).

Risk factors include early childhood sun exposure, people with multiple moles and those with skin types susceptible to sunburn. The first sign of melanoma is often a change in the size, shape or colour of a mole, although melanoma can also appear on the body as a new mole (Fig. 7.31). MM can be difficult to diagnose due to resemblance to moles. Early identification in their progression is essential and two commonly used checklists are used: the British seven-point checklist and the American ABCDE list.

The British Association of Dermatologists' seven-point list

This checklist consists of three major and four minor points:

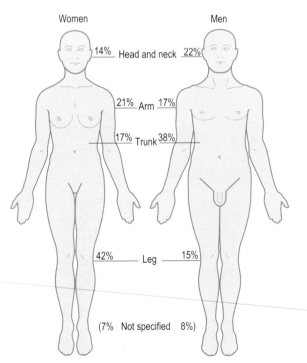

Fig. 7.30 Distribution of malignant melanoma

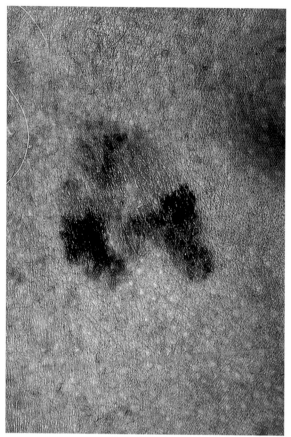

Fig. 7.31 Superficial spreading melanoma. Irregular in colour and shape. Reproduced from *Dermatology in Focus* by J Wilkinson et al, 2005, Churchill Livingstone, with permission

Major (scores 2):

1. Change in shape
2. Change in size
3. Change in colour

Minor (scores 1):

4. Largest diameter 7 mm or more
5. Inflammation
6. Oozing
7. Change in sensation (e.g. itch or irritation)

Any lesion should be suspected as MM if any major feature is present or there is a total score of 3 or more.

The ABCDE rule

In this checklist five points are used:

- Asymmetry – ordinary moles are usually symmetrical in shape. Melanomas are likely to be irregular or asymmetrical.
- Border – moles usually have a well-defined regular border. Melanomas are more likely to have an irregular border with jagged edges.

- Colour – moles are usually a uniform brown. Melanomas tend to have more than one colour. They may be varying shades of brown mixed with black, red, pink, white or a bluish tint.
- Diameter – moles are normally no bigger than the blunt end of a pencil (about 6 mm across). Melanomas are usually more than 7 mm in diameter.
- Evolution – the symmetry, border, colour or diameter of a mole has changed over time.

It is likely that patients will ask for advice and reassurance on skin lesions that they are concerned could be melanoma. It is essential that these people are given information, ideally both orally and written, regarding the changes that might subsequently suggest MM and should be instructed to seek medical help as soon as they notice changes.

NMSC

NMSC are the most common cancers in the UK. They are associated with older people, with the average age of diagnosis in the early 70s. The cancers are rarely fatal but can cause substantial morbidity. Both cancers commonly occur on skin surfaces that are exposed to a lifetime accumulation of UV radiation such as the hands, face and scalp. They are more common in people who have worked outdoors, in fair-skinned people and those living in tropical and subtropical climates. BCC and SCC vary in their appearance. SCC initially presents as raised lesions that exhibit a horny or scaly appearance; these later become non-healing lesions, often larger than 1 cm, which can ulcerate. BCC starts as a small translucent papule with obvious telangiectasia over the surface. Over time (growth can be very slow) the size of the papule increases and can ulcerate and crust over.

Conditions to eliminate

Actinic keratoses

Actinic keratoses is the most common premalignant skin condition and affects the same group of people as SCC, with approximately 1 in 1000 cases progressing to SCC. Lesions are generally flat, brown and rough to the touch and have well demarcated edges.

Seborrhoeic warts

These are benign flat or raised lesions that vary in colour. Initially, they take on the colour of the person's skin but gradually darken and range in colour from light brown to jet black (Fig. 7.20, page 211). They are more usual on the trunk and increase in incidence from 40 years onwards. Over time they can become wart-like and have a stuck-on waxy appearance. Occasionally, they can become inflamed, itchy or bleed but this is normally because they have been caught on clothing.

TRIGGER POINTS indicative of referral: Sunburn/damage

- Facial lesions in people over 40
- Lesions that have become itchy, irritated or are prone to bleeding
- Moles that have changed in size, shape or colour

Evidence base for over-the-counter medication

Avoidance measures

The most effective strategy for preventing skin damage/sunburn and reducing the chance of developing cancers is avoidance of UV light. Cancer Research UK has promoted a Sun Smart cancer prevention programme, which highlights the key sun avoidance measures that should be promoted to the public:

S – Spend time in the shade between 11 am and 3 pm
M – Make sure you never burn
A – Aim to cover up with a t-shirt, hat and sunglasses
R – Remember to take extra care with children
T – Then use factor 15+ sunscreen

It is also worth stressing to people that it is possible to burn on cloudy days.

Sunscreens

While sunscreens play an important role in sunburn protection, they should never replace minimising sun exposure. Sunscreens use the sun protection factor (SPF) system to indicate the level of protection against UV radiation. It is a measure of the protection from UVB radiation. This is calculated under experimental conditions using four times the amount of sunscreen usually applied by consumers. It is important that patients and consumers do not assume a linear increase in protection as the SPF increases. For example, a sunscreen with an SPF of 15 blocks 93% of UVB, whereas a doubling to SPF 30 only increases protection by 4% to 97%.

In the UK a controversial star rating also exists to indicate the level of protection offered against UVA relative to protection against UVB. A five star rating indicates the product has a balanced amount of UVA and UVB protection. The lower the star rating, the greater the protection offered against UVB compared to UVA.

Practical prescribing and product selection

Prescribing information relating to sunscreen products reviewed in the section 'Evidence base for over-the-counter medication' is discussed and summarised in Table 7.33; useful tips relating to patients asking for advice about protection from the sun are given in Hints and Tips Box 7.12.

All products should be applied 20 minutes before exposure to the sun, and reapplied every 2 to 4 hours and after swimming to ensure maximum protection. Standard practice until recently was to match skin type with the level of SPF protection the person required. However, this approach while preventing sunburn does not prevent long-term skin damage. Rather than selecting a specific sunscreen for skin type it is advocated that all white-skinned people should use a sunscreen with an SPF of at least 15 because this level of protection is effectively a sun block.

Chemical sunscreens

Chemical sunscreens work by absorbing UV energy and give protection against either UVA or UVB, although they tend to be more effective against UVB radiation. The majority of marketed products contain a combination of agents including benzophenones, cinnamates, dibenzoylmethanes and para-aminobenzoic acid. Para-aminobenzoic acid is now infrequently used, as it was often associated with contact sensitivity.

Table 7.33
Practical prescribing: Summary of sun protection products

Name of medicine	Use in children	Likely side effects	Drug interactions of note	Patients in whom care should be exercised	Pregnancy and breast-feeding
Chemical sunscreens	Infant upwards	Allergic reactions but may be linked to the vehicle and not the active ingredients	None	None	OK
Physical sunscreens		None, but may be cosmetically unacceptable			

HINTS AND TIPS BOX 7.12: SUN DAMAGE

Water-resistant sunscreens	These are claimed to be effective after immersion in water. However, studies have shown that sunscreen effectiveness decreases after water exposure. It would be prudent therefore to reapply sunscreens after swimming
Eye protection	Prolonged (over years) sun exposure can contribute to age-related macular degeneration. Therefore, wraparound sunglasses and lenses that effectively filter UV light should be worn
But what if the person has got sunburn?	Mild sunburn can be managed with a combination of topical cooling preparations, such as calamine and systemic analgesia
Medicine-induced photosensitivity	Piroxicam, tetracyclines, chlorpromazine, phenothiazines and amiodarone can cause pruritus and skin rash when the skin is exposed to natural sunlight. Protection from UVA radiation is particularly important for people taking phototoxic medications (e.g. tetracyclines) as UVA is not filtered by glass, unlike UVB radiation

Physical sunscreens

Physical sunscreens are opaque reflective agents and offer protection against UVA and UVB radiation. Examples of physical sunscreens include zinc and titanium oxide.

Further reading

Abbasi NR, Shaw HM, Rigel DS, et al. Early diagnosis of cutaneous melanoma: revisiting the ABCD criteria. JAMA 2004;292:2771–6.

Goodyear L. Skin conditions associated with the sun and heat. Pharm J 2001;266:892–7.

Kricker A, Armstrong BK, English DR, et al. Does intermittent sun exposure cause basal cell carcinoma? A case-control study in Western Australia. Int J Cancer 1995;60:489–94.

Wong JG, Feussner JR. Screening for melanoma. "Here's looking at you, kid." N C Med J 1994;55:142–5.

Web sites

Charities

The Skin Cancer Foundation: http://www.skincancer.org/

Cancer Research UK: http://www.cancerhelp.org.uk/default.asp

Cancer Bacup: http://www.cancerbacup.org.uk/Home

Guidance

Prodigy guidance: http://www.cks.library.nhs.uk/skin_cancer_suspected/view_whole_guidance

NICE guidance on skin tumours including melanoma: http://www.nice.org.uk/guidance/csgstim/?c=91528

SIGN guidance No. 72 – Cutaneous melanoma (July 2003): http://www.sign.ac.uk/guidelines/fulltext/72/index.html

British Association of Dermatologists' guidelines on cutaneous melanoma (2002): http://www.bad.org.uk/healthcare/guidelines/Cutaneous_Melanoma.pdf

General sites

Sunsmart website: http://www.sunsmart.com.au/

Cancer Council Australia: http://www.cancer.org.au/

Melanoma patients' information page: http://www.mpip.org/

Melanoma Research Foundation: http://www.melanoma.org/ and http://www.melanoma.com/

Self-assessment questions

The following questions are intended to supplement the text. Two levels of questions are provided: multiple choice questions and case studies. The multiple choice questions are designed to test factual recall and the case studies allow knowledge to be applied to a practice setting.

Multiple choice questions

7.1 Which medicine has *not* been proven to be efficacious in treating dandruff?

    a. Coal tar
    b. Cetrimide
    c. Ketoconazole
    d. Zinc pyrithione
    e. Selenium sulphide

7.2 Which form of psoriasis can be managed OTC?

    a. Guttate
    b. Pustular
    c. Plaque
    d. Seborrhoeic
    e. Erythrodermic

7.3 Which medicine is known to cause hair loss?

    a. Nifedipine
    b. Simvastatin
    c. Ranitidine
    d. Ibuprofen
    e. Warfarin

7.4 What symptom is least associated with athlete's foot?

    a. Itch
    b. Redness
    c. Involvement between the toes
    d. Scaling
    e. Odour

7.5 With which form of tinea infection are imidazoles ineffective?

    a. Athlete's foot
    b. Jock itch
    c. Infection involving the body
    d. Infection involving the nail
    e. Infection on the hand

7.6 A corn is caused by?

    a. Sweating feet
    b. Too much pressure caused by ill-fitting shoes
    c. Too little pressure caused by ill-fitting shoes

    d. Secondary bacterial infection of a verruca
    e. None of the above

7.7 In which condition is itching the least prominent?

    a. Allergic dermatitis
    b. Scabies
    c. Fungal infection
    d. Psoriais
    e. Lichen planus

7.8 What skin condition is characterised by silvery-white scaly lesions of salmon-pink appearance with well-defined boundaries?

    a. Contact dermatitis
    b. Rosacea
    c. Plaque psoriasis
    d. Seborrhoeic dermatitis
    e. Pityriasis versicolor

Questions 7.9 to 7.11 concern the following conditions:

    A. Dermatitis
    B. Plaque psoriasis
    C. Fungal infection
    D. Acne
    E. Cold sores

Select, from A to E, which of the above conditions:

7.9 Is characterised by itching and scaling

7.10 Often has prodromal symptoms prior to the rash appearing

7.11 Has a strong genetic link

Questions 7.12 to 7.14 concern the following medicines:

    A. Hydrocortisone cream
    B. Clotrimazole cream
    C. Posalfilin ointment
    D. Salicylic acid solution
    E. E45 cream

Select, from A to E, which of the above medicines:

7.12 Can be given to all patient groups *E*

7.13 Is contraindicated in pregnancy *C*

7.14 Should be used for no longer than 1 week
A

Questions 7.15 to 7.17: for each of these questions *one or more* of the responses is (are) correct. Decide which of the responses is (are) correct. Then choose:

A. If a, b and c are correct
B. If a and b only are correct
C. If b and c only are correct
D. If a only is correct
E. If c only is correct

Directions summarised

A	B	C	D	E
a, b and c	a and b only	b and c only	a only	c only

7.15 For the following statements about cradle cap which is/are true?

a. There is normally a family history
b. Ear and eye involvement is possible
c. The rash tends not to itch
C

7.16 Warts and verrucas are:

D
a. Caused by the human papilloma virus
b. Infections that never affect adults
c. Can develop into precancerous growths if left untreated

7.17 When supplying aciclovir, patients should be told to:

a. Use the product four times a day
E b. Apply once the rash has appeared
c. Wash their hands after application

Questions 7.18 to 7.20: these questions consist of a statement in the left-hand column followed by a statement in the right-hand column. You need to:

- decide whether the first statement is true or false
- decide whether the second statement is true or false

Then choose:

A. If both statements are true and the second statement is a correct explanation of the first statement
B. If both statements are true but the second statement is NOT a correct explanation of the first statement
C. If the first statement is true but the second statement is false
D. If the first statement is false but the second statement is true
E. If both statements are false

Directions summarised

	1st statement	2nd statement	
A	True	True	2nd statement is a correct explanation of the first
B	True	True	2nd statement is not a correct explanation of the first
C	True	False	
D	False	True	
E	False	False	

	First statement	Second statement
7.18	Benzoyl peroxide should be used to treat mild acne	It should be used for at least 6 weeks
	B	
7.19	Scabies is intensely itchy	The mites' faeces cause a hypersensitivity reaction
	A	
7.20	Minoxidil is used to treat hair loss	It works on over 80% of patients

Case study

CASE STUDY 7.1

Mr RJ and his 9-year-old son Jimmy want to buy something for Jimmy's verruca. Mr RJ thinks that Jimmy has had the verruca for about 4 to 6 weeks. He describes it as a circular discoloured piece of skin that looks like the verrucas he used to get.

a. What course of action are you going to take?

Try and question Jimmy directly. See if Jimmy knows how long the suspected verruca has been there. Ask if the lesion is causing any pain when walking. Instead of asking for further descriptions of what the lesion looks like and where it is positioned ask if you can actually look at the lesion. Remember to wash your hands before and after inspecting the foot.

On further questioning and examination you concur with the self-diagnosis of a verruca. The lesion is small (less than 0.5 cm in diameter) and causes no pain when direct pressure is applied.

b. What are you going to recommend?

A salicylic-acid based product is the most suitable product, and you recommend Bazuka after first making sure Jimmy is not diabetic.

Six weeks later Mrs J returns with Jimmy and demands to see the pharmacist. She says the stuff you recommended is rubbish and Jimmy's verruca is bigger than it was before!

c. How are you going to respond?

First, you must stay calm and not be defensive. Ask open questions to find out why Mrs J is unhappy; this approach will generally reveal what the problem is. Second, if the reason is not obvious then you must find out about compliance. Who has been responsible for applying the product? If the parents have told Jimmy to use it, has he been using the product correctly and at the correct dosage frequency? In addition, many patients have unrealistic expectations on how quickly the verruca will resolve with therapy. Did you tell them how long it would take before an effect will be seen? This is a vital piece of information to ensure patients realise that treatment is not a quick cure.

You find out that Mrs J has been applying the Bazuka and doing everything the instruction leaflet says. You inspect Jimmy's feet again and from what you can remember the lesion does look slightly larger.

d. Why might this be the case?

Salicylic acid is destructive in nature and if the product comes into contact with non-affected skin then it can damage the skin and appear to the patient that the lesion has indeed got bigger.

Mrs J wants to try Bazuka Extra Strength since the normal Bazuka isn't helping.

e. What are you going to do?

You must try to stress to Mrs J that she should continue with the normal Bazuka because 6 weeks of therapy is not long enough to make a decision to alter therapy.

Reluctantly, Mrs J accepts your advice and leaves the pharmacy promising she will try for a bit longer. One week later she presents a prescription for Cuplex gel for Jimmy.

f. What are you going to do?

It appears that Mrs J was not satisfied or convinced with your advice and has decided to see the GP. You do not know whether Mrs J told the GP about using an OTC product. You could ring the GP to tell him or her that Mrs J has been using a salicylic acid-based product already; however, this is likely to have little bearing on the outcome of product selection as Jimmy will still need to continue treatment with something for a few more weeks. The prescription should be dispensed and Mrs J counselled appropriately. It would be unprofessional to point out that Cuplex is unlikely to be any better than Bazuka.

When you hand Mrs Jenkins the Cuplex she mentions that the doctor said this was stronger than Bazuka and should do the trick.

g. How do you reply?

Be diplomatic and non-judgemental. It is likely that the GP knows that Cuplex is no better than Bazuka but if the parent is convinced that what she is now getting is superior to the previous product then her motivation to comply with directions might be better and hence the outcome for Jimmy will be eradication of the verruca. It might be worth asking the GP, next time you have a conversation, what his or her rationale for prescribing Cuplex was.

CASE STUDY 7.2

Ms AH is the mother of an infant son aged 4 months. She asks for your help in treating her son's flaky skin on his scalp. She says he has had the problem on and off for the last 6 weeks. She hasn't yet tried anything except baby shampoo, as recommended by the health visitor. However, she now wants a cream or something to get rid of the problem once and for all.

a. What further information do you require to be in a position to help her?

You need to know more about the severity of the problem, for example, whether any other parts of the baby's skin are affected. Does the baby appear to scratch at the rash and what were the previous episodes like? Were they the same as this time or different? Also is there a family history of atopy or other dermatological conditions in the family.
 You decide the child has cradle cap.

b. What treatment are you going to recommend?

The use of a mild tar-based product every other day until the scalp clears would be appropriate. In between using the tar-based product the mother should be instructed to use the baby shampoo.
 Ms AH returns to the pharmacy 2 weeks later with another of her children. Impressed that her son's scalp is now clear she wants some advice for her 7-year-old daughter. She has a sore on the corner of her mouth.

c. What further information do you require to be in a position to help her?

You need to know:

- *How long has the sore been present*
- *How the sore first developed*
- *What symptoms are associated with the sore*
- *The progression of the sore. Has it spread?*
- *Previous history of the rash and a family history*

You find out the sore appeared overnight and is now itchy. On inspection the lesion appears to be weeping a clear exudate.

d. What is the most likely diagnosis?

Based on this information the likely diagnosis is a cold sore.

e. What treatment, if any, are you going to recommend?

No treatment necessary but if the parent insists on therapy then any product could be given, although antiviral therapy is expensive and the cost difficult to justify. In addition, advice on minimising transmission could be given such as not sharing towels and trying to avoid kissing (e.g. mum and dad).

CASE STUDY 7.3

Mr RT, an elderly man, asks for some cream to help get rid of a rash he has over part of his chest. The following questions are asked, and responses received.

Information gathering	Data generated
Presenting complaint (possible questions)	
How long have you had the symptoms	Rash started 3 days ago
What does it look like	Red and angry
Where exactly	Started on his left side below his armpit and now spread under the arm pit
Other symptoms/provokes	Felt a bit unwell, slight loss of appetite & headache
Any itching or pain?	Some pain – rated as 4 on scale of 1 to 10
Additional questions	
Previous history of presenting complaint	None similar
Past medical history	Slight stroke 1 year ago. Hypertension controlled with medication Eczema, contact dermatitis +/–urticaria – to some plants

Information gathering	Data generated
Drugs (OTC, Rx and compliance)	Warfarin, bendroflumethiazide, Adalat LA Double base cream Occasional use of clobetasone (Eumovate) for dermititis
Allergies	Unknown
Social history	
Smoking Alcohol Drugs Employment Relationships	Wife died 6 months ago, finding it difficult to cope at times. Does not like to bother children who live locally. Feels very low
Family history	Not asked
On examination	Clusters of papules & vesicles unilaterally along dermatone affecting left chest and back

Diagnostic pointers with regard to symptom presentation

For skin rash seen on the trunk in the area observed then herpes zoster seems likely. The expected findings for questions when related to the possible conditions that could be confused with herpes zoster that are seen by community pharmacists are summarised below.

	Vesicles	Unilateral	Recurrent	Pain	Other symptoms
Herpes zoster	Yes	Yes	Unusual	Yes	Tingling/burning prior to eruption General malaise
Contact dermatitis	Possible	Yes	Yes	Possible	Itch
Herpes simplex	Yes	Yes	Yes	Yes	None of note
Eczema	Possible	Possible	Yes	Possible	Itch
Trauma	No	Possible	No	Yes	Should be an obvious cause

When this information is applied to that gained from our patient (next page) we see that his symptoms fit with herpes zoster.

CASE STUDY 7.3

7

	Vesicles	Unilateral	Recurrent	Pain	Other symptoms
Herpes zoster	✓	✓	✓	✓	✓
Contact dermatitis	✓	✓	✗	✗?	✗
Herpes simplex	✓	✓	✗	✓	✗
Eczema	✓	✓	✗	✗	✗
Trauma	✗	✓	✗	✓	✗

The patient could be given analgesics to help with pain but referred for possible antivirals (e.g. famciclover 250 mg tds for 7 days) and warned about postherpetic neuralgia. The patient also seems to be showing signs of depression and needs further investigation. It would be good practice, in this case, to try and speak with the GP to arrange an urgent appointment for the patient to treat the rash but also mention your concerns over the patient exhibiting signs of depressive illness.

Shingles (herpes zoster) information

Shingles is an acute infection caused by reactivation of latent varicella zoster virus. Following primary chickenpox infection, the virus lies dormant in the dorsal root ganglia of the spinal cord. When reactivated, it travels along the sensory nerve to affect one or more dermatomes, causing the characteristic shingles rash. Reactivation of the virus probably occurs following a decrease in cell-mediated immunity (e.g. with increasing age, HIV infection, illness).

CASE STUDY 7.4

Mr AC, a man in his late twenties/early thirties, presents with a very itchy rash on his left hand. He asks if you can give him a cream to stop the itching. The following questions are asked, and responses received.

Information gathering	Data generated
Presenting complaint (possible questions)	
How long have you had the symptoms	Few days
Rash anywhere else	No
Other symptoms/provokes	Not really – just really itchy!
Additional questions	No exposure to chemicals or new tasks involving hand work
Previous history of presenting complaint	No
Past medical history	Epileptic
Drugs (OTC, Rx and compliance)	Sodium valproate 500 mg bd. Well controlled
Allergies	None
Social history Smoking Alcohol Drugs Employment Relationships	Works for the NHS doing patient transports

Information gathering	Data generated
Family history	Dad has ezcema
On examination	Left hand and wrist very sore. Obvious red papules in places but look like they have been scratched (this is confirmed by patient)

Marked itching involving the hands is most likely to be scabies. However, other conditions are possible and are noted below:

Probability	Cause
Most likely	Scabies
Likely	Dermatitis, insect bites, pomphylox
Unlikely	Dermatitis herpetiformis

Using the information gained from questioning and linking this with known epidemiology, it should be possible to make a differential diagnosis.

Diagnostic pointers with regard to symptom presentation

The expected findings for questions when related to the different conditions that can be seen by community pharmacists are summarised below.

	Location other than hands and wrists	Lesion appearance	Itch	Positive family or social history
Scabies	Unusual	Red papules through to vesicles	Intense	Yes
Dermatitis	Often (depends on type of dermatitis)	Red scaling rash that might crust over due to scratching	Moderate to intense	No
Insect bites	Often	Red papules through to vesicles	Moderate to intense	Possible
Pomphylox	Unusual	Vesicles	Intense	No
Dermatitis herpetiformis	Usual	Red papules through to vesicles	Intense	No

When this information is applied to that gained from our patient (next page) we see that his symptoms most closely match scabies.

CASE STUDY 7.4

	Location other than hands and wrists	Lesion appearance	Itch	Positive family or social history
Scabies	✓	✓	✓ (intensity points more to scabies than other conditions)	✓ (occupation exposes person to higher risk)
Dermatitis	✗?	✗	✓	✗
Insect bites	✗	✓	✓	✗?
Pomphylox	✓	✗?	✓	✗
Dermatitis herpetiformis	✗	✓	✓	✗

Therapy could be started with permethrin cream, although it is expensive and referral to the GP might be considered. It is important to try and trace the contact from whom he has contracted scabies and also inform work.

Severe and extensive symptoms	✗
Suspected dermatitis herpetiformis	✗

Danger symptoms/signs (trigger points for referral)

As a final double check it might be worth making sure the person has none of the 'referral signs or symptoms'; this is the case with this patient.

Musculoskeletal conditions

Background

The musculoskeletal system comprises hard (bone and cartilage) and soft (muscles, tendons, ligaments) tissues. It is responsible for mobility and provides protection to vital structures. Most musculoskeletal problems occur as a result of injury or organic illness. The majority of patients presenting to a community pharmacist will have an acute and self-limiting problem, which will resolve spontaneously. Chronic conditions such as osteoarthritis will be encountered routinely when issuing prescriptions to patients.

The key role of the pharmacist when dealing with patients with a musculoskeletal problem is to establish the cause, its severity and whether it can be self-managed appropriately or requires further investigation.

General overview of musculoskeletal anatomy

The skeletal system of the human body is composed of 206 bones. At the point of contact between two or more bones an articulation (joint) is formed. This system of bones and joints maximises movement while maintaining stability. There are two basic types of joints:

- synovial joints: allow considerable movement (e.g. shoulder or knee)
- fibrocartilaginous joints: are completely immoveable (e.g. the skull) or permit only limited motion (e.g. spinal vertebrae).

Bones and joints cannot move by themselves. The integrity of the musculoskeletal system depends on the interaction between skeletal muscle and bones, and coordinated movement is only possible because of the way muscle is attached to bone. Tendons attach the end of the muscle to the bone or another structure upon which the muscle acts. To perform such a function tendons are composed of very dense fibrous tissue.

Joints require additional stability and support. Strong bands of fibrous tissue known as ligaments bind together bones entering a joint to provide this additional support and stability. It is often the integrity of the connecting structures that are damaged in a musculoskeletal injury. The simplified diagram of the medial aspect of the knee joint in Fig. 8.1 illustrates the relationship of the connective structures to the skeleton and musculature.

The knee joint is an example of a synovial joint. The femur, tibia and fibula do not touch each other because they are covered with articular cartilage and separated by the synovial cavity. The knee joint also contains bursae – small fluid sacs – that provide protection at points in the joint where friction or pressure is great. These can become inflamed, leading to bursitis.

History taking

Gaining an accurate history from the patient should provide enough information to determine if their injury is within the scope of a community pharmacist. By the very nature of musculoskeletal injuries, if someone manages to come into the pharmacy then the injury is

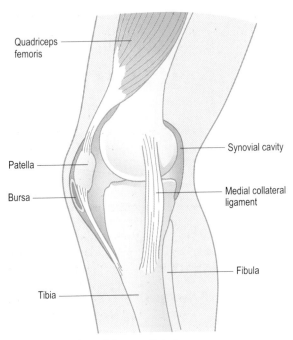

Fig. 8.1   The knee joint: medial view

Quadriceps femoris

Patella

Bursa

Tibia

Synovial cavity

Medial collateral ligament

Fibula

unlikely to be serious. Information gathering should concentrate on when the injury occurred, what precipitated the injury, the level of discomfort, any restriction in range of motion and whether the injury appears to be worsening, and finding out what expectations the patient has.

In general, any patient who presents with an injury that is causing extreme discomfort or the pain is worsening, adversely affects mobility and has been present for more than a week would probably be better managed by a GP or physiotherapist/sports therapist and referral should be made.

Acute low back pain

Background

Acute low back pain is self-limiting. Over 90% of patients will get better within 6 weeks, although up to two-thirds of patients will have a recurrence within 1 year after initial onset but fewer than 5% of patients go on to develop back pain classed as chronic (persists for more than 12 weeks).

Low back pain is extremely common. For example, in the US it is the fifth most common reason patients see a medical practitioner and in the UK 7 to 8% of all adult GP consultations are for low back pain. It is hardly surprising then that the economic burden to society is huge. In 2003/4, 5 million working days were lost in the UK, which equates to annual costs to employers of between £590 million and £624 million per annum.

Prevalence and epidemiology

Back pain is most common between the ages of 30 and 55 years with prevalence rates similar for men and women, although 50 to 90% of pregnant women develop low back pain. Studies and statistical data have shown that in developed countries 60 to 90% of adults will experience an episode of low back pain at some point in their adult lives. Back pain is most common in those with skilled manual, partly skilled and unskilled jobs. Occupational risk factors in developing back pain include those who perform heavy manual labour, frequent bending, twisting and lifting and people who remain in static positions for long periods of time such as truck and car drivers who drive long distances each year. Sports that involve excessive twisting, such as golf and gymnastics, can also lead to back pain.

Aetiology

In the majority of cases an exact cause cannot be determined for the patient's symptoms and is often referred to as simple, non-specific or uncomplicated low back pain. Pain originates from the lumbosacral region and is often mechanical in origin (Fig. 8.2), and includes problems caused by muscles, tendons, ligaments and discs. Contributory factors in the cause of low back pain are a general lack of fitness, occupational (as above) and psychosocial, for example, anxiety and depression. Serious underlying pathology is very rare with infection and malignancy accounting for less than 1% of cases.

Arriving at a differential diagnosis

The vast majority of patients (95%) who present in the pharmacy will have simple back pain that will, in time, resolve with conservative treatment. Bad posture when seated and poor lifting technique when performing day-to-day tasks such as cleaning or gardening are very common predisposing factors. The remaining cases will have back pain with associated nerve root compression. It is extremely unlikely that a pharmacist will encounter a patient with serious spinal pathology, such as infection or malignancy. However, pharmacists should be mindful that age can affect the diagnosis.

Taking a thorough history is of key importance when evaluating a patient with low back pain. Begin questioning the patient with traditional questions regarding the pain: location, radiation, evidence of trauma, the effect pain has on mobility and factors that aggravate or relieve the pain. Asking a number of symptom-specific questions will aid differential diagnosis (Table 8.1).

Clinical features of acute low back pain

Pain in the lower lumbar or sacral area is usually described as aching or stiffness. Depending on the cause, pain

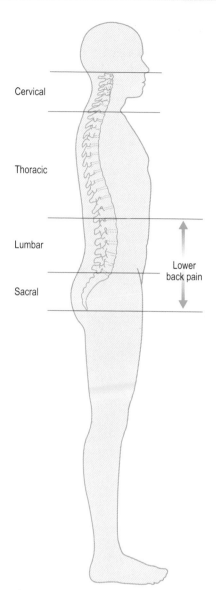

Fig. 8.2 Location and distribution of lower back pain: L4/L5, pain radiates down outer calf and onto the top of the foot; L5/S1, pain radiates to the outside and sole of the foot

might be localised (e.g. lumbosacral strains following physical activity) or more diffuse (e.g. from postural backache after sitting incorrectly for a prolonged period). In cases of acute injury the symptoms come on quickly and there will be a reduction in mobility.

Conditions to eliminate

Causes of low back pain not related to back pathophysiology

It must be remembered that acute illness, for example colds and influenza, can give rise to generalised aching or pain. Likewise pre-rash pain associated with shingles

and referred pain from abdominal organs (e.g. pyleone-phritis) can present as low back pain. A careful history of the presenting symptoms should enable exclusion of such conditions.

Sciatica

Sciatica typically occurs in the healthy middle-aged adult. Pain is acute in onset and radiates to the leg. Pain starts in the lower back and as it intensifies radiates into the lower extremity. Disc herniation usually involves those between L4–L5 and L5–S1 vertebrae (see Fig. 8.2), although most occur between L5 and S1. If disc hernia-tion is minimal, pain is characterised by being dull, deep and aching. It is usually felt in the upper part rather than the lower part of the leg and spreads from the lumbar spine. If the disc ruptures or herniates under strain then the pain is usually lancinating in quality, shooting down the leg like an electric shock. Valsalva movements, for example coughing, sneezing or straining at stool, often aggravate pain. Referral is needed for confirmation of the diagnosis. GPs can perform a straight-leg raising test whereby the pain of sciatica can be induced by elevating the leg of the patient when lying down. Prognosis is good, although improvement and recovery is often slower than in low back pain alone.

Malignancy

Malignancy is very rare; it is more prevalent in patients over 50, although rates are still low – 0.14% in patients under 50 and 0.56% in those over 50. History of sig-nificant weight loss, presence of anaemia, general malaise, night pain and failure to improve over a 4-week period warrant referral for further evaluation.

Infection

Infection is a rare cause of back pain. Presence of fever is the most suggestive historical feature for infection, although pain tends to worsen with activity.

Chronic causes of low back pain

Patients in whom pain lasts longer than 12 weeks are said to suffer from chronic back pain. In the context of low back pain pharmacists should only manage acute problems; however, patients will present with chronic symptoms and seek advice, especially on drug manage-ment. The following section highlights degenerative joint disease as it is the most common cause of chronic low back pain in people older than 50.

Osteoarthritis

Associated with advancing age, osteoarthritis affects up to one-third of people aged over 65 and is twice as common in women. It can be localised to a single joint or involve multiple joints and most commonly affects the

Table 8.1
Specific questions to ask the patient: Back pain

Question	Relevance
Age	• Under 15: although back pain is commonly reported in children, children do have a higher incidence of identifiable and potentially serious causes, for example, spondylolysis, malignancy and Scheuermann's disease (although pain is experienced in upper back and neck). Also recent studies have linked weight of their book bags to back pain. It would seem prudent to refer all children unless backache is associated with recent participation in sport • 15 to 30: prolapsed disc, trauma, fractures and pregnancy most likely • 30 to 50: degenerative joint disease (osteoarthritis), prolapsed disc and malignancy most likely • Older than 50: patients are more likely to have serious underlying disorders such as osteoporosis, malignancy and metabolic bone disorders (Paget's disease)
Location	• Pain that radiates into the buttocks, thighs and legs implies nerve root compression. If pain is felt below the knee, this is highly suggestive of sciatica
Onset	• Low back pain that is acute and sudden in onset is likely to be muscle strain in the lumbosacral region and not serious. However, acute low back pain in the elderly should be referred as even slight trauma can result in compression fractures • The patient will normally remember performing some recent exertion (playing sport, gardening, etc) or say the pain started when they bent forward • Low back pain that is insidious in onset should be viewed with caution
Restriction of movement	• People with disc herniation usually have difficulty in sitting down for long periods • Mechanical causes of pain are exacerbated by physical activity and relieved by rest • Systemic causes of back ache are usually worse with rest and disturb sleep
Weakness or numbness	• Progressive muscle weakness must be referred for further evaluation

hands, knees, hips, neck and low back. It is thought that an imbalance of synthesis and degradation of cartilage is responsible for the disease, which affects the whole joint. It is characterised by pain of insidious onset that progressively increases over months or years and is exacerbated by exertion and relieved by rest. Stiffness in the affected joint occurs typically in the morning and after prolonged rest but usually only lasts for 15 to 30 minutes.

Inflammatory arthropathies

These include ankylosing spondylitis and psoriatic arthritis. Spondylitis is characterised by thinning or loss of elasticity of the discs that cushion the vertebrae of the spine, and is the commonest cause of chronic low back pain in the middle-aged and elderly. It is more common in men and tends to run in families. Patients commonly have marked stiffness on awakening and pain that alternates from side to side of the lumbar spine. Exercise relieves the pain but it is made worse by bending, lifting and prolonged sitting in one position (e.g. long car journeys).

TRIGGER POINTS indicative of referral:
Low back pain

Symptoms/signs	Possible danger/reason for referral
Fever	Infection
Pain that radiates away from lower back area	Sciatica
Young or older people (<20 and >55 years old) Numbness Persistent and progressively worsening pain Weight loss Feeling unwell	Possible sinister spinal pathology
Bowel or bladder incontinence	Cauda equina syndrome (rare and very unlikely to be seen by a pharmacist)

Symptoms/signs	Possible danger/reason for referral
Back pain from structures above the lumbar region	Outside scope of community pharmacist
Failure of symptoms to improve after 4 weeks	Requires further investigation as pain becoming subacute (approx. 6 weeks duration) and requires medical intervention

Evidence base for over-the-counter medication

Pharmacists can appropriately treat patients with uncomplicated acute low back pain. Recommendations made here take into account UK guidelines issued by Prodigy, which follow the 2004 European Guidelines for the management of acute simple low back pain in primary care.

The goal of treatment is to provide relief from symptoms and a return to normal mobility.

Conservative treatment

Bed rest was once widely prescribed for patients with low back pain. However, it is now widely accepted that prolonged bed rest is counterproductive and the latest Cochrane review (Hagen et al 2004) has consolidated this position. In the previous Cochrane review (Hagen et al 2000) the authors concluded: 'advice to rest in bed, compared to advice to stay active, would at best have small effects, and at worst might have small harmful effects, for those with acute LBP'. The latest Cochrane review now states: 'people with acute low back pain who are advised to rest in bed have a little more pain and a little less functional recovery'. In conclusion, the authors state that rest in bed is less effective than advice to stay active.

Analgesics (paracetamol, aspirin, NSAIDs, e.g. ibuprofen)

All systemic analgesics when prescribed as monotherapy have proven efficacy in pain relief at standard doses. However, the use of NSAIDs for 7 to 10 days is widely advocated. A review by van Tulder (2000) investigating NSAID use in low back pain concluded that NSAIDs, regardless of which specific NSAID was used, were effective for short-term symptomatic relief. It should be noted that this Cochrane review was withdrawn in March 2006, although subsequent randomised controlled trials (RCTs)

have found broadly similar findings to the Cochrane review.

Compound analgesics (paracetamol/codeine, aspirin/codeine or paracetamol/dihydrocodeine)

It is recognised that combination analgesics with high doses of opioids are effective in acute and chronic pain. However, in the UK, codeine and dihydrocodeine can only be prescribed OTC provided their respective maximum strengths do not exceed 1.5% and the maximum dose does not exceed 20 or 10 mg respectively. In practice, this equates to commercially available products with a maximum dose of 12.8 mg of codeine and 7.46 mg of dihydrocodeine. At these doses their pain-killing effect has been called into question and a number of papers have concluded that OTC doses are too low to produce statistically significant reductions in pain compared to single agents. However, the opioid dose might be sufficient to cause side effects such as constipation. Elderly patients are particularly susceptible to opioid side effects and might, in rare circumstances, experience drowsiness even at OTC doses.

Caffeine

A number of proprietary products contain caffeine in doses ranging from 15 to 110 mg. It has been claimed that caffeine enhances analgesic efficacy but evidence is lacking to substantiate these claims. They might have a mild stimulant effect and should therefore be avoided before going to bed.

Topical NSAIDs

Topical NSAIDs have been available OTC in the UK since ibuprofen was deregulated in 1988. Since then, a number of other NSAIDs have been deregulated from prescription only control. Ibuprofen has subsequently been further deregulated to General Sales List status allowing patients greater access with less control on their sale. Yet controversy has surrounded, and to some extent still does, the effectiveness of topical NSAIDs. For NSAIDs to work they must penetrate the skin, be absorbed into tissues and be in sufficiently high concentration to inhibit COX enzymes. Experimental results suggest that NSAIDs do penetrate the skin but peak plasma concentrations are greatly lower than oral NSAIDs (approximately 5% of oral plasma levels).

Prior to 1998 publications such as *MeReC* and the *Drug and Therapeutics Bulletin* stated that although several trials had shown topical NSAIDs to be more effective than placebo, the quality of this evidence was poor. Subsequently, in 1998 Moore et al published a systematic review of the safety and effectiveness of topical NSAIDs in acute and chronic pain conditions involving over 10 000 patients from 86 trials. The review included all

NSAIDs available OTC. Positive outcomes were defined as 50% pain relief after 1 week for acute conditions. The review concluded that topical NSAIDs were effective and had a lower incidence of side effects than the same drugs taken orally.

However, a number of bodies involved in formulary development produced guidelines subsequent to the Moore review that still questioned topical NSAID use and publications such as the current *British National Formulary* (edition 54) are still guarded with their opinion stating: 'topical NSAIDs may provide some slight relief of pain in musculoskeletal conditions'.

In 2004, an updated systematic review of Moore et al was published (Mason et al 2004). This review had stricter inclusion criteria than Moore et al, only accepted randomised double-blind trials and included trials published since the previous review. Findings showed NSAIDs to be significantly better than placebo in 19 of the 26 trials reviewed with an NNT (number needed to treat) of 3.8; ketoprofen was found to be significantly better than other topical NSAIDs.

Rubefacients

Rubefacients (also known as counter irritants) have been incorporated in topical formulations for decades. They cause vasodilation, producing a sensation of warmth that distracts the patient from experiencing pain. It has also been hypothesised that increased blood flow might help disperse chemical mediators of pain, although this is unsubstantiated. Numerous chemicals are listed as being rubefacients. Bandolier (http://www.ebandolier.com) produced a detailed summary of topical analgesics and usefully reviewed what constituted a rubefacient. Until recently, evidence has been lacking for their effectiveness but a systematic review published in the BMJ (Mason et al 2004) looked at the efficacy of rubefacients containing salicylates. Three trials (n=182) investigating their effect in acute conditions were reviewed. Salicyclates were found to be significantly better than placebo with a NNT of 2.1. Although the NNT is low it should still be interpreted with caution as it was derived from only 182 patients. Further trials are needed to substantiate the findings by Mason.

Capsaicin

Two POM products in the UK have been granted licences for post-herpetic neuralgia and painful diabetic neuropathy (Axsain, capsaicin 0.075%) and symptomatic relief in osteoarthritis (Zacin, capsaicin 0.025%). Clinical efficacy has been proven for both products when used to treat chronic pain. While these are not available OTC, a number of OTC products do contain capsaicin (e.g. Balmosa (0.035%), Ralgex cream (0.12%) and stick (1.96%)) at concentrations equivalent to or higher than those found in the POM products. Although no evidence exists for these products in relieving acute low back pain it would

seem a reasonable supposition that they might show similar effects. Trials are therefore needed to determine if OTC products are effective.

Enzymes

Heparinoid and hyaluronidase are included in a number of products. Theoretically, they are supposed to disperse fluids in swollen areas, reducing swelling and bruising, but this is unproven.

Summary on topical products

Current evidence points to topical rubefacients and NSAIDs being effective in treating acute musculoskeletal conditions such as low back pain. NSAIDs have the greatest body of evidence and should be recommended as first-line therapy, and salicylate-containing rubefacients reserved for patients who have had hypersensitivity reactions to topical NSAIDs or take oral NSAIDs.

Complementary therapies

Back pain accounts for more visits to a complementary practitioner than any other pain condition. In one study, 10% of people complaining of back pain had visited a complementary practitioner (osteopath, chiropractor, acupuncturist).

A limited, but growing body of clinical evidence exists to assess whether complementary therapies are effective. In light of the growing public interest and the expanding volume of literature, four Cochrane reviews have been conducted on heat and cold therapy (2006), herbal remedies (2006), acupuncture (2005) and massage (2002) respectively.

Herbal remedies

Several herbal medicines are promoted as treatments for various types of pain, some of which have been tested for the relief of symptoms of low back pain. In the 2006 Cochrane review, three active constituents were reviewed; *Harpagophytum procumbens* (Devil's Claw), *Salix alba* (White Willow Bark) and *Capsicum frutescens* (Cayenne). Devil's Claw (standardised daily dose of 50 mg or 100 mg harpagoside) reduced pain more than placebo and a standardised daily dose of 60 mg was equally as effective as 12.5 mg of Rofecoxib (Vioxx, and now withdrawn from the market). Similarly, Willow Bark (standardised daily dose of 120 mg and 240 mg of salicin) was also more effective than placebo and 240 mg of salicin was as effective as 12.5 mg of Vioxx. Cayenne (as a plaster) reduced pain more than placebo. It therefore appears that these products can be used as viable alternatives to conventional medicine.

Acupuncture

The available evidence for acupuncture in acute low back pain does not support its use, although if used in chronic back pain acupuncture is more effective for pain relief than no treatment in the short term.

Massage therapy

Eight RCTs were identified for the review. Overall, the review concluded that massage might be beneficial in non-specific back pain when combined with exercise and education. However, the results were less convincing for acute low back pain and insufficient evidence exists to recommend this as a credible treatment for acute low back pain.

Superficial heat and cold

Applying heat or cold to superficial musculoskeletal injuries such as non-specific back pain is a popular lay recommendation. These range from hot water bottles, heat pads and infra-red lamps to ice packs. A 2006 Cochrane review identified nine trials that met their inclusion criteria (six trials involved heat and three trials cold therapy). The authors concluded that many of the studies were of poor methodological quality but evidence exists that continuous heat wrap therapy reduces pain and disability in the short term to a small extent. No conclusions could be drawn on cold therapy due to the limited nature of the three trials reviewed.

Glucosamine

Although glucosamine is not used for acute low back pain it is widely advertised to the general public as a treatment for osteoarthritis. Glucosamine is naturally found in the body, especially in cartilage, tendons and ligaments, and must be synthesised by the body because significant amounts are not found in the diet. Its active form, D-glucosamin, is used in the manufacture of glycoaminoglycan, a precursor to cartilage tissue. Early reviews of glucosamine (1999) reported favourable decreases in pain and increases in joint function. However, more recent reviews (Towheed 2005) have questioned these conclusions. Taking into consideration new studies the overall benefit of glucosamine is approximately 50% less than previously thought (pain reduction of 28% compared to 60% and function 21% compared to 33%).

Chondroitin

Early research into the benefit of chondroitin in reducing pain and improving functionality in people with osteoarthritis showed chondroitin to be beneficial. Recent research that involved larger trials has shown no significant benefit. Patients should be advised that if they use chondroitin the benefits are likely to be modest at best, and if they want to use a natural product then glucosamine would be a better choice.

Summary

Based on the evidence, patients with acute low back pain should be encouraged to keep active and be given a 7-day course of a systemic NSAID unless contraindicated. Topical NSAIDs could also be recommended for those patients in whom side effects need to be minimised, for example, elderly patients or patients who have experienced GI side effects with previous NSAID use. Alternatively, a salicylate rubefacient could be substituted for NSAID intolerant patients. The only complementary therapy that appears to have credible evidence is the herbal remedies and their use might be justified.

Compound analgesics should be avoided, although patients might perceive they are getting a stronger painkiller and the placebo response of such medicines should not be underestimated.

Practical prescribing and product selection

Prescribing information relating to systemic analgesics reviewed in the section 'Evidence base for over-the-counter medication' is discussed and systemic proprietary products summarised in Table 8.2; useful tips relating to systemic analgesics are given in Hints and Tips Box 8.1.

Paracetamol

Paracetamol is the safest analgesic. It can be given to all patient groups, has no significant drug interactions and side effects are very rare. Patients with low back pain will benefit most from taking paracetamol regularly at its maximum dose of eight tablets per day. It is the drug of choice in pregnancy and breast-feeding.

Aspirin

Unlike paracetamol, aspirin is associated with problems in its use. Children under 16 should avoid any products containing aspirin (although children with low back pain should be referred). It can cause gastric irritation and is associated with gastric bleeds, especially in the elderly. For this reason, aspirin should not be given to this patient group or any patient with a history of peptic ulcer. In a small minority of asthmatic patients, aspirin can precipitate shortness of breath, therefore any asthmatic who has previously had a hypersensitivity reaction to aspirin should avoid it. It should be avoided in patients taking warfarin as bleeding time is increased. Aspirin is best avoided in pregnancy because adverse effects to the mother and foetus have been reported. It should also be avoided in breast-feeding.

Ibuprofen

Ibuprofen should be used as first-line therapy unless the patient is contraindicated from using an NSAID. Adults should take 200 to 400 mg (one or two tablets) three times a day, although most patients will need the higher dose of 400 mg three times a day. Ibuprofen is best avoided in certain patient groups, such as the elderly,

Table 8.2
Systemic proprietary analgesics available OTC (excludes paediatric formulations)

Product	Aspirin	Paracetamol	Ibuprofen	Codeine	Other	Children
Alka-Seltzer Original	324 mg					>16 years
Alka-Seltzer XS	267 mg	133 mg			Caffeine 40 mg	>16 years
Alka Rapid Crystals	500 mg					>16 years
Anadin Extra Tablets/ Soluble Tablets	300 mg	200 mg			Caffeine 45 mg	>16 years
Anadin Ibuprofen			200 mg			>12 years
Anadin Paracetamol		500 mg				>6 years
Anadin Original	325 mg				Caffeine 15 mg	>16 years
Anadin Ultra			200 mg			>12 years
Anadin Ultra Double Strength			400 mg			>12 years
Askit Powders	530 mg				Aloxiprin 140 mg Caffeine 110 mg	>16 years
Aspro Clear	300 mg					>16 years
Aspro Clear Maximum Strength	500 mg					>16 years
Care ibuprofen tablets			200 mg			>12 years
Caprin Tab	300 mg					>16 years
Codis 500	500 mg			8 mg		>16 years
Cuprofen			200 mg			>12 years
Cuprofen Maximum Strength			400 mg			>12 years
Cuprofen Plus			200 mg	12.8 mg		>12 years
Disprin & Disprin Direct	300 mg					>16 years
Disprin Extra	300 mg	200 mg				>16 years
Galprofen Ibuprofen long-lasting capsules			200 mg			>12 years
Feminax		500 mg		8 mg		>12 years
Hedex		500 mg				>6 years
Hedex Extra		500 mg			Caffeine 65 mg	>12 years
Hedex Ibuprofen			200 mg			>12 years
Ibufem			200 mg			>12 years
Librofem			200 mg			>12 years
Mandafen			400 mg			>12 years
Mandanol		500 mg				>6 years
Manorfen			200 mg			>12 years

Table 8.2 continued

Product	Aspirin	Paracetamol	Ibuprofen	Codeine	Other	Children
Migrafen			200 mg			>12 years
Nurofen Tabs, Meltlets, liquid cap, caplets, Recovery, Tension Headache & Migraine Pain			200 mg			>12 years
Nurofen Back Pain SR Caps			300 mg			>12 years
Nurofen Plus			200 mg	12.8 mg		>12 years
Nurse Sykes Powders	165 mg	120 mg			Caffeine 60 mg	>16 years
Obifen			400 mg			>12 years
Obimol		500 mg				>12 years
Panadol Tabs, Soluble		500 mg				>6 years
Panadol Caps and Actifast		500 mg				>12 years
Panadol Extra Tabs & Extra Soluble Tabs		500 mg			Caffeine 65 mg	>12 years
Panadol Night Pain		500 mg			Diphenhydramine 25 mg	>12 years
Panadol Ultra		500 mg		12.8 mg		>12 years
Paracet Tabs & Caps		500 mg				>6 years for tabs & >12 years for caps
Paracodol Soluble		500 mg		8 mg		>6 years
Paracodol Tabs & Caps		500 mg		8 mg		>12 years
Paradote		500 mg			Methionine 100 mg	>12 years
Paramol Tabs, Soluble tabs		500 mg			Dihydrocodeine 7.46 mg	>12 years
Phensic	325 mg				Caffeine 22 mg	>16 years
Propain		400 mg		10.0 mg	Caffeine 50 mg Diphenhydramine 5 mg	>12 years
Propain Plus		400 mg		10 mg	Caffeine 30 mg Doxylamine 5 mg	
Solpadeine Plus Tabs, Caps & Soluble Tabs		500 mg		8 mg	Caffeine 30 mg	>12 years
Solpadeine Max		500 mg		12.8 mg		>12 years
Solpadeine migraine			200 mg	12.8 mg		>12 years
Solpadeine headache Tabs, sol Tabs		500 mg			Caffeine 65 mg	>12 years

table continues

Table 8.2 continued

Product	Aspirin	Paracetamol	Ibuprofen	Codeine	Other	Children
Solpaflex			200 mg	12.8 mg		>12 years
Solpadeine Headache Tabs, Soluble Tabs		500 mg			Caffeine 65 mg	>12 years
Syndol		450 mg		10 mg	Caffeine 30 mg Doxylamine 5 mg	>12 years
Ultramol		500 mg		8 mg	Caffeine 30 mg	>12 years
Veganin		500 mg		8 mg	Caffeine 30 mg	

HINTS AND TIPS BOX 8.1: ASPIRIN IN CHILDREN

Children and aspirin	Aspirin-taking in children has been linked to Reye's syndrome, a rare syndrome in which encephalopathy occurs and if not diagnosed early can lead to death
	Until October 2002 advice from the CSM stated that no child under 12 should take aspirin. However, due to wide availability of aspirin and other safer treatment choices it was decided to simplify the advice in the interest of public health and raise the age to children under 16. Many parents might not be aware of the age restriction for aspirin and it is important that pharmacists remind parents

because they are more prone to GI bleeds and have reduced renal function, and patients with a history of peptic ulcers and those patients with asthma who are hypersensitive to aspirin or any other NSAID. However, it appears to be safe in pregnancy and breast-feeding.

For the majority of patients, ibuprofen is well tolerated, although gastric irritation is a well-recognised side effect. It can interact with many medicines and although none of these interactions are truly significant, ibuprofen can increase the risk of lithium and methotrexate toxicity, and enhance the anticoagulating effect of warfarin. In such circumstances an alternative should be recommended.

Topical NSAIDs

Topical NSAIDs provide an alternative to those patients who should avoid systemic NSAID therapy. They have fewer side effects than systemic therapy with the most commonly reported adverse events being skin reactions (maculopapular rash or itching) at the site of application. Low plasma levels probably explain their low incidence of adverse systemic effects. A review published in the BMJ (Evans et al 1995) involving over 23 000 people over a 5-year period found no association between topical NSAIDs and upper gastrointestinal bleeding.

Topical NSAIDs come in a range of formulations, including cream, gel, spray and mousse. Ibuprofen is the market leader, although other NSAIDs are available and include piroxicam, diclofenac, ketoprofen, felbinac, sali-cylic acid and benzydamine. Table 8.3 highlights all commercially available NSAIDs and summarises their prescribing information.

Rubefacients (e.g. Balmosa, Deep Heat, Radain B and Ralgex ranges)

Rubefacients should be avoided in young children and most manufacturers state they should not be used in children under 5 or 6 years of age. They have no drug interactions and side effects are localised to excessive irritation at the site of application. The majority of products contain two or more compounds, although most contain nicotinates and/or salicylates. Other compounds in rubefacients include menthol, camphor, capsaicin and turpentine oil.

Further reading

Bueff HU, Van Der Reis W. Low back pain. Prim Care 1996;23:345–64.

Deyo RA, Weinstein JN. Low back pain. N Engl J Med 2001;344:363–70.

Evans JM, McMahon AD, McGilchrist MM, et al. Topical non-steroidal anti-inflammatory drugs and admission to hospital for upper gastrointestinal bleeding and perforation: a record linkage case-control study. BMJ 1995;311:22–6.

French SD, Cameron M, Walker BF, et al. Superficial heat or cold for low back pain. The Cochrane Database of

Table 8.3
Proprietary topical NSAID analgesics available OTC

Product	Formulation	Strength	Dosage	Children
Ibuprofen				
Care	Gel	5 & 10%	qds	>14 years
Cuprofen	Gel	5%	tds-qds	>12 years
Deep Relief	Gel	5%	tds	>12 years
Fenbid	Gel	5%	Up to qds	>14 years
Ibugel	Gel	5%	No dose stated	>12 years
Ibuleve	Gel, spray, mousse	5%	tds-qds	>12 years
Ibuleve Maximum Strength	Gel	10%	tds	>12 years
Ibuleve Mousse	Mousse	5%	No dose stated	>12 years
Ibuspray	Spray	5%	No dose stated	>12 years
Mentholatum	Gel	5%	tds	>14 years
Nurofen and Nurofen Maximum Strength	Gel	5 & 10%	qds	>14 years
Phorpain & Phorpain Forte	Gel	5% & 10%	No dose stated	>12 years
Proflex	Cream	5%	tds-qds	>12 years
Radian B ibuprofen gel	Gel	5%	tds	>14 years
Other NSAIDs				
Difflam (benzydamine)	Cream	3%	tds but max of six times	No lower age limit stated
Feldene P (piroxicam)	Gel	0.5%	tds-qds	>12 years
Movelat (mucopolysaccharide polysulpahate & salicylic acid)	Cream and gel	0.2% & 2.0%	qds	>12 years
Oruvail (Ketoprofen)	Gel	2.5%	tds	>12 years
Traxam (Felbinac)	Gel	3%	bd-qds	>12 years
Voltarol Emulgel (Diclofenac)	Gel	1.16%	tds-qds	>12 years

Systematic Reviews 2006, issue 1. Oxford: Update Software.

Furlan AD, van Tulder MW, Cherkin DC, et al. Acupuncture and dryneedling for low back pain. The Cochrane Database of Systematic Reviews 2005, issue 1. Oxford: Update Software.

Furlan AD, Brosseau L, Imamura M, Irvin E. Massage for low-back pain. The Cochrane Database of Systematic Reviews 2002, issue 2. Oxford: Update Software.

Gagnier JJ, vanTulder M, Berman B, Bombardier C. Herbal medicine for low back pain. The Cochrane Database of Systematic Reviews 2006, issue 2. Oxford: Update Software.

Hagen KB, Hilde G, Jamtvedt G, Winnem M. Bed rest for acute low back pain and sciatica. The Cochrane Database of Systematic Reviews 2004, issue 4. Oxford: Update Software.

Koes BW, van Tulder MW, Thomas S. Diagnosis and treatment of low back pain. BMJ 2006;332:1430–4.

Mason L, Moore RA, Edwards, JE, et al. Topical NSAIDs for acute pain: a meta-analysis. BMC Fam Pract 2004;5:10.

Mason L, Moore RA, Edwards JE, et al. Systematic review of efficacy of topical rubefacients containing salicylates for the treatment of acute and chronic pain. BMJ 2004;328:995–8.

Maniadakis A, Gray A. The economic burden of back pain in the UK. Pain 2000;84:95–103.

Moore RA, Tramer MR, Carroll D, et al. Qualitative systematic review of topically applied NSAIDs. BMJ 1998;316:333–8.

Reichenbach S, Sterchi R, Scherer M, et al. Chondroitin for osteoarthritis of the knee or hip. Ann Intern Med 2007;146:580–90.

Towheed TE, Maxwell L, Anastassiades TP, et al. Glucosamine therapy for treating osteoarthritis. The Cochrane Database of Systematic Reviews 2005, issue 2. Oxford: Update Software.

van Tulder MW, Scholten RJPM, Koes BW, Deyo RA. Non-steroidal anti-inflammatory drugs for low-back pain. The Cochrane Database of Systematic Reviews 2000, issue 2. Oxford: Update Software.

Web sites

European guidelines on the prevention and treatment of low back pain: http://www.backpaineurope.org

BackCare – the charity for healthier backs: http://www.backcare.org.uk/

The National Ankylosing Spondylitis Society: http://www.nass.co.uk/

BMJ article on sciatica (June 2007): http://www.bmj.com/cgi/content/extract/334/7607/1313

Activity-related/sports-related soft tissue injuries

This section will discuss common conditions affecting the shoulder, elbow, knee, ankle and foot.

Background

Muscle, tendons, ligaments, fascia and synovial capsules are all soft tissue structures. Damage to any of these structures will result in pain and/or inflammation. The pharmacist will encounter patients with soft tissue injuries, although the majority of patients present to a GP, physiotherapist or casualty department. In a number of small studies, most respondents did not consider the pharmacist as a source of advice or help, although the minority who had consulted a pharmacist were satisfied with the advice received. This suggests that pharmacists could play a greater role in managing patients with activity-/sport-related problems.

Prevalence and epidemiology

Most injuries are as a direct result of physical activity or accident. Prevalence is therefore higher in people who actively participate in sports and injuries involving the lateral ligaments of the ankle account for 25% of all sports injuries. The knee is another common site of injury.

Aetiology

The aetiology of soft tissue injury depends on the structures affected. Sprains are caused by forcing a joint into an abnormal position that overstretches or twists ligaments, and can vary from damage of a few fibres to complete rupture. Strains involve tearing of muscle fibres, which can be partial or complete and are usually a result of overexertion when the muscle is stretched beyond its usual limits.

Arriving at a differential diagnosis

Patients will often state they have sprained or strained something. It is important to confirm their self-diagnosis as these terms are often used interchangeably. Sprains and strains can be graded according to the severity of the injury, but this is of little practical value because it has no therapeutic consequence. The major role of the pharmacist is to determine if the patient can manage the injury or whether referral is needed. This will be primarily based on questions asked (Table 8.4) of the patient but, even without an intimate knowledge of joint anatomy, limited physical examination can be performed to help decide if referral is necessary.

Clinical features of soft tissue injury

In general patients will present with pain, swelling and bruising. The extent and severity of symptoms will be determined by the severity of the injury.

Shoulder-specific conditions

The shoulder provides the greatest range of motion of any joint. It is a very mobile and complex interconnected structure (Fig. 8.3); consequently, there are a number of commonly encountered shoulder injuries, such as frozen shoulder, impingement syndromes and rotator cuff syndrome. The prevalence of shoulder-related problems is uncertain, although estimates range from 4 to 20% with rotator cuff syndrome accounting for up to 70% of shoulder problems.

Within the confines of the community pharmacy, the patient can be asked to perform certain arm movements that will allow the range of motion of the shoulder to be determined (Fig. 8.4). Patients who show marked loss of motion should be referred.

Rotator cuff syndrome

The rotator cuff refers to the combined tendons of the scapula muscles that hold the head of the humerus in place. Rubbing of these tendons causes pain. It is most often seen in patients over the age of 40 and is associated with repetitive overhead activity. Pain tends to be worse at night and might disturb sleep. Reaching behind the back also tends to worsen pain. Also, the patient cannot normally initiate abduction.

Table 8.4
Specific questions to ask the patient: Soft tissue injuries

	Relevance
When did it happen and when did the patient present	• The closer these two events are the more likely the patient will be suffering from a serious problem that is outside the remit of the pharmacist, unless the injury was sustained in close proximity to the pharmacy and the patient has asked for first aid
Presenting symptoms	• Marked swelling, bruising and pain occurring straight after injury is suggestive of more serious injury and referral to casualty for X-rays and further tests is needed
Nature of injury	• If an injury occurred in which impact forces were great then fracture becomes more likely • Sudden onset, associated with a single traumatic event suggests a mechanical problem such as tendon/ligament tearing • If the person has a foot injury and is unable to bear their full weight while walking then referral is needed
Range of motion	• If the affected joint shows marked reduction in normal range of motion this requires referral for fuller evaluation
Nature of pain	• Referred pain suggests nerve root compression involvement, for example, a shoulder injury in which pain is also felt in the hand • Pain that is insidious in onset and progressive is more likely to be due to some form of degenerative disease and requires referral
Age of patient	• *Children*: Bones are softer in children and therefore more prone to greenstick fractures (fracture of the outer part of the bone) and should be referred to exclude such problems • *Elderly*: Risk factors for fracture, such as osteoarthritis and osteoporosis is higher in the elderly

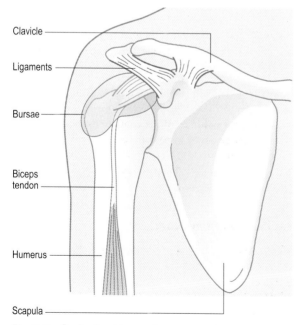

Fig. 8.3 Basic shoulder anatomy

Frozen shoulder

This term is used to describe the shoulder when it has marked restriction in all the major ranges of motion. It is a relatively uncommon cause of shoulder pain accounting for 2% of cases. It often occurs without warning or explanation and can vary in severity from day to day. NSAIDs could be offered but if symptoms fail to respond to treatment after 5 days then referral for alternative treatment and physiotherapy should be considered.

Elbow-specific conditions

In primary care, pharmacists are only likely to see three elbow problems: tennis elbow (lateral epicondylitis), golfers' elbow (medial epicondylitis) and student's elbow (bursitis).

Tennis elbow is characterised by pain and tenderness felt over the outer aspect of the elbow joint that might also spread up the upper arm. The patient should have a history of gradually increasing pain and tenderness. If the patient tries to extend the wrist against resistance then pain increases. In comparison, the pain of golfer's elbow is noticed on the inner side of the elbow and can

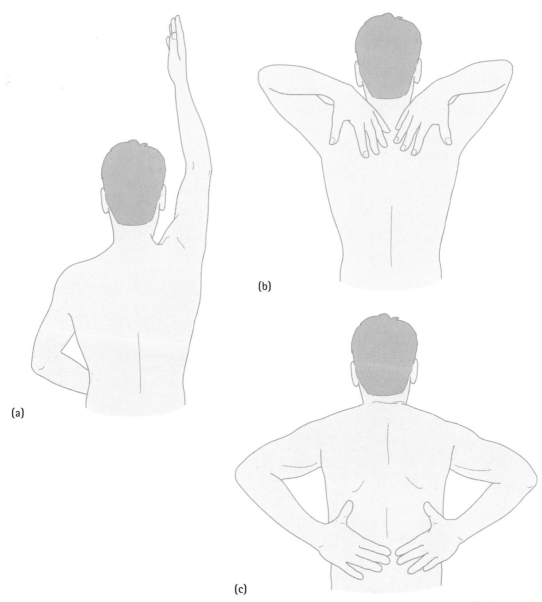

(a)

(b)

(c)

Fig. 8.4　Determining the range of motion of the shoulder: (a) ask the patient to raise the arm as if going to ask a question at school; (b) ask the patient to touch the back of the neck with both hands; (c) ask the patient to touch the back of the scapulae with both hands.

radiate down the forearm. Both names are misleading as these conditions are usually related to a repetitive activity, which can include sports activity.

Knee-specific conditions

The knee is the largest joint in the body and is subject to extreme forces. Unsurprisingly, it is one of the most common sites of sport injuries, especially among footballers. To help maintain stability the knee has three main pairs of ligaments: the medial collateral ligament, which connects the femur to the tibia; the lateral collateral ligament, which connects the femur to the fibula; and

the anterior cruciate ligament, which prevents the tibia from sliding forward on the femur (Fig. 8.5).

Ligament damage

This is most often seen in footballers. Find out from the patient how the injury occurred. If the injury occurred when twisting this implies damage to the medial meniscus (incomplete rings of cartilage that promote joint stability) as the medial collateral ligament is attached to the meniscus and forces applied to the ligament result in tears of the meniscus. This is less serious than damage to the anterior cruciate ligament, which usually occurs

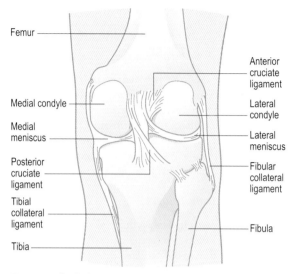

Fig. 8.5 Basic knee anatomy

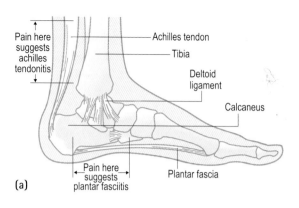

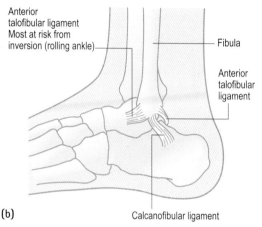

Fig. 8.6 Basic anatomy of the ankle: (a) medial view; (b) lateral view.

when the person receives a blow to the back of the knee. The former can usually respond to NSAIDs and physiotherapy, whereas the latter can take months to heal and might stop people from playing competitive sport.

Runner's knee (chondromalacia)

Most commonly noted in recreational joggers who are increasing their mileage, for example, training to run a marathon. It develops insidiously with pain being the predominant symptom. Pain can be aggravated by prolonged periods of sitting down in the same position or climbing stairs. Treatment depends on the severity of pain but NSAIDs can be tried if the pain is mild, to total rest and stopping running if severe.

Ankle and foot-specific conditions

The majority of injuries involve sprained ankles whether through sporting activity or just as a result of accidents.

Ankle sprains

The ankle acts as a hinge joint permitting up and down motion. Three sets of ligaments provide stability to the joint: the deltoid, lateral collateral and syndesmosis. The majority of ankle sprains involve the lateral ligamentous structures due to inversion of the joint leading to injury (Fig. 8.6). Patients usually describe an accident when they 'went over their ankle'. Most patients will walk with a limp because the ankle cannot support their full weight.

Achilles tendon injuries

Injuries to the structures associated with the Achilles tendon are usually seen in runners or athletes involved in jumping sports. Inflammation of bursae or the Achilles tendon itself will manifest with similar symptoms. Pain is felt behind the heal, just above the calcaneus, and progressively worsens the longer the injury lasts. It often occurs when runners increase their mileage or run over hilly terrain. Depending on the severity of the injury, treatment could be anything from NSAIDs, complete rest or having a cast fitted. If the injury is recent in onset and pain not too severe the pharmacist could suggest NSAID therapy and rest. If this fails then the person should be referred.

Plantar fasciitis

The plantar fascia extends from the calcaneus to the middle phalanges of the toes allowing toes to flex. Runners are most prone to plantar fasciitis, although it can affect older people. Patients will present with tenderness and pain felt along the plantar surface of the foot and heel. Pain is insidious and progressively worsens, which can limit activity.

Common muscle strains

Thigh strains

Tears of the quadriceps (front of the thigh) and hamstring (back of the thigh) are very common. Patients will not always be able to recall a specific event that has caused the strain. Pain and discomfort is worsened when the patient tries to use the muscle but daily activities can usually be performed. RICE (see below) followed by NSAID treatment will usually resolve the problem; however, referral is needed if daily activities are compromised.

Conditions to eliminate

Delayed onset muscle soreness

This is a common problem and follows unaccustomed strenuous activity. For example, the patient might describe playing football for the first time in a long while or just having started going to aerobic classes. Pain is felt in the muscles, which feel stiff and tight. Pain peaks within 72 hours. Patients should be encouraged to properly stretch prior to exercising to minimise the problem. No treatment is necessary.

Shin splint syndrome

Recreational runners and people unaccustomed to regular running can experience pain along the front of the lower third of the tibia. Pressing gently on this area will cause considerable pain. It is caused by over stretching the tibial muscle and is usually precipitated by running on hard surfaces. Pain is made worse by continued running or climbing stairs. Treatment involves running less frequently or for shorter distances and NSAID therapy for approximately 1 week.

Bursitis

Bursae can become inflamed, which leads to accumulation of synovial fluid in the joint. Housemaid's knee and student's elbow are such examples. Clinically, joint swelling is the predominant feature with associated pain and local tenderness.

Stress fractures

These are most commonly associated with the foot. Patients experience a dull ache along the affected metatarsal shaft that changes to a sharp ache behind the metatarsal head. It is often seen in those patients that have a history of increased activity or a change in footwear.

Gout

Acute attacks of gout are exquisitely painful, with patients reporting that even bedclothes cannot be toler-

ated. Approximately 80% of cases affect the big toe. Gout is more prevalent in men, especially over the age of 50.

Carpal tunnel syndrome

At the base of the palm is a 'tunnel' through which the median nerve passes; this narrow passage between the forearm and hand is called the carpal tunnel. If the median nerve becomes trapped, it can cause numbness and tingling in the hand. Often the patient will wake in the night with numbness and tingling pain that radiates to the forearm, and sometimes extends to the shoulder.

Repetitive strain injury

This condition, also termed chronic upper limb pain syndrome, often results after prolonged periods of steady hand movement involving repeated grasping, turning and twisting. The predominant symptom is pain in all or one part of one or both arms. Usually the person's job will involve repetitive tasks such as keyboard operations.

 TRIGGER POINTS indicative of referral: Soft tissue injury

- Acute injuries that show immediate swelling and severe pain
- Children under 12 and elderly patients
- Decreased range of motion in all direction involving the shoulder
- Excessive range of movement in any joint (may suggest major ligament disruption)
- Patients unable to bear any weight on an injured ankle/foot
- Suspected fracture
- Treatment failure

Evidence base for over-the-counter medication and practical prescribing and product selection

Prescribing information relating to medication for soft tissue injuries is the same as for acute low back pain (see pages 249–254). However, non-drug treatment plays a vital and major role in the treatment of soft tissue injuries. Standard advice follows the acronym RICE:

Rest: Rest allows immobilisation, enhancing healing and reducing blood flow

Ice   Ice should be applied while the injury feels warm to the touch. Apply until the skin becomes numb and repeat at hourly intervals. Bags of frozen peas wrapped in a towel are ideal to use on the injury as they conform to body shape and provide even distribution of cold

Compression — A crepe bandage provides a minimum level of compression. Tubular stockings (e.g. Tubigrip) are convenient and easy to apply but fail to give adequate compression

Elevation — Ideally the injured part should be elevated above the heart to help fluid drain away from the injury

Further reading

Calmbach WL, Hutchens M. Evaluation of patients presenting with knee pain: Part II. Differential diagnosis. Am Fam Physician 2003;68:917–22.

Donnelly AE, Maughan RJ, Whiting PH. Effects of ibuprofen in exercise induced muscle soreness and indices of muscle damage. Br J Sports Med 1990;24:191–5.

Kayne S, Reeves A. Sports care and the pharmacist – an opportunity not to be missed. Pharm J 1994;253:66–7.

Knill-Jones R. Survey of activity in Scottish sports medicine centres. Performance 1989;1:4.

Murrell GA, Walton JR. Diagnosis of rotator cuff tears. Lancet 2001;357:769–70.

Polisson RP. Sports medicine for the internist. Med Clin N Am 1986;70:469–89.

Spiegel TM, Crues JV. The painful shoulder: diagnosis and treatment. Prim Care 1988;15:709–24.

West SG, Woodburn J. Pain in the foot. BMJ 1995;310:860–4.

Web sites

Society of Sports Therapists: http://www.society-of-sports-therapists.org

The Repetitive Strain Injury Association: http://www.rsi.org.uk/index.asp

Self-assessment questions

The following questions are intended to supplement the text. Two levels of questions are provided; multiple choice questions and case studies. The multiple choice questions are designed to test factual recall and the case studies allow knowledge to be applied to a practice setting.

Multiple choice questions

8.1 Which of the following is not used in topical formulations for musculoskeletal disorders?

- a. Nicotinates
- b. Hyaluronidase
- c. Choline
- d. Menthol
- e. Capsaicin

8.2 Which of the following statements is true of osteoarthritis?

- a. Morning stiffness usually lasts less than 30 minutes
- b. Pain is eased by movement
- c. Pain is usually worst in the morning
- d. Osteoarthritis commonly affects small joints
- e. Inflammation is a key pathological finding

8.3 Which of the following patients would *not* be at increased risk of developing gastrointestinal problems while taking NSAIDS?

- a. A patient taking Pariet
- b. An elderly patient
- c. A patient suffering from *H. pylori* infection
- d. A patient with asthma
- e. A patient with gastro-oesophageal reflux disease (GORD)

8.4 Vertebrae involved in sciatica are:

- a. L1–L2
- b. L2–L3
- c. L3–L4
- d. L4–L5
- e. None of the above

8.5 Which ligament is most often damaged in a sprained ankle?

- a. Cruciate ligament
- b. Deltoid ligament
- c. Medial collateral ligament
- d. Posterior talofibular ligament
- e. Anterior talofibular ligament

8.6 A strain is said to affect which structure?

- a. Tendon
- b. Ligament
- c. Bursa
- d. Muscle   "muscle strain"
- e. Cartilage

8.7 From the following list, what common name is given to inflammation of the bursa?

- a. Golfer's elbow
- b. Student's elbow
- c. Tennis elbow
- d. Repetitive strain injury
- e. Shin splints

8.8 In which of the following conditions does pain often wake the patient?

- a. Rotator cuff syndrome
- b. Frozen shoulder
- c. Hamstring strain
- d. Plantar fasciitis
- e. Housemaid's knee

Questions 8.9 to 8.11 concern the following groups of people:

- A. Runners/joggers
- B. Footballers
- C. Squash players
- D. Occasional gardeners
- E. Swimmers

Select, from A to E, which of the above groups of people are more prone to:

8.9 Anterior cruciate ligament damage

8.10 Plantar fasciitis

8.11 Tennis elbow

Questions 8.12 to 8.14 concern the following OTC medications:

A. Feldene P Gel
B. Codis tablets — under 16 not to be given – codiene
C. Panadol tablets 6-12yrs.
D. Radian B cream – children not recommended
E. Voltarol emulgel

Select, from A to E, which of the above medicines

8.12 Can only be given to children older than 16 B

8.13 Has no evidence of efficacy d. working?

8.14 May cause constipation B

Questions 8.15 to 8.17: for each of these questions *one or more* of the responses is (are) correct. Decide which of the responses is (are) correct. Then choose:

A. If a, b and c are correct
B. If a and b only are correct
C. If b and c only are correct
D. If a only is correct
E. If c only is correct

Directions summarised

A	B	C	D	E
a, b and c	a and b only	b and c only	a only	c only

8.15 Which of the following measures should be recommended to a patient who has just suffered an acute soft tissue injury?

a. Heat and massage of the affected area
b. Elevation of the affected area
c. Compression of the affected area by means of an elastic bandage or support

8.16 Acute low back pain is characterised by:

a. Insidious onset and progressively worsening pain
b. Radiating pain towards the thoracic vertebrae
c. Decreased mobility
E.

8.17 Children under 12 with a soft tissue injury should be referred to the GP because:

a. 'RICE' is only suitable for adults
b. OTC medication is contraindicated
c. More prone to greenstick fractures than adults

Questions 8.18 to 8.20: these questions consist of a statement in the left-hand column followed by a statement in the right-hand column. You need to:

- decide whether the first statement is true or false
- decide whether the second statement is true or false

Then choose:

A. If both statements are true and the second statement is a correct explanation of the first statement
B. If both statements are true but the second statement is NOT a correct explanation of the first statement
C. If the first statement is true but the second statement is false
D. If the first statement is false but the second statement is true
E. If both statements are false

Directions summarised

	1st statement	2nd statement	
A	True	True	2nd statement is a correct explanation of the first
B	True	True	2nd statement is not a correct explanation of the first
C	True	False	
D	False	True	
E	False	False	

	First statement	*Second statement*
8.18	Carpal tunnel syndrome causes hand numbness	Medial nerve impingement results in symptoms
8.19	Low back pain with associated fever should be referred	Malignancy is the likely cause
8.20	NSAIDs are the mainstay of systemic treatment for soft tissue injuries	They should be used for 7 to 10 days. If symptoms do not improve, referral is needed

Case study

CASE STUDY 8.1

Mrs BB, a 69-year old women, hobbles into your pharmacy, supported by her husband. She has just slipped off the pavement edge and believes she has sprained her ankle.

a. To ascertain if referral is necessary, describe the questions you would ask Mrs BB?

Find out exact nature of pain and its location. It is likely that the anterior talofibular ligament has been damaged. Symptoms that would warrant referral are severe pain in any bone prominence, if Mrs BB is unable to walk unsupported for at least four steps and marked swelling and bruising occurred straight after the fall. Mrs BB should be told to go to casualty if these symptoms are present.

You decide that Mrs BB has indeed sprained her ankle but referral is unnecessary. Mrs BB asks to purchase some OTC analgesia to alleviate her pain. Her regular medication is as follows:

- Bendroflumethiazide 2.5 mg od: used to treat hypertension. Taken for 5 years
- Fybogel sachets, 1 bd: taken for 4 years for constipation
- Lansoprazole 15 mg od: maintenance therapy in treatment of GORD associated with hiatus hernia.

b. Which OTC systemic analgesics would be most suitable for Mrs BB. Explain how you arrived at your choice and why you eliminated others.

Aspirin: can cause GI disturbance; Mrs BB has GORD, therefore, contraindicated.

Ibuprofen: NSAIDs can cause fluid retention and Mrs BB has hypertension. However, this is unlikely to be clinically significant, especially if NSAIDs are recommended for only a few days. Like aspirin, ibuprofen can cause GI disturbances.

Codeine: Cannot be bought as a single agent. Combinations with aspirin need to be avoided. Paracetamol and codeine combinations could be offered but the codeine content is likely to cause constipation, which Mrs BB is already being treated for. Therefore, codeine is likely to worsen her already existing constipation. Finally, OTC analgesic combinations have been shown not to significantly reduce pain compared to monotherapy. This leaves paracetamol as the medicine of choice for Mrs BB.

Mrs BB asks if she should also use a topical preparation on her ankle.

c. Describe the range of topical preparations available to treat soft tissue injuries and which would be suitable to recommend to Mrs BB, giving the reasons for your decision(s).

Rubefacients contain essential oils, salicylates, nicotinates, capsicum, camphor, terpentine and menthol. They provide warmth to the injury site, except menthol and camphor, which are cooling. These can be recommended to Mrs BB.

Ideally recommend a product with no salicylate present, as there is a low risk of systemic absorption and gastric irritation.

Topical NSAIDs: relatively low doses reach the bloodstream and there is therefore less risk of GI problems than with systemic NSAIDs. Use of topical NSAIDs are unlikely to cause side effects if used for short periods of time (5 to 10 days) and could be given to Mrs BB even though she has GORD. However, she should be told that if she experiences any indigestion-type symptoms to stop using the product.

8

CASE STUDY 8.2

Mr JD, a 47-year old male, asks you for something for low back pain. On questioning you find out the following:

Information gathering	Data generated
Presenting complaint (possible questions)	
What symptoms have you got/describe the pain	Pain described as aching and dull and spreads to bottom on the right-hand side
How long have you had the symptoms	Came on about 2 days ago. Woke up with the pain
Where is the pain	Pain is diffuse over low back
Any other symptoms	No other symptoms
When do you get the symptoms	Constant
Does the pain move anywhere	Top of the bum (as above)
Does anything make the symptoms better/worse	Pain is made worse if sitting over a period of long time
Additional questions asked	Cannot remember doing anything to precipitate it. Severity: 5/6 out of 10
Previous history of presenting complaint	No
Past medical history	No past medical history
Drugs (OTC, Rx and compliance)	Esomeprazole 1 od for last year to help with indigestion
Allergies	

Information gathering	Data generated
Social history	
Smoking	Works in an office
Alcohol	No lifestyle changes
Drugs	
Employment	
Relationships	
Family history	Not asked
On examination	Not performed

Epidemiology dictates that the most likely cause of back pain seen in primary care for all ages is related to physical activity. However, other conditions are possible and are noted below:

Probability	Cause
Most likely	Simple back pain associated with physical activity
Likely	Nerve root compression (e.g. sciatica), pregnancy (not applicable in this case)
Unlikely	Osteomyelitis, ankylosing spondylitis
Very unlikely	Malignancy

Diagnostic pointers with regard to symptom presentation

The following page summarises the expected findings for questions when related to the different conditions that can be seen by community pharmacists.

Continued

CASE STUDY 8.2

	Age	Radiation of pain	Onset	Absence of systemic or neurological signs	Precipitating factors
Simple back pain	All adults	No	Acute	Yes	Yes
Sciatica	>30 years	Yes (buttocks and leg)	Acute	Yes	Yes
Osteoarthritis	>30 years but more common with increased age	No	Chronic	Yes	No
Osteomyelitis	All ages	No	Acute	No	No
Ankylosing spondylitis	>50 years	Yes (side-to-side of back)	Chronic	Yes	No
Malignancy	>50 years	No	Chronic	No	No

When this information is applied to that gained from our patient (below) we see that his symptoms most closely match sciatica. Acute onset and radiation are very suggestive of this condition despite there being no obvious cause.

	Age	Radiation of pain	Onset	Absence of systemic or neurological signs	Precipitating factors
Simple back pain	✓	✗	✓	✓	✗
Sciatica	✓	✓	✓	✓	✗
Osteoarthritis	✓	✗	✗	✓	✓
Osteomyelitis	✓	✗	✓	✗	✓
Ankylosing spondylitis	✗?	✓	✗	✓	✓
Malignancy	✗?	✗	✗	✗	✓

Danger symptoms/signs (trigger points for referral)

As a final double check it might be worth making sure the person has none of the 'referral signs or symptoms'; this is the case with this patient. Referred pain (see below) is usually an indication to refer the patient. However, NSAIDs could usually be given while the patient waits to see a GP but as he takes a proton pump inhibitor it would be best to recommend paracetamol.

Fever	✗
Pain that radiates away from lower back area	✓
Failure of symptoms to improve after 2 weeks	N/A
Young or elderly people	N/A
Numbness	✗
Persistent and progressively worsening pain	✗
Bowel or bladder incontinence	✗
Back pain from structures above the lumbar region	✗

Answers to multiple choice questions

1 = c	2 = a	3 = d	4 = d	5 = e	6 = d	7 = b	8 = a	9 = b	10 = a
11 = c	12 = b	13 = d	14 = b	15 = c	16 = e	17 = e	18 = a	19 = c	20 = b.

Paediatrics

Background

A number of conditions are encountered much more frequently in children than the rest of the population. It is these conditions that this chapter focuses on. A small number of conditions that affect all age groups but are often associated with children are not included, for example, middle ear infection. Such conditions are covered in other chapters and where appropriate will be cross-referenced to the relevant sections within the text.

History taking

In the majority of cases pharmacists will be heavily dependent on getting details about the child's problem from their parents or an adult responsible for the child's welfare. This presents both benefits and problems to the pharmacist. Parents will know when their child is not well and asking the parent about the child's general health will help to determine how poorly the child actually is. Additionally, a child who is running around and lively is unlikely to be acutely ill and referral to a GP is less likely. The major problem faced by all healthcare professionals is the difficulty in gaining an accurate history of the presenting complaint. This poses difficulties in assessing the quality and accuracy of the information as children find it hard to articulate their symptoms. If the child can be asked questions, these often have to be posed in either closed or leading formats to elicit information.

As a rule of thumb, any child who appears visibly ill should always be seen by the pharmacist and referral might well be needed, whereas children who are acting normally and appear generally well will normally not need to see the GP and can be managed by the pharmacist.

Head lice

Background

Humans act as hosts to three species of louse; *pediculosis capitis* (head lice), *pediculosis corporis* (body lice) and *pediculosis pubis* (pubic lice). In this section only head lice are discussed.

Prevalence and epidemiology

Head lice affect all ages but are much more prevalent in children aged 4 to 11 years, especially girls. Studies conducted in schools show wide variation of current lice infestation ranging from 4 to 22% of pupils. Head lice can occur at any time and do not show any seasonal variation. Most parents will have experienced a child who has head lice, or received letters from school alerting parents to head lice infestation within the school.

Aetiology

Head lice can only be transmitted by head-to-head contact. Fleeting contact will be insufficient for lice to be transferred between heads. Once transmitted lice begin to reproduce. The adult louse lives for approximately 1 month. Throughout this time the female louse lays several eggs at the base of the hair shaft each night. Eggs hatch after 6 to 9 days, leaving the egg case attached to the hair shaft (known as a 'nit'). In the course of maturing to adulthood the young louse – the nymph – undergoes three moults. Shortly after maturing, the female louse is sexually mature and able to mate.

Arriving at a differential diagnosis

Most parents will diagnose head lice themselves or be concerned that their child has head lice because of a recent local outbreak at school. Occasionally, parents will also want to buy products to prevent their child contracting head lice. It is the role of the pharmacist to confirm the self-diagnosis and stop inappropriate sales of products. It should also be remembered that an itching scalp in children is not always due to head lice and other causes should be eliminated. Asking a number of symptom-specific questions should enable a diagnosis of head lice to be easily made (Table 9.1).

Clinical features of head lice

Unless live lice have been found, most patients will present with scalp itching. Itching is caused by an aller-

gic response of the scalp to the saliva of the lice and can take weeks to develop. However, only a third of patients experience itching. Head lice are most commonly found in the occipital and auricular areas.

Conditions to eliminate

Dandruff

Dandruff can cause irritation and itching of the scalp. However, the scalp should be dry and flaky. Skin debris might also be present on clothing.

Seborrhoeic dermatitis

Typically, seborrhoeic dermatitis will affect areas other than the scalp, most notably the face and nappy area. If only scalp involvement is present then the child might complain of severe and persistent dandruff. In infants the patient will have large yellow scales and crusts of the scalp (cradle cap).

 TRIGGER POINTS indicative of referral: Head lice

- Parents who find cost of treatment prohibitive

 Table 9.1
Specific questions to ask the patient: Head lice

Question	Relevance
Have live lice been seen	• The presence of live lice is diagnostic. Pharmacists can advise patients on how best to check for infection. Currently, both wet and dry combing are advocated Dry combing: 1. Straighten and untangle the dry hair using an ordinary comb 2. Once the hair moves freely, switch to a detection comb. Starting from the back of the head, comb from the scalp down to the end of the hair 3. After each stroke examine the comb for live lice 4. Continue to comb all the hair in sections until the whole head has been combed This process can take 5 or more minutes in people with shoulder length hair Wet combing: Wash the hair with a normal shampoo Apply hair conditioner Repeat steps 1 to 4 as for dry combing Rinse out the conditioner Wet combing is more time consuming than dry methods and both should be performed on all family members
Empty egg shells (nits)	• This does not constitute evidence of current infection. This is a common misconception held by the general public and the pharmacist must ensure that parents seeking treatment have observed live lice • Egg shells are not removed by using insecticides. Patients need to be reassured that the presence of egg shells does not mean treatment failure
Presence of itching	• Itching is not always present in head lice. Inspection of the scalp should be made to check for signs of dandruff, psoriasis or seborrhoeic dermatitis

Evidence base for over-the-counter medication

Treatment options include insecticides, wet combing and dimeticone. All treatments available in the UK have shown clinical effectiveness; however, it is difficult to assess which treatment is most effective as very few comparative trials have been performed and insecticidal resistance varies from region to region. No treatment is 100% effective and failure has been linked to poor adherence with each treatment regime. Of the treatment approaches, insecticides have been most studied. These include malathion, permethrin and pyrethrin. Cure rates of 70 to 80% are reported with insecticides in recent clinical trials. Resistance to insecticides is a serious problem and appears to be increasing. Wet combing is therefore an alternative treatment option because there are no contraindications to its use and insecticidal resistance is not an issue. However, cure rates are reported to be only 50 to 60% and adherence to the treatment schedule is a factor, with rates reported to be as low as 50% (Roberts et al 2000).

Dimeticone is a recent introduction to the UK market. Its inclusion in treatment options seems to stem from one robust trial conducted by Burgess et al (2005). Dimeticone was compared against phenothrin with cure rates determined at days 9 and 14. Dimeticone was shown to have comparable cure rates to phenothrin (69% compared to 78%). The study has been criticised for using dry detection methods and using different detection days (days 5 and 12 as recommended by the department of health); however, a further trial in 2007 supports the 2005 trial results. In the latter study, 4% dimeticone lotion, applied for 8 hours or overnight was compared to 0.5% malathion liquid applied for 12 hours or overnight. The results found dimeticone was significantly more effective than malathion, with 30/43 (69.8%) participants cured using dimeticone compared with 10/30 (33.3%) using malathion.

Other non-insecticidal methods of eradication are also promoted. These include herbal remedies such as tea tree oil or essential oils (e.g. Lyclear SprayAway) No evidence exists on the effectiveness of tea tree oil and this should

not be recommended until such time that data support its use.

In summary, treatment used will be driven by individual preference, the patient's medical history and previous exposure to treatment regimes. Wet combing (available as bug busting kits) is time consuming and requires patient motivation but is helpful in areas of high insecticidal resistance. Insecticides and dimeticone are simpler to use than bug-busting kits and appear to have higher cure rates. The July 2007 edition of the *Drug and Therapeutics Bulletin* recommended dimeticone as first-line therapy for those parents that did not want to use conventional insecticides.

Practical prescribing and product selection

Prescribing information relating to medicines for head lice reviewed in the section 'Evidence base for over-the-counter medication' is discussed and summarised in Table 9.2; useful tips relating to patients presenting with head lice are given in Hints and Tips Box 9.1. All regimes have to be used more than once: insecticides have to be repeated 7 days after first application (this is based on expert opinion, as the second application is intended to kill nymphs emerging from eggs that have survived the first application); wet combing every 4 days for at least 2 weeks; and dimeticone repeated after 7 days.

All products can be used on children older than 6 months. Insecticides should be avoided in pregnant and breast-feeding women. When applying the products, particular attention should be paid to the areas behind the ears and at the nape of the neck, as these areas are where lice are most often found.

Permethrin (Lyclear Crème Rinse – see Hints and Tips Box 9.1 for suitability)

Before application the hair should be washed with a mild shampoo and towelled dry. Enough Lyclear should be applied to the hair to ensure the hair and scalp is thoroughly saturated. It should be left on the hair for 10 minutes before rinsing the hair thoroughly with water. One bottle is sufficient for shoulder length hair of average

---

Table 9.2
Practical prescribing: Summary of medicines for head lice

Name of medicine	Use in children	Likely side effects	Drug interactions of note	Patients in whom care should be exercised	Pregnancy and breast-feeding
Permethrin	>6 months	Irritation of scalp (rare)	None	Asthmatic patients and those with scalp conditions should avoid alcohol-based products	OK, but malathion has less safety data
Phenothrin					
Malathion					
Dimeticone				None	OK

HINTS AND TIPS BOX 9.1: HEAD LICE

Who to treat?	Only those individuals with an active head lice infestation should be treated
Products for prevention	Prevention of lice using insecticides is not advocated and the patient should be counselled on when treatment is required
Lotion, liquid, mousse or shampoo?	Do not recommend shampoos. The concentration of insecticide will be too low to ensure eradication because the shampoo is diluted by water. In addition they have a much shorter contact time with the hair and scalp compared to lotions and liquids This advice is also given in edition 55 of the *British National Formulary* for Lyclear crème rinse as contact time is lower than currently recommended A liquid product is the most suitable formulation for very young children and asthmatics
Treatment failure	It is recommended that detection combing is performed 2 to 3 days after treatment to confirm success or failure of treatment. If no lice live are found, this should be repeated again 1 week after the first detection combing
Myths	Public misconceptions about head lice need to be dispelled • Head lice are not only associated with dirty hair • Head lice do not only affect children • Children should not be kept off school

---

thickness. It might rarely cause scalp reddening and irritation.

Phenothrin (Full Marks)

Full Marks is available as liquid, lotion or mousse. Liquids and lotions are rubbed into the scalp until all the hair and scalp is thoroughly moistened and then allowed to dry naturally. They should be applied as close to the base of the hair and scalp as possible. Twelve hours later the hair should be shampooed in the normal way. Most parents find it easier and more convenient to apply the solution before bedtime and leave on overnight. The mousse is applied to dry hair at several points on the scalp and massaged into the scalp, ensuring no part of the scalp is left uncovered. After 30 minutes the hair can be washed with normal shampoo.

Malathion (e.g. Derbac-M, Prioderm, Quellada-M, Suleo-M)

Malathion is available as liquid, lotion or shampoo. Liquids and lotions are applied in exactly the same manner as Full Marks products.

Shampoos, if used (see Hints and Tips Box 9.1), should be applied to wet hair and left on for 5 minutes before rinsing. After rinsing the process should be repeated. Two further treatment courses then have to be applied at 3-day intervals.

Two products (Prioderm lotion and Suleo-M) have an alcoholic base and should be avoided in asthmatics and small children because they might precipitate bronchospasm. Like permethrin, skin irritation has been reported on application but is rare.

Dimeticone 4% Lotion (Hedrin)

Hedrin is applied to dry hair and the scalp ensuring that the scalp is fully covered. The lotion should be spread evenly from the hair root to the tips. It should be left on for a minimum of 8 hours (overnight is preferable) before being rinsed off.

Further reading

Burgess IF, Brown CM, Peock S, et al. Head lice resistant to pyrethroid insecticides in Britain. BMJ 1995;311:752.

Burgess IF, Brown CM, Lee PN. Treatment of head louse infestation with 4% dimeticone lotion: randomised controlled equivalence trial. BMJ 2005;330:1423-5.

Burgess IF, Lee PN, Matlock G. Randomised, controlled, assessor blind trial comparing 4% dimeticone lotion with 0.5% malathion liquid for head louse infestation, 2007. PLoS ONE 2(11): e1127. doi:10.1371/journal.pone.0001127.

Dodd CS. Interventions for treating headlice. Cochrane Database of Systematic Reviews 2006, issue 4 (status withdrawn Issue 2, 2007, pending update).

Effectiveness matters. NHS Centre for Reviews and Dissemination 1999;4(1).

Hill N, Moor G, Cameron, MM, et al. Single blind, randomised, comparative study of the Bug Buster kit and over the counter pediculicide treatments against head lice in the United Kingdom. BMJ 2005;331:384-7.

Roberts RJ, Casey D, Morgan DA, Petrovic M. Comparison of wet combing with malathion for treatment of head lice in the UK: a pragmatic randomised controlled trial. Lancet 2000;356:540-4.

[Anonymous] Treating head louse infections. Drug Ther Bull 1998;36:45-6.

Thomas DR, McCarroll L, Roberts R. Surveillance of insecticide resistance in head lice using biochemical and molecular methods. Arch Dis Child 2006;91:777-8.

Web sites

Prodigy topic review: http://www.cks.library.nhs.uk/head_lice/about_this_topic

Clinical Evidence: http://www.clinicalevidence.com

Community Hygiene Concern: http://www.chc.org/bugbusting/

Pediculosis.com: http://www.pediculosis.com/intro.html

Once a week – take a peek: http://www.onceaweektakeapeek.com/

Threadworm (Enterobius vermicularis)

Background

Worm infections are extremely common both in the developed and developing world. In Western countries the most common worm infection is threadworm (known in some countries as pinworm), which is a condition that causes inconvenience and embarrassment rather than one that causes morbidity. Social stigma surrounds the diagnosis of threadworm. This belief is unfounded as infection occurs in all social strata. The patient might benefit from reassurance from the pharmacist, explaining that the condition is very common and is nothing to be ashamed or embarrassed about.

Prevalence and epidemiology

Threadworm is the most common helminth infection throughout temperate and developed countries. This is primarily due to threadworm transmission not being soil or waterborne, unlike other helminth infections. Threadworm prevalence is difficult to establish due to the high number of people who self-medicate or are asymptomatic. However, UK prevalence rates have been estimated at 20% in the community, rising to 65% in institutionalised settings. Threadworms are much more common in school or preschool children than adults, because of their inattention to good personal hygiene.

Aetiology

Eggs are transmitted to the human host primarily by the faecal-oral route (autoinfection) but also by retroinfec-tion and inhalation. Faecal-oral transmission involves eggs lodging under fingernails, which are then ingested by finger sucking after anal contact. Retroinfection occurs when larvae hatch on the anal mucosa and migrate back into the sigmoid colon. Finally, threadworm eggs are highly resistant to environmental factors and can easily be transferred to clothing, bed linen and inanimate objects (e.g. toys) resulting in dust-borne infections. Once eggs are ingested, duodenal fluid breaks them down and releases larvae, which migrate into the small and large intestines. After mating, the female migrates to the anus, usually at night, where eggs are laid on the perianal skin folds, after which the female dies. Once laid, eggs are infective almost immediately. Transmission back into the gut can then take place again via one of the three mechanisms outlined above and so the cycle is perpetuated.

Arriving at a differential diagnosis

Threadworm diagnosis should be one of the more simple conditions to diagnose. Patients who are not asymptomatic generally present with very specific symptoms.

Clinical features of threadworm

Night-time perianal itching is the classic presentation (caused by the mucus produced by females when laying eggs). However, patients might experience symptoms ranging from a local 'tickling' sensation to acute pain. Any child with night-time perianal itching is almost certain to have threadworm. Itching can lead to sleep disturbances resulting in irritability and tiredness the next day. Diagnosis can be confirmed by observing threadworm on the stool, although they are not always visible.

Complicating factors such as excoriation and secondary bacterial infection of the perianal skin can occur due to persistent scratching. The parent should be asked if the perianal skin is broken or weeping.

Conditions to eliminate

Other worm infections

Roundworm and tapeworm infections are encountered occasionally. However, these infections are usually contracted by adults when visiting poor and developing countries.

Contact irritant dermatitis

Occasionally, dermatitis can cause perianal itching especially in adults. If there is no recent family history of threadworm or there is no visible sign of threadworm on the faeces then dermatitis is possible.

> **TRIGGER POINTS indicative of referral:**
> **Threadworm**
>
> * Medication failure
> * Secondary infection of perianal skin due to scratching

Evidence base for over-the-counter medication

Mebendazole and piperazine are available OTC for the treatment of threadworm. There is a large body of evidence to support the effectiveness of mebendazole in roundworm infections but for other worm infections, including threadworm, there is a less evidence showing consistently high cure rates. For threadworm, cure rates between 60 and 82% for single-dose treatment of mebendazole have been reported.

Piperazine appears to have less evidence supporting its effectiveness than mebendazole. One study has compared piperazine to mebendazole and found mebendazole to have a higher cure rate than piperazine, although the number of patients in the trial was low.

The difference in cure rates might be, in part, due to their respective mechanisms of action. Mebendazole inhibits the worm's uptake of glucose thus killing it, whereas piperazine paralyses the worm. To optimise worm clearance from the gut one piperazine formulation also contains senna. However, if paralysis wears off then the worm might be able to migrate back into the colon and thus treatment would fail.

Practical prescribing and product selection

Prescribing information relating to medicines for threadworm reviewed in the section 'Evidence base for over-the-counter medication' is discussed and summarised in Table 9.3; useful tips relating to patients presenting with threadworm are given in Hints and Tips Box 9.2.

Treatment should ideally be given to all family members and not only the patient with symptoms, as it is likely that other family members will have been infected even though they might not show signs of clinical infection. A repeated dose 14 days later is often recommended to ensure worms maturing from ova at the time of the first dose are also eradicated.

Mebendazole and piperazine should be avoided in pregnancy because foetal malformations have been reported but appear safe in breast-feeding. Patients should be advised to practise hygiene measures. If treatment is absolutely essential, piperazine has been used, although this should not be in the first trimester.

Mebendazole (e.g. Ovex, Pripsen Mebendazole)

The dose for adults and children over 2 is a single tablet. Young children might prefer to chew the tablet and it has been formulated to taste of orange. Side effects reported include abdominal pain, diarrhoea and rash but are very rare. It does interact with cimetidine, increasing mebendazole plasma levels but this is of little clinical

Table 9.3
Practical prescribing: Summary of medicines for threadworm

Name of medicine	Use in children	Likely side effects	Drug interactions of note	Patients in whom care should be exercised	Pregnancy and breast-feeding
Mebendazole	>2 years	Abdominal pain, rash	Phenytoin and carbamazepine	None	Avoid in pregnancy; OK in breast-feeding
Piperazine	>3 months	Diarrhoea, rash	None	None	

HINTS AND TIPS BOX 9.2: THREADWORM

Hygiene measures	Complementary to drug treatment is the need for strict personal hygiene
	Nails should be kept short and clean. Careful washing and nail scrubbing prior to meals and after each visit to the toilet is essential to prevent autoinfection
	Bed linen should be washed frequently, ideally every day although this might not be practical
	Underwear should be worn underneath night clothes to prevent scratching
	On awakening the patient should have a bath or shower paying particular attention to washing around the anus
	Damp dusting and daily vacuuming are recommended to remove eggs

9

consequence. However, phenytoin and carbamazepine decrease mebendazole plasma levels and the dose of mebendazole may need to be increased.

Piperazine (e.g. Pripsen Piperazine Phosphate Powder)

Piperazine is available as sachets that also contain senna. They can be given from 3 months of age upwards. The dose should be given in the morning (for adults the dose is recommended to be taken at night). From 3 months to 1 year, half a 5 mL spoonful should be taken, for children aged 1 to 6 years the dose is one 5 mL spoonful and for children over 6 years (and adults) one sachet should be taken. The sachets can be taken in water or milk.

A number of side effects have been reported with piperazine but all are rare and generally are of GI origin such as diarrhoea or allergic reactions, for example, rash.

Further reading

Albonico M, Smith PG, Hall A, et al. A randomized controlled trial comparing mebendazole and albendazole against ascaris, trichuris and hookworm infections. Trans R Soc Trop Med Hyg 1994;88:585-9.

Rafi S, Memon A, Billo AG. Efficacy and safety of mebendazole in children with worm infestation. J Pak Med Assoc 1997;47:140-1.

Russell LJ. The pinworm, Enterobius vermicularis. Prim Care 1991;18:13-24.

Sorensen E, Ismail M, Amarasinghe DK, et al. The efficacy of three anthelmintic drugs given in a single dose. Ceylon Med J 1996;41:42-5.

Zaman V. Other gut nematodes. In: Weatherall DJ, Ledingham JGG, Warrell DA (eds) Oxford textbook of medicine. Oxford: Oxford Univeristy Press, 1987.

Web sites

Prodigy guidance: http://www.cks.library.nhs.uk/threadworm/about_this_topic

Article in the Pharmaceutical Journal (Sept. 2006) on parasitic worm infections: http://www.pjonline.com/editorial/20060916/cpd/p343parasiticworm.html

Division of parasitic diseases: http://www.cdc.gov/ncidod/dpd/parasites/pinworm/default.htm

Colic

Background

There is no universally agreed definition of colic. A widely used definition is that proposed by Wessel (1954) and has come to be known as the 'rule of threes'. Wessel proposed that an infant could be considered to have colic if it cries for more than 3 hours a day for more than 3 days a week for more than 3 weeks. However, the definition by Wessel is arbitrary and few parents are willing to wait 3 weeks to see if the infant meets the criteria for colic. As a result the third criterion is usually dropped in the clinical setting. In addition, some authors have defined crying for as little as 90 minutes per day as excessive. Regardless of which definition is used, persistent crying is a cause of stress and anxiety to parents.

Prevalence and epidemiology

Owing to no universally accepted definition of colic its prevalence is difficult to determine, and estimates vary widely from 3 to 40% dependent on which definition is used. Studies reporting lower figures strictly applied Wessel's criteria, while higher figures used wider definitions. It is likely that prevalence falls between the two extremes and affects 10 to 20% of infants.

Colic starts in the first few weeks of life and usually resolves by the age of 3 to 5 months.

Aetiology

The cause of colic is poorly understood. Two theories are currently favoured. Firstly, it is a disorder of the GI tract, where painful contractions cause excessive crying, and might be caused by allergy to cow's milk. Secondly, it might stem from emotional and behavioural problems in the mother brought on by a difficult temperament of the infant as a possible explanation for inadequate parental reactions.

Arriving at a differential diagnosis

It is difficult to determine if the baby is considered to have colic or is just crying excessively, as the diagnosis of the condition is dependent on qualitative descriptions. However, the term colic is often wrongly applied to any infant who cries more than usual. Asking a number of symptom-specific questions should enable a diagnosis of colic to be made (Table 9.4).

Clinical features of colic

Excessive crying and inconsolable crying are obvious clinical features. Pain may be mild, merely causing the child to be restless in the evenings or severe resulting in rhythmical screaming attacks lasting a few minutes at a time, alternating with equally long quiet periods in which the child almost goes to sleep, before another attack starts. Attacks appear to be more common in the early evening, giving rise to the name 6 pm colic. However, both normal infant crying and the crying in colic peak in the late afternoon and early evening and this is therefore of limited value. The infant will be healthy and thriving.

Table 9.4
Specific questions to ask the patient: Colic

Question	Relevance
Cry quality	• High-pitched crying, often associated with facial flushing, drawing up the legs and fist clenching are common in colic
History of crying	• Excessive crying is not isolated and will have been present for some time. Acute infections are normally sudden in onset and the baby will not exhibit a long-standing history of excessive crying

Conditions to eliminate

Acute infection

Colic and acute infections of the ear or urinary tract can present with almost identical symptoms. However, in acute infection the child should have no previous history of excessive crying and have signs of systemic infection such as fever.

Intolerance to cow's milk protein

Colicky pain in infants is sometimes due to intolerance to cow's milk protein. This is far less common than generally believed but should be considered if the infant is failing to thrive.

Gastro-oesophageal reflux disease (GORD)

GORD can present with excessive crying, although this is normally accompanied by visible regurgitation.

TRIGGER POINTS indicative of referral: Colic

- Infants that are failing to put on weight
- Medication failure
- Overanxious parents

Evidence base for over-the-counter medication

Parents of the infant should be reassured that symptoms will subside over time and that their child will not be harmed by the symptoms. Most parents will be seeking some form of medical treatment but products have limited effect. Treatments include simeticone, lactase enzymes

and low-lactose milk formulas. Gripe mixtures are commercially available but have no evidence base and should not be recommended.

Simeticone is reported to have antifoaming properties, reducing surface tension and allowing easier elimination of gas from the gut by passing flatus or belching. It is widely used yet has very limited evidence of efficacy. Of three trials reported, only one found a small improvement in the number of crying attacks. This trial was small (n = 26) and suffered from methodological flaws and so results should be viewed with caution.

Lactase enzymes

Lactase breaks down lactose present in milk to glucose and galactose. This reduction in lactose concentration is reported to improve colic symptoms but four small trials investigating its effect were inconclusive.

Summary

Although evidence for simeticone and lactase enzymes is not strong it would seem unreasonable not to let parents try either for a trial period of a week if they are finding it difficult to cope. If no response is seen then referral to the GP for an alternative formula feed would be advisable.

Practical prescribing and product selection

Prescribing information relating to simeticone is discussed and summarised in Table 9.5; useful tips relating to colic are given in Hints and Tips Box 9.3.

Simeticone (e.g. Infacol and Dentinox)

Simeticone is pharmacologically inert; it has no side effects, drug interactions or precautions in its use and can therefore be safely prescribed to all patients. It should be given with or just after each feed. Products contain different strengths of simeticone; however, the dose administered to a child is almost equivalent, for example, Infacol 0.5 to 1 mL (20 to 40 mg) and Dentinox 2.5 mL (21 mg).

Lactase enzyme (Colief)

The dose of Colief differs depending on whether the baby is formula or breast-fed: if breast-feeding, four drops should be added to a small amount of expressed milk and the baby breast-fed as normal; if using an infant formula then the feed should be made up as usual and four drops added to warm, but not hot, formula. If making the formula up in advance then two drops of Colief should be added and stored in the fridge for 4 hours.

Table 9.5
Practical prescribing: Summary of medicines for colic

Name of medicine	Use in children	Likely side effects	Drug interactions of note	Patients in whom care should be exercised	Pregnancy and breast-feeding
Simeticone	Infant upwards	None	None	None	Not applicable
Lactase					

HINTS AND TIPS BOX 9.3: COLIC

Review feeding technique	Before recommending a product it is worth checking feeding technique. Underfeeding the baby can result in excessive sucking resulting in air being swallowed leading to colic-like symptoms. Additionally, the teat size of the bottle should be checked. When the bottle is turned upside down the milk should drop slowly from the bottle

Further reading

Barr RG, Lessard J. Excessive crying. In: Bergman AB (ed) 20 common problems in paediatrics. New York: McGraw-Hill, 2001.

Garrison MM, Christakis DA. A systematic review of treatments for infant colic. Pediatrics 2000;106:184–90.

Lucassen PL, Assendelft WJ, Gubbels JW, et al. Effectiveness of treatments for infantile colic: systematic review. BMJ 1998;316:1563–9.

Wessel MA, Cobb JC, Jackson EB, et al. Paroxysmal fussing in infancy, sometimes called 'colic'. Paediatrics 1954;14:421–4.

Web sites

Prodigy guidance: http://www.cks.library.nhs.uk/colic_infantile

CRY-SIS:http://www.cry-sis.org.uk

General site on colic: http://www.colichelp.com/

Atopic dermatitis

Background

Atopic dermatitis is a chronic non-infective inflammatory skin condition that is characterised by an itchy red rash. It usually starts within the first 6 months of life and predominantly affects young children. The majority (60 to 70%) of patients will 'grow out' of the condition by their early teens. However, in a small number of patients in whom atopic dermatitis persists into adulthood the condition becomes chronic. Atopic eczema can impair the quality of life of patients and their families, with itching and sleep loss having a major effect.

Prevalence and epidemiology

The prevalence of atopic dermatitis is unclear. Rates vary from country to country. In the UK prevalence rates have been rising, and it now affects 15 to 20% of children, although over 80% are reported to have mild disease. The condition usually presents in infants aged between 2 and 6 months, but it can occur in older children. Upward of 60% of children will have onset within the first year, rising to 80% within the first 5 years. Atopic dermatitis is much less common in adults affecting only 1 to 3% of people.

Aetiology

Atopic dermatitis has a strong genetic component, although the precise genetic cause is unknown. Two-thirds of people with the disease have a family history of atopic eczema, asthma or hayfever. Atopic eczema is present in approximately 80% of children where both parents are affected and in 60% if one parent is affected. In addition, a number of environmental factors have been implicated in the development or worsening of the condition and include certain foods (e.g. diary products), stress, extremes of heat and humidity and irritants such as detergents and chemicals.

Arriving at a differential diagnosis

To help with diagnosis, criteria-based protocols are available, for example, those produced by the *British Journal of Dermatology* and NICE, which state atopic dermatitis can be diagnosed if the person has had an itchy skin condition (Fig. 9.1) in the past 12 months plus three or more of the following:

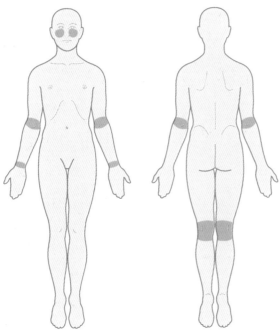

Fig. 9.1 Typical distribution of atopic dermatitis

- onset before age of 2 years (Fig. 9.2)
- history of dry skin
- history of eczema in the skin creases (and also the cheeks in children under 10 years)
- visible flexural eczema (inside elbows, behind knees (Fig. 9.3) or involvement of the cheeks/forehead and outer limbs in children under 4 years)
- personal history of other atopic disease

Asking a number of symptom-specific questions should enable a diagnosis of atopic dermatitis to be made (Table 9.6).

Clinical features of atopic dermatitis

A typical presentation of a child with atopic dermatitis is an irritable, scratching child with dermatitis of varying severity. Itching is the predominant symptom, which can induce a vicious cycle of scratching, leading to skin damage, which in turn leads to more itching – the so-called itch scratch itch cycle. The child might have had the symptoms for some time and the parent has often already tried some form of cream to help control the itch and rash. Scratching can lead to broken skin, which can become infected. There is a tendency to a dry sensitive skin even in those who have 'grown out' of the disease.

Conditions to eliminate

Seborrhoeic dermatitis

Seborrhoeic dermatitis in infants typically occurs in the first 6 months. Itching is generally not present and the

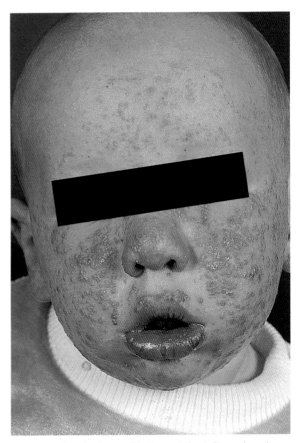

Fig. 9.2 Atopic dermatitis in an infant. Reproduced from *Dermatology: An Illustrated Colour Text* by D J Gawkrodger, 2008, Churchill Livingstone, with permission

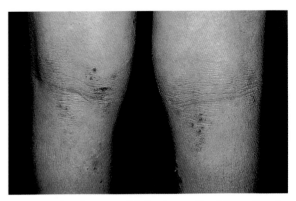

Fig. 9.3 Atopic dermatitis in the popliteal fossa (bend of knee). Reproduced from *Dermatology: An Illustrated Colour Text* by DJ Gawkrodger, 2008, Churchill Livingstone, with permission

condition usually spontaneously resolves after a few weeks and seldom recurs. It usually affects the scalp, face and nappy area. Large yellow scales and crusts often appear on the scalp and are often referred to as cradle cap (see Fig. 7.10, p. 194).

Table 9.6
Specific questions to ask the patient: Atopic dermatitis

Question	Relevance
Is itching present	• Atopic dermatitis is classically associated with intense itching • Psoriasis and seborrhoeic dermatitis are not usually associated with itching
Distribution of rash	• Varies according to age (see Fig. 9.1) but in infants the nappy area is not involved and is a useful distinction between atopic dermatitis and seborrhoeic dermatitis
Age of child	• Presentation varies with age • Babies: facial involvement (the cheeks) is common along with patchy red scaly lesions on the wrists and hands (see Fig. 9.2) • Toddlers and older children: the antecubital (in front or at the bend of the elbow), popliteal fossae (behind the knee) and ankles are more commonly involved (see Fig. 9.3)
Family history of atopy	• If a parent has eczema, hayfever or asthma then the likelihood of atopic dermatitis rises

Psoriasis

Psoriasis can be mistaken for atopic dermatitis because the rash is erythematous and can occur on parts of the body such as the scalp, elbows and knees, which is a common location for atopic dermatitis in older children. However, the rash is raised, has well-defined boundaries with a silvery-white scaly appearance and itch, if present, is mild.

Herpes simplex complications

Sufferers from atopic dermatitis are susceptible to the herpes simplex virus. If herpes is suspected the patient should be referred quickly for aciclovir. For further information on herpes simplex the reader is referred to Chapter 7, page 223.

TRIGGER POINTS indicative of referral: Atopic dermatitis

- Children with widespread or severe dermatitis
- Child requiring steroid therapy or medication failure
- Presence of secondary infection (weeping and crusting lesions)

Evidence base for over-the-counter medication

The mainstay of treatment for atopic dermatitis consists of avoiding potential irritants, managing dry skin, controlling itching and using topical corticosteroids to treat flare-ups. Unfortunately, the latter option is not available OTC because licence restrictions mean that only children over the age of 10 can be given OTC corticosteroids.

Avoiding irritants

Where practical, factors that worsen eczema should be avoided. The use of highly perfumed soaps and detergents should be discouraged and replaced with soap substitutes (e.g. Alpha Keri, Neutrogena, Dove). Patients should be told to have lukewarm not hot baths because in some patients hot water can aggravate the problem. In addition, a bath additive should be used (e.g. Balneum, Oilatum, Emulsiderm) to help hydration of the skin.

Emollients

It is believed that emollients add moisture to the skin and repair the lipid barrier function while also helping to prevent penetration by irritants and decrease the need for steroids. Despite a lack of high-quality randomised controlled trials, emollients are well established as first-line treatment for atopic eczema. In addition, no trials appear to have addressed whether one emollient is superior to another in treating atopic eczema. Patients might have to try several emollients before finding one that is most effective for their skin.

Antihistamines

There appear to be no clinical trial data on the use of sedative antihistamines for reducing pruritus in atopic dermatitis; however, they are often prescribed to children to help with itching. Additionally, they can also help prevent night-time scratching.

Corticosteroids

A substantial body of evidence exists for corticosteroids in controlling all types of dermatitis, including atopic dermatitis. If the symptoms warrant corticosteroid therapy then the patient needs to be referred to the GP. Usually mild steroids such as hydrocortisone (1 to 2.5%), preferably in an ointment base, should be prescribed twice daily.

Practical prescribing and product selection

Prescribing information relating to medicines for atopic dermatitis reviewed in the section 'Evidence base for over-the-counter medication' is discussed and summarised in Table 9.7; useful information regarding emollients containing lanolin is given in Hints and Tips Box 9.4.

Emollients

There are a plethora of emollient products marketed and which one a patient uses will be dictated by patient response and acceptability. All emollients should be regularly and liberally applied with no upper limit on how often they can be used. All are chemically inert and therefore can be safely used from birth upwards. For a summary of emollient products see Table 7.32 (page 231).

Sedating antihistamines

Although no sedating antihistamine products, except hydroxyzine (POM), have a specific product licence for the treatment of pruritus, they are frequently prescribed by GPs and could be given OTC. However, it must be remembered that if recommended then the person concerned is acting outside the product licence and will be therefore liable for any clinical consequence associated with the use of the product. The doses that can be given for the various sedating antihistamines are listed below.

Chlorphenamine (Piriton)

Chlorphenamine can be given from the age of 1 year. Children up to the age of 2 years should take 2.5 mL of syrup (1 mg) twice a day. For children aged between 2 and 5 the dose is 2.5 mL (1 mg) three or four times a day and those over the age of 6 should take 5 mL (2 mg) three or four times a day.

Clemastine (Tavegil)

Clemastine is taken twice a day by children over the age of 1 year. Those aged between 1 and 3 should take 250 to 500 µg, children aged between 3 and 6 should take 500 µg and for those over 6 the dose is 500 µg to 1 mg.

Table 9.7
Practical prescribing: Summary of medicines for atopic dermatitis

Name of medicine	Use in children	Likely side effects	Drug interactions of note	Patients in whom care should be exercised	Pregnancy and breast-feeding
Emollients	Birth onwards	None	None	None	Not applicable
Sedating antihistamines Chlorphenamine	>1 year	Sedation	Increased sedation with opioid analgesics, anxiolytics, hypnotics and antidepressants. However, it is unlikely a child will be taking such medicines	None	Not applicable
Clemastine	>1 year				
Cyproheptadine	>2 years				
Promethazine	>2 years				

HINTS AND TIPS BOX 9.4: ATOPIC DERMATITIS

Lanolin-containing emollients	Emollients that contain lanolin (e.g. Keri Lotion and E45) should be avoided as they are known to cause sensitisation
Applying emollients	They are best applied when the skin is moist, for example, during bath times. Bath additives will make the bath slippery so care should be taken when getting the child out Apply as frequently as possible The more oily the emollient the more effective it tends to be

Tavegil is only available as 1 mg tablets and so dosing in young children is difficult.

Cyproheptadine (Periactin)

Children between 2 and 6 should take 2 mg (half a tablet) and for children over 7 the dose is 4 mg (one tablet) two or three times a day.

Promethazine (Phenergan Elixir 5 mg/5 mL and 10 mg and 25 mg tablets)

Children between 2 and 5 years should take 5 to 15 mg (5 to 15 mL) daily in one to two divided doses and for those over 5 the dose is 10 to 25 mg daily in one to two divided doses.

Further reading

Brown S, Reynolds NJ. Atopic and non-atopic eczema. BMJ 2006;332:584-8.

Clark C, Hoare C. Making the most of emollients. Pharm J 2001;266:227-9.

Web sites

Prodigy guidance: http://www.cks.library.nhs.uk/eczema_atopic

NICE Atopic dermatitis (eczema) – topical steroids (August 2004): http://www.nice.org.uk/guidance/TA81/?c=91528

Management of atopic eczema in primary care, article in ePrescriber, Sept 2003: http://www.escriber.com/Assets/EscriberDownloads/Images/14-18%20eczema%20rev.pdf

MeReC Bulletin: http://www.npc.co.uk/MeReC_Bulletins/2003Volumes/Vol14no1.pdf

National Eczema Society: http://www.eczema.org/

General dermatology site: http://www.dermatologist.co.uk/index.html

---

Fever

Background

Fever is simply a rise in body temperature above normal. Normal oral temperature is 37°C (98.6°F), plus or minus 1°C, although rectal temperature is about 0.5°C higher and underarm temperature 0.5°C lower than oral temperature. During the course of 24 hours minor fluctuations in temperature are observed. Fever is often classified as being either mild (up to 39°C) or high (above 39°C).

In a practice setting, for those aged under 5 years of age, the best temperature to take is under the arm using an electronic or chemical dot thermometer. Infrared tympanic thermometers are also advocated (NICE guidance No. 47, May 2007) but a systematic review by Dodd et al (2006) questioned their reliability. Using forehead strip thermometers is popular because it is easy, but these should not be used as they are unreliable.

Prevalence and epidemiology

Fever is a common symptom of many conditions, and in children viral and to a lesser extent bacterial causes are most commonly implicated. It has been reported that fever is probably the commonest reason for a child to be taken to a doctor.

Aetiology

Body temperature is regulated closely because temperature changes can significantly alter cellular functions and, in extreme cases, lead to death. Thermoregulation is a balance between heat production and heat loss. Cellular metabolism produces heat and this means that energy – in the form of heat – is produced continually by the body. This heat production is lost through the skin by radiation, evaporation, conduction and convection. The thermoregulation centre located in the hypothalamus controls the whole process. When body temperature reaches its 'set point' (approximately 37°C) mechanisms to lose or conserve heat are activated. When a person suffers from a fever this suggests that there is some defect in the temperature regulating control system. In fact the system is functioning normally but with an adjusted higher 'set point'. This process is complex but involves the production of pyrogens (fever-causing substances) that alter the set point.

Arriving at a differential diagnosis

The parent, in nearly every instance, will diagnose fever in the child. This is usually a subjective perception by the parent that the child feels warm or is off colour. The importance of the parent's perception should not be underestimated or dismissed if the child's temperature has not been taken. Many healthcare professionals often place too much value on an empirical figure when in many instances the look of the child is more important than the height of the fever. Asking a number of symptom-specific questions should enable the pharmacist to treat or refer the child with fever (Table 9.8).

Additionally, NICE recommend using a 'traffic light' system to assess the risk of serious disease (Table 9.9). In a pharmacy setting any child that show symptoms or signs of intermediate (amber) or high (red) risk should be referred to the GP.

Clinical features of fever

A child with fever will generally be irritable, off his or her food and seek greater parental attention. Other signs that might be seen include facial flushing and shivering.

Table 9.8
Specific questions to ask the patient: Fever

Question	Relevance
How old is the child	• Children under 3 months should be referred automatically because diagnosis can be very difficult and serious complications can arise
How poorly is the child	• The parent will know how poorly the child is relative to normal behaviour. A child might have a high temperature but appear relatively normal whereas a child with a mild temperature might be quite poorly
Associated symptoms	• Viral upper respiratory tract infections are usually accompanied by one or more symptoms including cough, cold or sore throat • Glandular fever is usually accompanied by fatigue and lymph node enlargement (usually teenagers) • If no other symptoms are present it suggests a bacterial infection, often a urinary tract infection

Table 9.9
Assessment of the seriousness of fever*

	Green – low risk	Amber – intermediate risk	Red – high risk
Colour	Normal colour of skin, lips and tongue	Pallor reported by parent/carer	Pale/mottled/ashen/blue
Activity	Responds normally to social cues Content/smiles Stays awake or awakens quickly Strong normal cry/not crying	Not responding normally to social cues Wakes only with prolonged stimulation Decreased activity No smile	No response to social clues Appears ill to the pharmacist Unable to rouse or if roused does not stay awake Weak, high-pitched or continuous cry
Respiratory		Nasal flaring 6–12 months, RR >50 breaths/ minute >12 months, RR 40 breaths/minute	Grunting RR >60 breaths/minute
Hydration	Normal skin and eyes Moist mucous membranes	Dry mucous membrane Poor feeding in infants CRT ≥3 seconds Reduced urine output	Reduced skin turgor
Other	NONE of the amber or red signs or symptoms	Fever ≥5 days Swelling of a limb/joint	0–3 months ≥38°C 3–6 months ≥39°C Non-blanching rash Neck stiffness Bulging fontanelle Seizures

CRT, capillary refill time; RR, respiration rate
*Table adapted from NICE. CG 47 Feverish illness in children: assessment and initial management in children younger than 5 years. London: National Institute for Health and Clinical Excellence, 2007. Reproduced with permission. Guidelines are accurate at time of going to press. Latest guidelines are available at http://www.nice.org.uk/CG47

Conditions to eliminate

Upper respiratory tract infections

It is rare for upper respiratory tract infections to present with fever alone. Cough, cold or sore throat are usually present. Treatment can be offered and referral is generally not needed unless secondary bacterial infection is suspected; earache symptoms might suggest this.

Roseola infantum (sixth disease)

Roseola infantum is probably caused by a neurodermotropic virus and is most prevalent in children under 1 year of age. Onset is with a sudden high fever (40°C) that usually subsides by the third or fourth day once the rash, which blanches when pressed, appears on the trunk and limbs. The condition is self-limiting.

Glandular fever

Glandular fever is most commonly seen in young adults rather than children but any patient who has a long-standing history of fatigue and a low fever (<38.5°C) should be referred for further evaluation. Further information can be found on page 283.

Urinary tract infection

One of the most common causes of fever in children is urinary tract infection. Often the child will present only with fever. Other symptoms can be present and include irritability, poor feeding, vomiting or abdominal pain. Referral is needed.

Medicine-induced fever

A number of medicines can elevate body temperature and should be considered if no other cause can be determined. Penicillins, cephalosporins, macrolides, tricyclic antidepressants, anticonvulsants and anti-inflammatory medicines, when associated with hypersensitivity, have all been associated with increasing temperature.

Meningitis

Meningitis should be considered in any child with fever and non-blanching rash, especially if the child looks ill and has other symptoms such as severe headache, photophobia, lethargy, drowsiness and neck stiffness. However, non-blanching rash is often seen late in symptom presentation so children with fever who exhibit decreased levels of consciousness or neck stiffness must be referred.

Pneumonia

Children who exhibit increased respiration rates and fever must be referred for further evaluation by the GP as pneumonia is a possibility.

! TRIGGER POINTS indicative of referral: Fever

- Any feverish child under 3 months old
- Fever accompanied by no other symptoms
- Fever of 5 days or longer
- Febrile convulsion/seizures
- Joint swelling
- Non-blanching rash
- Obviously ill child or child who fails to respond to stimuli
- Signs of dehydration (see Table 9.9)
- Stiff neck
- Temperature of 39°C or higher in children aged 3 to 6 months old

Evidence base for over-the-counter medication

Paracetamol and ibuprofen have been used for many years to treat fever in children. A number of recent reviews have looked at pharmacological and non-pharmacological intervention in reducing temperature. Two reviews by Meremikwu et al (2002, 2003) looked at the effect of paracetamol and tepid sponging in reducing fever. Conclusions from both reviews were guarded in stating they were effective, due to the small number of trials reviewed that met their inclusion criteria. This of course does not mean to say that these approaches are ineffective but that better, larger trials are required, although Watts et al (2001) concluded sponging does not seem to have a long-term effect. A further review by Perrott et al (2004) compared paracetamol and ibuprofen and concluded that single doses of ibuprofen were superior to paracetamol.

Alternating paracetamol with ibuprofen has also been advocated as a strategy to reduce fever, though evidence is lacking to recommend this as a credible option.

NICE guidance recommends that routine use of antipyretics should be avoided, although if deemed necessary, either paracetamol or ibuprofen can be used. They also state that they should be used as monotherapy and not alternated.

Practical prescribing and product selection

Prescribing information relating to medicines for fever reviewed in the section 'Evidence base for over-the-counter medication is discussed and summarised in Table 9.10; useful tips relating to patients presenting with fever are given in Hints and Tips Box 9.5.

Paracetamol (e.g. Calpol, Disprol, Medinol)

Paracetamol is available as liquid, soluble tablets, sachets and melt tabs, although the most frequently purchased formulation is liquid. In addition, paracetamol

Table 9.10
Practical prescribing: Summary of medicines for fever

Name of medicine	Use in children	Likely side effects	Drug interactions of note	Patients in whom care should be exercised	Pregnancy and breast-feeding
Paracetamol	>3 months Note: paracetamol from 2 months for post immunisation pyrexia	None	None	None	N/A
Ibuprofen		GI disturbances		Children with known hypersensitivity to NSAIDs	

HINTS AND TIPS BOX 9.5: FEVER

Drinking fluids	Children should be told to drink additional fluid to prevent dehydration, as a fever will make them sweat more than usual

antihistamine combinations (Medised for children – containing diphenhydramine) are available. Children should be given paracetamol every 4 to 6 hours, with a maximum of four doses in 24 hours. Children over 3 months to 1 year of age should be given 60 to 120 mg (2.5 to 5 mL of the paediatric version), while for those aged between 1 and 5 years the dose is 120 to 250 mg (5 mL of a paediatric version or 5 mL of Calpol 6 Plus or Medinol Over 6). For children over the age of 6 the dose is 250 to 500 mg (5 to 10 mL of Calpol 6 Plus or Medinol Over 6). Paracetamol has no commonly occurring side effects, does not interact with any medicines and so can be safely taken by all children.

Ibuprofen (e.g. Calprofen)

Ibuprofen can be given to children over 3 months old. The *British National Formulary* dosage (which is different to some proprietary products) is infants 3 to 6 months weighing more than 5 kg: 2.5 mL (50 mg) three times a day, those aged 6 months to 1 year: 2.5 mL (50 mg) three to four times a day. All children over 1 year can take three doses in 24 hours; those aged between 1 and 3 should take 5 mL (100 mg), children aged 4 to 6 years should take 7.5 mL (150 mg), children aged 7 to 9 should take 10 mL (200 mg) and children aged 10 to 12 should take 15 mL (300 mg).

Ibuprofen can cause gastrointestinal side effects such as nausea and diarrhoea and also interacts with many other medicines, although those medicines that interact with ibuprofen are very unlikely to be taken by children. Any child who has previously taken an NSAID and had an allergic reaction to it should avoid ibuprofen.

Further reading

Dodd SR, Lancaster GA, Craig JV, et al. Sensitivity and specificity of aural compared with rectal thermometers: a meta-analysis. J Clin Epidemiol 2006;59(4):354-7.

Meremikwu M, Oyo-Ita A. Paracetamol for treating fever in children. Cochrane Database of Systematic Reviews 2002, issue 2.

Meremikwu M, Oyo-Ita A. Physical methods for treating fever in children. Cochrane Database of Systematic Reviews 2003, issue 2.

Nowak TJ, Handford AG. Essentials of pathophysiology. New York: McGraw-Hill, 2000.

Perrott DA, Piira T, Goodenough B, Champion GD. Review: efficacy and safety of acetaminophen vs ibuprofen for treating children's pain or fever: a meta-analysis. Arch Pediatr Adolesc Med 2004;158:521-6.

Watts R, Robertson J, Thomas G, and review panel. The nursing management of fever in children. A systematic review. Adelaide: Joanna Briggs Institute for Evidence Based Nursing and Midwifery, 2001.

Web sites

NICE Guidance 47: http://guidance.nice.org.uk/CG47

The Joanna Briggs Institute for Evidence Based Nursing & Midwifery: http://www.joannabriggs.edu.au/best_practice/BPISfever.php

General site on fever: http://www.nlm.nih.gov/medlineplus/fever.html

Infectious childhood conditions

Background

A number of infectious diseases are more prevalent in children than the rest of the population. Many of these diseases are now vaccine preventable and the provision of immunisation programmes has almost eradicated them from developed countries. However, some conditions have no vaccine or incomplete vaccine cover is provided, which means contraction of the disease is still possible. This usually results in the child suffering from mild symptoms from which a full and speedy recovery is made but in some circumstances, for example meningitis, infection can result in death. In addition, media coverage over the safety of the triple vaccine for measles, mumps and rubella has seen vaccination rates fall, despite the overwhelming evidence showing that the MMR vaccine is the safest way to protect against these diseases (http://www.mmrthefacts.nhs.uk/library/research.php). This raises the possibility of children contracting these diseases and recent outbreaks in Western countries have been recorded (http://www.mmrthefacts.nhs.uk/worldmap/mmr.php). Mention of measles, mumps and rubella is therefore made at the end of this section for completeness.

Meningitis

Meningitis is usually caused by bacterial or viral infection. Viral meningitis is much more common than bacterial meningitis but, thankfully, viral infections are much less serious than bacterial causes. The peak incidence of contracting meningitis is between 6 and 12 months, and over 90% of all cases occur before the age of 5.

Signs and symptoms are non-specific in the early stages of the disease and are similar to flu. Symptoms range from fever to nausea, vomiting, headache and irritability. Symptoms can develop quickly, in a matter of hours, and be unpredictable, especially in infants and young children. Symptoms of fever, lethargy, vomiting and irritability are common in children aged between 3 months and 2 years. In infants, floppiness and dislike of being handled are also common features. Symptoms that are more common in older children include severe headache, stiff neck and photophobia. Any child who experiences pain at the back of the neck when moving their chin to their chest must be immediately referred.

In the latter stages of the disease a petechial or purpuric non-blanching rash characteristically develops in meningococcal infection.

The number of cases in the UK is now at its lowest ever level due to the introduction of two vaccines into the UK vaccination schedule. The Hib vaccine was introduced in 1992 (active against *Haemophilus influenzae)* and the meningococcal C conjugate vaccine was introduced in 1999 (active against serogroup C *Meningococcus).*

Glandular fever (infectious mononucleosis)

Glandular fever is caused by the Epstein-Barr virus and is most commonly seen in patients aged between 15 and 24. In Western countries it is rare in children under 5 and less frequent in those aged between 5 and 14.

It is transmitted from close salivary contact and is also known as the kissing disease and has an incubation period of 4 to 7 weeks. Symptoms are vague but characterised by fatigue, headache, sore throat and swollen and tender lymph glands. A macular rash can also occur in a small proportion of patients. The symptoms tend to be mild but can linger for many months.

Chicken pox

Chicken pox is very common and is probably the most likely infectious childhood rash to be seen in community pharmacy. It is the primary infection observed when the patient contracts the varicella zoster virus and is transmitted either by droplet infection or by contact with vesicular exudates. The incubation period ranges from 10 to 20 days and prior to the rash developing the patient might experience up to 3 days of prodromal symptoms that could include fever, headache and sore throat. The rash typically begins on the face and scalp, and spreads to the trunk and limbs. Initially, the rash appears as small red lumps that rapidly develop into vesicles, which crust over after 3 to 5 days. New lesions tend to occur in crops of three to five for the first 4 days so that at its height of infectivity lesions appear in all stages of development (Fig. 9.4). The vesicles are often extremely itchy and secondary bacterial infection due to the vesicles being

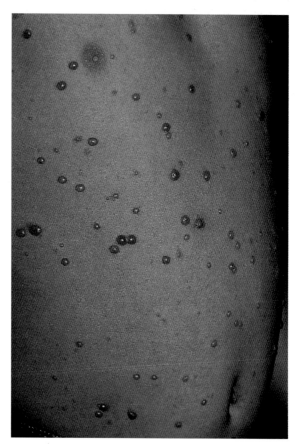

Fig. 9.4 Chicken pox. Reproduced from *Color Atlas of Dermatology* by G White, 2004, Churchill Livingstone, with permission

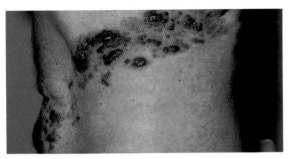

Fig. 9.5 Typical dermatomal distribution of herpes zoster. Reproduced from *Dermatology in Focus* by J Wilkinson et al, 2005, Churchill Livingstone, with permission

scratched is not unusual. Chicken pox is highly contagious, from a few days prior to the onset of rash until all lesions have crusted over. Re-infection results in people suffering from shingles (Fig. 9.5). A vaccination has been available since the mid 1990s and has shown to be 70 to 90% effective. It is part of standard vaccination schedules in countries such as the USA and Australia but currently not the UK.

Molluscum contagiosum

Caused by a pox virus, molluscum contagiosum is usually transmitted by indirect contact, for example, sharing towels, although it is not very contagious. The face and axillae are common sites of infection. Lesions generally appear in crops as pink pearl-like spots usually less than 0.5 cm in diameter. All lesions have a central punctum that is a diagnostic feature (Fig. 9.6). Confusion should not arise with other conditions other than viral warts (for further information on warts see Chapter 7, page 209). The condition will spontaneously resolve but if the parent or child is anxious then referral to the GP should be made because liquid nitrogen can be used to remove the lesions.

Impetigo

Impetigo is caused by a bacterial infection, most notably *Staphylococcus aureus* or S*treptococcus pyogenes*. It presents mainly on the face, around the nose and mouth. It usually starts as a small red itchy patch of inflamed skin that quickly develops into vesicles that rupture and weep. The exudate dries to a brown, yellow sticky crust (Fig. 9.7). It is contagious and children should be kept off school until the rash clears. General hygiene measures should include not sharing towels, which will help to stop household contacts contracting the infection. The child's nails should be kept short to stop him or her from scratching the lesions. Treatment involves topical or systemic antibiotics (e.g. fusidic acid or flucloxacillin), which currently are not available OTC in most Western

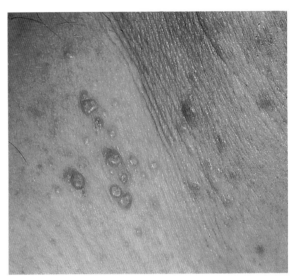

Fig. 9.6 Molluscum contagiosum. Reproduced from *Dermatology: An Illustrated Colour Text* by D J Gawkrodger, 2008, Churchill Livingstone, with permission

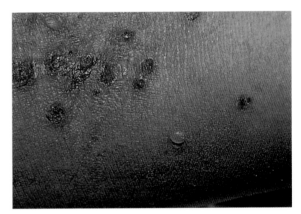

Fig. 9.7 Impetigo. Reproduced from *Color Atlas of Dermatology* by G White, 2004, Churchill Livingstone, with permission

countries but topical formulations are likely to be deregulated in the future.

Measles

Since 1968 all infants in the UK have routinely been offered vaccination against measles. It is caused by the paramyxo virus and spread by droplet inhalation. It is the most dangerous of childhood diseases because of the complications that can occur. Approximately 7% of patients develop respiratory complications such as otitis media and pneumonia but encephalitis is seen in about one in every 600 to 1000 cases of measles.

Measles has an incubation period of between 7 to 14 days, which is then followed by 3 or 4 days of prodromal symptoms where the child will have a fever, head cold, cough and conjunctivitis. On the inner cheek and gums small white spots are visible, like grains of salt and are known as Koplik's spots; these are diagnostic for measles. A blotchy red rash appears around the ears before moving on to the trunk and limbs. Immediate referral to the GP is needed.

German measles (rubella)

Rubella is caused by an RNA virus and spread by either close personal contact or airborne droplets. It is less contagious than measles and if contracted many people suffer from mild symptoms and the infection passes undiagnosed. After the incubation period of 14 to 21 days the child experiences up to 5 days of prodromal symptoms, which include cold-like symptoms and swollen glands in the neck before a rash appears on the face that quickly moves on to the trunk and extremities. The rash tends to be pinpoint and macular. The biggest threat posed by rubella is to women in early pregnancy, as foetal damage is possible.

Mumps

Mumps is caused by a paramyxo virus and is transmitted by airborne droplets from the nose and throat. It is the least contagious of the childhood diseases and requires close personal contact before infection can occur. There is an incubation period of 16 to 21 days followed by fever; this is followed by swelling of one or both parotid glands and the child will experience pain when the mouth is opened.

Mumps is much more unpleasant if contracted as an adult and in 20 to 30% of men the disease affects the testicles, with a serious infection possibly causing sterility. The most serious complication from mumps is meningitis.

To aid in differential diagnosis of childhood conditions see Table 9.11.

> ### Web sites
> NHS sites: http://cks.library.nhs.uk/chickenpox and http://www.immunisation.nhs.uk/
> Charities: http://www.meningitis.org and http://www.meningitis-trust.org

Nappy rash

Background

Nappy rash (also known as nappy dermatitis or diaper rash) is a non-specific term used to describe inflammatory eruptions in the nappy area.

Prevalence and epidemiology

The incidence and prevalence of nappy rash is difficult to determine because of variability between studies. Nappy rash is most commonly seen between 6 and 12 months of age and in one UK study 25% of infants aged under 1 month had an episode of nappy rash.

Aetiology

Nappy rash is caused by a number of contributory factors. Friction and maceration of the skin are key to its cause. This is compounded by excessive heat and moisture combined with the effect of faecal and urinary enzymes when in prolonged contact with the skin (faeces breakdown produces ammonia and is considered a contributory cause, as ammonia is only an irritant when in contact with damaged skin). Greater exposure of skin surfaces to moisture impairs the skin's barrier function and makes the skin more susceptible to secondary infection.

Arriving at a differential diagnosis

The diagnosis is straightforward although identifying the cause is slightly more difficult. There are four forms of nappy rash encountered and Table 9.12 highlights the key differences between symptom presentation. One of the roles of the pharmacist is to assess the severity of the rash. Prodigy guidance separates nappy rash into either mild (faint to definite pink rash covering less than 10% of the nappy area with or without a few scattered papules, with or without slight scaling and dryness) or moderate/severe (covers more than 10% of the nappy area, with or without papules, oedema or ulceration). The severity of the rash will influence treatment.

Clinical features of irritant nappy rash

Irritant nappy rash is by far the most common form. The rash affects primarily the buttocks (i.e. the area in contact with the irritant) but can involve the lower abdomen and upper thighs. The flexures, which are protected from exposure, are usually spared.

Conditions to eliminate

Secondary infections

An environment that is wet and warm is an ideal breeding ground for opportunistic infection. Most commonly, secondary infections are caused by *Candida albicans*, but other pathogens such as *Staphylococcus aureus* are involved. Candidiasis is associated with satellite lesions (i.e. away from the main skin involvement). The lesions tend to be papular or pustular.

Table 9.11
Differential diagnosis of childhood conditions

	Measles	German measles	Meningitis	Glandular fever	Chicken pox	Molluscum contagiosum	Mumps	Impetigo
Prodromal stage								
Fever	Yes	No	Yes	Yes	Yes, in older individuals	No	Yes	No
Swollen glands	No	Yes	No	Yes	No	No	Yes	No
Cold-like symptoms	Yes	Yes	No	No	No	No	No	No
Other signs	Koplik's spots*	Malaise	Lethargy, stiff neck, vomiting, photophobia	Malaise & headache	Malaise & headache	None	None	None
Rash								
Location	Ears & face progressing to trunk & limbs	Face moving quickly to trunk	Trunk and limbs	Trunk	On trunk & face, rarely on extremities	Face and axillae	N/A	Facial area especially around nose & mouth
Character	Maculopapular	Macules, often pinpoint by 2nd day	Purplish blotches. Do not blanch	Maculopapular About 10% have rash	Lesions discrete and appear in crops	Pink pearl-like spots with central punctum*		Vesicles that exude forming yellow crusts
Epidemiology								
Age group most affected	Children & adolescents	Children under 12	90% before age of 5	15- to 24-year-olds most at risk	Very common in children	Young children	Children under 12	School-aged children

*Diagnostic.

Table 9.12
Differences in symptom presentation among the four causes of nappy rash

	Irritant	Candidal	Seborrhoeic	Psoriasiform
Flexure involvement	No	Yes	Yes	Yes
Satellite lesions	No	Yes	No	No
Other sites involved	No	Yes	Yes	Yes
Rash description	Red raw	Bright red and well demarcated	Shiny/greasy	Often no scaling present

HINTS AND TIPS BOX 9.6: NAPPY RASH

Preventative measures	Leave the nappy off for as long as possible each day
	Avoid using soaps for cleaning
	Washed nappies should be thoroughly rinsed to ensure that they do not contain residues of soap and detergent
	Change nappies as soon as they have been soiled

Seborrhoeic dermatitis

Seborrhoeic dermatitis presents as a rash, which is bright red and confluent. The flexures are not spared and the rash can take on a diffuse, red, shiny or greasy look. It is common for other sites to be involved, such as the scalp and face.

Psoriasiform nappy eruptions

Infants usually develop this form of nappy rash within the first 4 months of life. It presents as well demarcated erythematous plaques that can show scaling which resembles psoriasis. Involvement away from the nappy area is common and affects the limbs, face and scalp. A small proportion (approximately 10%) of infants go on to develop psoriasis.

TRIGGER POINTS indicative of referral: Nappy rash

- OTC treatment failure
- Severe rash requiring corticosteroids

Evidence base for over-the-counter medication

Little in the way of evidence exists to support current recommendations. Management centres on skin care of the nappy area by reducing skin irritation – either by removing occlusion or changing the nappy frequently; or applying a protective layer of barrier cream and reducing the inflammation and/or eliminating infection.

Barrier creams are designed to rehydrate and soothe the skin. A number of chemical constituents are formulated into barrier creams, including silicone, antiseptics and protectorants. Many proprietary products are available and often consist of a combination of ingredients. Secondary infection with *Candida* can be treated with imidazole products.

Practical prescribing and product selection

Products marketed as barrier creams/protectorants can be given to all children. They should be applied to all skin surfaces, including the skin folds after each nappy change. They have no side effects, although some products do contain potential sensitising agents and it is best to patch test an area of skin before application. Commonly prescribed products include Draoplene, Metanium and Sudocrem.

Mild cases of nappy rash can be managed with good skin care routines (see Hints and Tip Box 9.6) and the use of barrier creams. For more severe cases, in general those that are secondarily infected, the use of an imidazole twice a day combined with barrier creams is recommended. Where the child is distressed and there are obvious signs of inflammation then referral is needed for steroids.

Further reading
Baer EL, Davies MW, Easterbrook KJ. Disposable nappies for preventing napkin dermatitis in infants. Cochrane Database of Systematic Reviews 2006, issue 3.

Web sites
Prodigy guidance: http://cks.library.nhs.uk/nappy_rash

Self-assessment questions

The following questions are intended to supplement the text. Two levels of questions are provided: multiple choice questions and case studies. The multiple choice questions are designed to test factual recall and the case studies allow knowledge to be applied to a practice setting.

Multiple choice questions

9.1 The common name of nits refers to:
  a. An adult head louse
  b. An immature head louse
  c. Live eggs
  d. Egg cases
  e. None of the above

9.2 Which antihistamine has a licence for pruritus?

  a. Chlorphenamine
  b. Clemastine
  c. Cyproheptadine
  d. Hydroxyzine
  e. Azatadine

9.3 A low grade fever is defined as a temperature of?

  a. Less than 36.5°C
  b. Less than 37.5°C
  c. Less than 38.5°C
  d. Less than 39.5°C
  e. Less than 40.5°C

9.4 Which patient group should avoid using alcoholic insecticides?

  a. Patients with asthma
  b. Patients with coeliac disease
  c. Patients with hypertension
  d. Patients with peptic ulcer
  e. Epileptic patients

9.5 Fever in children with no associated symptoms or signs is usually due to:

  a. Gastroenteritis
  b. Urinary tract infection
  c. Upper respiratory tract infection
  d. Bacterial tonsillitis
  e. Impetigo

9.6 What is the usual age at which children present with atopic dermatitis?

  a. In the first month of life
  b. Before 6 months

  c. Before 1 year
  d. Before 2 years
  e. Before 5 years

9.7 Mebendazole can be given to patients from what age?

  a. 1
  b. 2
  c. 3
  d. 4
  e. 5

9.8 How many days after initial treatment should a second application of insecticide be used to eradicate head lice?

  a. 3
  b. 5
  c. 7
  d. 10
  e. 14

Questions 9.9 to 9.11 concern the following conditions:

A. Chicken pox
B. Measles
C. German measles
D. Glandular fever
E. Impetigo

Select, from A to E, which of the above conditions:

9.9 Is often caused by *Staphylococcus* E

9.10 Is characterised by a vesicular rash A

9.11 Is transmitted by close salivary contact D

Questions 9.12 to 9.14 concern the following medicines:

A. Piperazine
B. Mebendazole
C. Permethrin
D. Dimethicone
E. Brompheniramine

Select, from A to E, which of the above medicines:

9.12 Is associated with sedation *E*

9.13 Is contraindicated in pregnancy *b*

9.14 Causes abdominal pain *b*

Questions 9.15 to 9.17: for each of these questions *one or more* of the responses is (are) correct. Decide which of the responses is (are) correct. Then choose:

A. If a, b and c are correct
B. If a and b only are correct
C. If b and c only are correct
D. If a only is correct
E. If c only is correct

Directions summarised

A	B	C	D	E
a, b and c	a and b only	b and c only	a only	c only

9.15 Colic is generally due to:

   a. The teat hole being too large
   b. Swallowing air when being breast-fed
   c. Being given too much food

9.16 Atopic dermatitis can be defined as itchy skin plus:

   a. History of dry skin
   b. Flexural eczema
   c. A personal history of other atopic disease

9.17 Which statement(s) about head lice treatment is/are true

   a. Shampoos are not as effective as lotions
   b. Alcoholic lotions are suitable for all patients
   c. They can be used prophylactically

Questions 9.18 to 9.20: these questions consist of a statement in the left-hand column followed by a statement in the right-hand column. You need to:

● decide whether the first statement is true or false
● decide whether the second statement is true or false

Then choose:

A. If both statements are true and the second statement is a correct explanation of the first statement
B. If both statements are true but the second statement is NOT a correct explanation of the first statement
C. If the first statement is true but the second statement is false
D. If the first statement is false but the second statement is true
E. If both statements are false

Directions summarised

	1st statement	2nd statement	
A	True	True	2nd statement is a correct explanation of the first
B	True	True	2nd statement is not a correct explanation of the first
C	True	False	
D	False	True	
E	False	False	

	First statement	Second statement
9.18	Emollients are the mainstay of treatment of atopic dermatitis	Products with lanolin should be avoided
9.19	Oral temperature is the most accurate measure of temperature	Normal body temperature is 37°C
9.20	Measles is vaccine preventable	It is usually given as a triple vaccine

Case study

Ms JP, a young mother of two children, comes into the pharmacy one afternoon clutching a letter from the children's primary school. The letter says that there is a head lice outbreak and instructs parents to treat their children for head lice.

a. How do you respond?

You need to find out if her children actually have head lice or if she is trying to buy a product to stop them getting head lice. She should be told that products cannot be bought to prevent her children contracting head lice and she should inspect their heads regularly, and only when live lice are found should a product be bought. Ms JP should be told how to inspect her children's hair for signs of head lice.

Ms JP returns to the pharmacy 4 days later and says her youngest daughter does now have head lice. She is 5 and suffers from no medical problems.

b. What product are you going to recommend?

Insecticides or dimeticone would be acceptable treatment options. Patient acceptability will primarily drive choice of product.

c. What patient factors will influence your recommendation?

If the child has broken scalp skin then an alcoholic product should be avoided because irritation and stinging may occur. Additionally, very long hair might require more than one bottle of product.

Ms JP says she is not very keen on using chemicals on her daughter's hair. She has heard that you can use conditioner and that will get rid of the problem.

d. How do you respond?

Ms JP is probably referring to the 'bug busting' technique. She should be told that the effectiveness of bug busting is lower than using chemicals but can be tried if she really does not want to use insecticides. You should stress that it is very important to adhere to the regimen, as poor compliance with the bug busting method is probably why it has been shown to be less effective.

Alternatively, you could recommend dimeticone. Although few trials have been conducted at present, cure rates are comparable, if not higher than with insecticides.

Ms JP then asks you whether her older daughter, Samantha, should also be treated even though she has not got head lice.

e. What do you say?

Only those with a live lice infestation should be treated. Ms JP should be asked to keep checking Samantha's hair on a regular basis.

9

CASE STUDY 9.2

Mr PB is looking after his grandson for the weekend. He asks for some advice because he has noticed a rash on his grandson's body and wants something to help get rid of it.

a. What do you need to know?

You need to know:

- *The location of rash*
- *What the rash looks like*
- *When the rash appeared*
- *Associated symptoms such as itch*
- *General health of the child*
- *If the child has a temperature*
- *What, if any, symptoms the child had before the rash appeared*
- *The age of his grandson*

All Mr PB is able to tell you is that his grandson has been with him for the last day and he only noticed the rash this morning when he was dressing him. He is 4 years old and the rash is on his chest and back; Mr PB describes them as spots. He thinks it is probably itchy because he saw his grandson scratching this morning.

b. What do you think could be the problem?

Without seeing the child and the rash it is always difficult to make a differential diagnosis from

information from a third party, but it appears the child might have chicken pox.

c. Are there any further questions you could ask the man to confirm your diagnosis?

Further questions you could ask are:
- *Are the spots coming out in groups?*
- *Have any of the spots turned into little blisters?*
- *Has he been exposed to other children with chicken pox?*

Mr PB is unsure and concerned that his grandson is OK.

d. What could you do?

It appears that his grandson is not poorly and unless he deteriorates there is probably no need to call out the GP. You could recommend an antihistamine to help with the itching and reassure him that his grandson will be OK, but if he becomes poorly the GP should be called out. You also tell him that the rash fits the description of chicken pox but without seeing the rash you cannot be sure. It would therefore be useful if you could see the child or if the child could be seen by someone over the next couple of days to confirm your suspicions.

CASE STUDY 9.3

Mrs JR, the mother of a 2-month-old girl asks for help with her baby, as she seems to be crying all the time. On questioning you find out the following.

Information gathering	Data generated
Presenting complaint (possible questions)	
Describe symptoms	Baby cries and will not be consoled, even after feeding, burping and nappy changes. Brings knees to her chest as she cries
How long had the symptoms	About a month but just not getting better. Usually worse in the evening
Severity of pain/distress of child	Difficult to say but she is obviously worse than other babies she knows about
Other symptoms/ provokes	As above
Any symptoms previous	Has always had stints where she has cried a lot, but is just far worse in the last month
Additional questions	Baby is bottle-fed Baby is gaining weight satisfactorily. No stomach distension and baby is passing stool adequately
Previous history of presenting complaint	As above
Past medical history	Has bought Woodwards Gripe mixture last week on advice of a relative. This seems to have had no effect

Information gathering	Data generated
Drugs (OTC, Rx and compliance)	Woodwards Gripe mixture
Allergies	NKA
Social history	
Smoking	Mother has changed
Alcohol	formula milk twice in the
Drugs	last month. Mother is
Employment	frustrated and appears
Relationships	tired
Family history	None for presenting complaint
On examination	N/A

This case obviously relates to whether the baby has colic. It is difficult to determine if the baby is considered to have colic or is just excessively crying, as the diagnosis of the condition is dependent on qualitative descriptions. Other conditions can cause prolonged crying and are listed below.

Probability	Cause
Most likely	Colic
Likely	Acute infection
Unlikely	GORD, intolerance to cow's milk protein

Diagnostic pointers with regard to symptom presentation

The following page summarises the expected findings for questions when related to the different conditions that can be seen by community pharmacists.

9

CASE STUDY 9.3

	History	Weight gain	Systemic symptoms	Inconsolability
Colic	Weeks	OK	No	Yes
Infection	Days/hours	OK	Yes	Yes?
GORD	Weeks	OK	No	No
Intolerance to cow's milk protein	Weeks	Poor	No	No

When this information is applied to that gained from our patient (below) we see that everything points to a diagnosis of colic. To further eliminate GORD, questions asked about regurgitation could be asked and also the duration of crying.

	History	Weight gain	Systemic symptoms	Inconsolability
Colic	✓	✓	✓	✓
Infection	✗	✓	✗	✓?
GORD	✓	✓	✓	✗
Intolerance to cow's milk protein	✓	✗	✓	✗

Reassure the parent that symptoms are transient. Although something has already been tried it is probably worth starting with a simeticone (Infacol) or Colief for 1 week. If that fails to help then refer.

Danger symptoms/signs (trigger points for referral)

As a final double check it might be worth making sure the baby has none of the 'referral signs or symptoms'; this is the case with this patient.

Infants that are failing to put on weight	✗
Medication failure (yes, but product of doubtful efficacy)	?
Overanxious parents	✗

Specific product requests

Background

Many patients will present in the pharmacy requesting a specific product rather than wanting advice on symptoms. They might have seen the product advertised on the television or been told to purchase it from their doctor. Regardless of the reason why they are asking for the product, it is the responsibility of the pharmacist to ensure that the patient receives the most appropriate therapy. This chapter therefore deals with situations where patients ask for a particular product or class of product but the pharmacist needs to elicit more information from the patient before complying with the request.

Motion sickness

Background

Motion sickness is a symptom complex that is characterised by nausea, pallor, vague abdominal discomfort and occasionally vomiting. Symptoms of fatigue, weakness and inability to concentrate can also be observed prior to nausea. Over prolonged exposure to motion, symptoms tend to resolve. For example, seasickness at the beginning of a voyage disappears over time – a characteristic called adaptation or habituation. Pharmacists are frequently asked to recommend a product, especially by anxious parents. Motion sickness can affect any individual and involve any form of movement, from moving vehicles to fairground rides.

Prevalence and epidemiology

The exact prevalence of motion sickness is unknown. Children between the ages of 2 and 12 are most commonly affected and it tends to affect women more than men. However, certain sectors of the population understandably show a higher prevalence rate than the normal population, for example naval crew and pilots.

Aetiology

It is widely believed that motion sickness results from the inability of the brain to process conflicting information received from sensory nerve terminals concerning movement and position, the sensory conflict hypothesis. Motion sickness can occur when motion is expected but not experienced, or the pattern of motion differs from that previously experienced.

Evidence base for over-the-counter medication

First-generation antihistamines (cyclizine, cinnarizine, meclozine and promethazine) and the anticholinergic hyoscine are routinely recommended to prevent motion sickness. All have shown various degrees of effectiveness, with hyoscine consistently proving the most effective (Spinks et al 2004).

Non-pharmacological approaches to the prevention of motion sickness using acupressure are also available OTC. Bruce et al (1990) investigated the use of Sea Band acupressure bands versus hyoscine and placebo. Eighteen healthy volunteers were subjected to simulated conditions to induce motion sickness. The findings showed that while hyoscine exerted a preventative effect, Sea Bands were no more effective than placebo. Further trials have confirmed these findings, although one small trial by Stern et al (2001) reported positive findings. Further trials are needed as acupressure has shown positive effects for nausea and vomiting associated with pregnancy.

Practical prescribing and product selection

Prescribing information relating to medicines for motion sickness reviewed in the section 'Evidence base for over-the-counter medication' is discussed and summarised in Table 10.1. They are most effective when given prior to exposure and products should be selected based on matching the length of the journey with the

duration of action of each medicine (see Hints and Tips Box 10.1).

Antihistamines

Antihistamines used in products for motion sickness are first-generation H_1 antagonists and are associated with sedation. They therefore have the same side effects, interactions and precautions in use as other first-generation antihistamines used in cough and cold remedies. For further information see Chapter 1, page 9.

Cyclizine (Valoid)

Cyclizine is prescribed very rarely. It is subject to abuse by drug misusers and many pharmacies do not stock it. If taken, adults and children over 12 should take one

Table 10.1
Practical prescribing: Summary of medicines for travel sickness

Name of medicine	Use in children	Likely side effects	Drug interactions of note	Patients in whom care should be exercised	Pregnancy and breast-feeding
Cyclizine (Valoid)	>6 years	Dry mouth, sedation	Increased sedation with alcohol, opioid analgesics, analgesics, anxiolytics, hypnotics and antidepressants	Angle-closure glaucoma, prostate enlargement	Standard references state OK, although some manufacturers advise avoidance
Cinnarizine (Stugeron 15)	>5 years				
Meclozine (Sea-Legs)	>2 years				
Promethazine (Avomine)	>5 years				
Hyoscine Joy-rides	>3 years	Dry mouth, sedation	Increased anticholinergic side effects with TCAs and neuroleptics	Angle-closure glaucoma, prostate enlargement	Avoid if possible
Kwells	>10 years				
Kwells Kids	>4 years				

HINTS AND TIPS BOX 10.1: TRAVEL SICKNESS

How to minimise motion	Planes – sit over the wing Ships – sit in the middle close to the water line Cars – sit in the front Avoid rear-facing seats in any form of transport Focus on stationary objects Avoid alcohol or overeating before journeys
Dry mouth problems	Many people will complain of a dry mouth with travel sickness medicines. This is easily overcome by sucking a sweet, which will stimulate saliva production
Matching up length of journey with product	Hyoscine should be recommended for journeys up to 4 hours; cinnarizine for journeys over 4 hours but less than 8 hours; and promethazine and meclozine for journeys longer than 8 hours

tablet (50 mg) three times a day. The dose for children over the age of 6 is half the adult dose.

Cinnarizine (Stugeron)

Adults and children over 12 should take two tablets 2 hours before travel. The dose can be repeated every 8 hours (one tablet) if needed. For children aged between 5 and 12 the dose is half the adult dose.

Meclozine (Sea-Legs)

Adults and children over 12 years should take two tablets (25 mg) 1 hour prior to travel; however, as activity lasts 24 hours the dose can be taken the night before travel. Children aged between 6 and 12 years should take half the adult dose (one tablet, 12.5 mg) and for children over 2, half a tablet (6.25 mg) should be taken. The dose can be repeated every 24 hours if needed.

Promethazine (Avomine)

Avomine can be given for both prevention and treatment of travel sickness. For prevention, adults and children over the age of 10 should take one tablet at least 1 or 2 hours before travel. For treatment, one tablet should be taken as soon as sickness is felt followed by a second tablet the same evening. For children over 5 the dose should be half that of the adult dose in both prevention and treatment. Promethazine is also available as Phenergan, and can be given to children from the age of 2 years.

Hyoscine

Hyoscine can be taken either orally (e.g. Joy-rides and Kwells) or transdermally (scopolamine patches – although these were discontinued in September 2006). Products should be taken 20 to 30 minutes before the time of travel; because they have a short half life they have a short duration of action and the dose might therefore have to be repeated on journeys longer than 4 hours. Anticholinergic side effects are more obvious than with antihistamines and it does interact with other medicines that have anticholinergic side effects and should therefore not be co-prescribed. Because hyoscine hydrobromide crosses the blood–brain barrier, it can cause sedation. It appears to be safe in pregnancy, although the manufacturers state it should be avoided.

Joy-rides

Joy-rides can be given from age 3 upwards. Children aged between 3 and 4 years should take half a tablet (75 µg) and no more than one tablet (150 µg) in 24 hours. Children between the age of 4 and 7 should take one tablet (150 µg) with a maximum of two tablets (300 µg) in 24 hours and children aged between 7 and 12 should take one to two tablets.

Kwells

Kwells can only be given to children aged 10 and over. Children over 10 should take half to one tablet. For adults the dose is one tablet. The dose can be repeated every 6 hours when needed. Tablets should be taken 30 minutes before travel.

Kwells Kids

Kwells Kids contain half the amount of hyoscine (150 µg) of Kwells and are marketed at children under the age of 10, although older children can take them. Children aged between 4 and 10 should take half to one tablet. Like Kwells, the dose can be repeated every 6 hours when needed and be taken 30 minutes before travel.

Further reading

Bruce DG, Golding JF, Hockenhull N, et al. Acupressure and motion sickness. Aviat Space Environ Med 1990;61:361–5.

Dahl E, Offer-Ohlsen D, Lillevold PE, et al. Transdermal scopolamine, oral meclizine and placebo in motion sickness. Clin Pharmacol Ther 1984;36:116–20.

Klocker N, Hanschke W, Toussaint S, et al. Scopolamine nasal spray in motion sickness: a randomised, controlled and crossover study for the comparison of two scopolamine nasal sprays with oral dimenhydrinate and placebo. Eur J Pharm Sci 2001;13:227–32.

Pingree BJ, Pethybridge RJ. A comparison of the efficacy of cinnarizine with scopolamine in the treatment of seasickness. Aviat Space Environ Med 1994;65:597–605.

Spinks AB, Wasiak J, Villanueva EV, Bernath V. Scopolamine for preventing and treating motion sickness. Cochrane Database of Systematic Reviews 2004, issue 3.

Stern RM, Jokerst MD, Muth ER, Hollis C. Acupressure relieves the symptoms of motion sickness and reduces abnormal gastric activity. Altern Ther Health Med 2001;7:91–4.

Emergency hormonal contraception

Background

Emergency hormonal contraception (EHC) is one of only a handful of deregulated products that targets preventative healthcare and fits in with UK government public health policy. Like other Western countries, the UK has high teenage pregnancy rates and associated high abortion rates.

The intention of UK government policy on making EHC available through pharmacies was to improve access for patients requiring EHC at times when other providers might be closed, for example, at weekends and evenings. This policy appears to have been effective. Since its launch in the UK in 2001 the percentage of EHC provided through community pharmacies has steadily increased.

Pharmacy supply is now (2005/6 figures) the most popular route with 45% through a pharmacy, compared to 30% via a doctor and 25% from a family planning clinic.

In the UK, 86% of women classed as being 'at risk' of becoming pregnant use at least one form of contraception. The pill and the condom are the most popular methods of contraception (38 and 34% respectively), but in younger women (16 to 29 years) the pill is used by almost 80%. Despite most women using contraception, the number of unwanted pregnancies in young women (under 18) in the UK over the period 1998 to 2005 has remained relatively constant, although abortion rates have risen over the same period. Condom failure accounts for almost half of all requests for EHC, followed by missed pills (approximately 20%).

Studies have shown that most women have heard of EHC (>90%), although their knowledge on when it can be taken and its effectiveness is lower, for example, less than half of women are aware of how long the EHC remains effective and less than two-thirds are aware that it is most effective the sooner it is taken after intercourse.

Aetiology

The active ingredient in EHC is levonorgestrel. Its exact mechanism of action is not clear and it appears to have more than one mode of action at more than one site. It is thought to work mainly by preventing ovulation and fertilisation if intercourse has taken place in the preovulatory phase, when the likelihood of fertilisation is the highest. It is also suggested that it causes endometrial changes that discourage egg implantation.

Evidence base for over-the-counter medication

The effectiveness of levonorgestrel is hard to establish because many women will not become pregnant regardless of whether EHC is taken or not. However, in head-to-head trials levonoergestrel when compared against the Yuzpe regimen (Schering PC4) found the progestogen only regime to prevent 86% of expected pregnancies when treatment was initiated within 72 hours compared to 57% with PC4. Levonorgestrel is more effective the earlier it is taken after unprotected sex; it prevents 95% of pregnancies if taken within 24 hours of unprotected sex, 85% between 24 and 48 hours, and 58% if used within 48 to 72 hours. In addition to being more effective than the Yuzpe method, trials have shown levonorgestrel to have a more favourable side effect profile, with lower incidences of nausea and vomiting.

Some concerns were raised over women abusing EHC as a result of its greater accessibility once deregulated. This appears to have been unfounded as the 2005/6 omnibus survey found that only 5% of women had used EHC in the past year and is consistent with previous years' findings.

Practical prescribing and product selection

Prescribing information relating to EHC is discussed and summarised in Table 10.2.

Assessing patient suitability

Prior to any sale or supply of EHC the pharmacist has to be in a position to determine if the patient is suitable to take the medicine. To do this an assessment has to be made on the likelihood that the patient is pregnant:

- First, has the patient had unprotected sex, contraceptive failure or missed taking contraceptive pills in the last 72 hours?
- EHC can only be given to patients who present within 72 hours. If more than 72 hours have elapsed but less than 120 hours (5 days) then the patient can have an intrauterine device fitted.
- Is the patient already pregnant? Details about the patient's last period should be sought. Is the period late, and if so how many days late? Was the nature of the period different or unusual. If pregnancy is suspected a pregnancy test could be offered.
- When and how many pills were missed? The Royal College of Obstetricians and Gynaecologists have produced guidelines (2006) on when EHC is offered:

Table 10.2
Practical prescribing: Summary of medicines for emergency hormonal contraception

Name of medicine	Use in children	Likely side effects	Drug interactions of note	Patients in whom care should be exercised	Pregnancy and breast-feeding
Levonelle One Step	>16 years	Nausea	Anticonvulsants, rifampicin, griseofulvin, St John's wort and ciclosporin	Conditions in which Levonelle absorption may be impaired, for example, Crohn's disease	Not applicable

Who is eligible?	Only patients over the age of 16 can be supplied with Levonelle, although family planning services, doctors and pharmacists acting under a patient group direction can supply EHC to patients under 16
Do you have to supply EHC?	The supply of EHC is at the discretion of each pharmacist and some, for religious beliefs, might choose not to supply EHC. However, the patient should be advised on other local sources of supply so that she can access the service

- For combined pills – if three or more 30 to 35 μg ethinylestradiol or two or more 20 μg ethinylestradiol tablets have been missed in the first week of pill taking and unprotected sex occurred during the first week or in the pill-free week.
- For progestogen only pills – if one or more pills have been missed or taken >3 hours late (>12 hours late for Cerazette) and unprotected sex has occurred in the 2 days following this.

A number of useful checklists have been produced and are used in practice. Many pharmacists ask patients to complete one of these forms, instead of asking potentially embarrassing questions in the pharmacy. Additionally, the manufacturer has an on-line form that patients can complete, print off and bring to the pharmacy (http://www.levonelle.co.uk/output/Page37.asp).

Once the details of the form are completed, the pharmacist can decide whether EHC can be supplied to the patient.

is available, that patients taking these medicines are best referred to the GP. In such circumstances, increasing the dose of Levonelle is commonly practised (although not licensed). If this is not the preferred option then an alternative form of EHC can be given, for example, an intrauterine device.

In December 2006, the Royal Pharmaceutical Society of Great Britain (RPSGB) issued new guidance on advanced sale of EHC following announcements from the British Pregnancy Advisory Service (BPAS), Marie Stopes International and the Faculty of Family Planning and Reproductive Health Care and the Royal College of Obstetricians supporting advance supply. The RPSGB states that EHC can be supplied in advance but pharmacists must consider the clinical appropriateness of a supply. They should decline repeated requests for advance supply and advise patients to use more reliable methods of contraception.

Levonelle One Step

Levonelle should be taken as soon as possible after unprotected sex or contraceptive failure (see Hints and Tips Box 10.2). The dose consists of a single tablet (levonorgestrel 1500 μg). About 1 in 5 patients experience nausea but only 1 in 20 go on to vomit. If the patient vomits within 3 hours of the first dose she should be advised that a further supply of EHC would be needed. Taking EHC can affect the timing of the next menstrual period and patients should be told that their period might be earlier or later than usual. However, if the period is different from normal or more than 5 days late then she should be advised to have a pregnancy test. A number of medicines do, theoretically, interact with Levonelle, most notably those that are enzyme inducers and include anticonvulsants, rifampicin, griseofulvin and St John's wort, although the clinical significance of the interactions appear low as only a handful of drug interaction reports have been received by the manufacturers. It seems prudent, until such time that more substantial evidence

Further reading

Piaggio G, von Hertzen H, Grimes DA, et al. Timing of emergency contraception with levonorgestrel or the Yuzpe regimen. Task Force on Postovulatory Methods of Fertility Regulation. Lancet 1999;353:721.

Task Force on Postovulatory Methods of Fertility Regulation. Randomised controlled trial of levonorgestrel versus the Yuzpe regimen of combined oral contraceptives for emergency contraception. Lancet 1998;352:428–33.

Web sites

British Pregnancy Advisory Service: http://www.bpas.org

Brook Advisory Centres: http://www.thebabyregistry.co.uk/advice/b/bac.htm

Family Planning Association: http://www.fpa.org.uk

Marie Stopes International: http://www.mariestopes.org.uk

Prodigy: http://www.cks.library.nhs.uk/contraception_emergency

Bayer site: http://www.levonelle.co.uk/output/page1.asp

Nicotine replacement therapy

Background

Smoking represents the single greatest cause of preventable illness and premature death worldwide. Smoking kills approximately 114 000 people each year in the UK; putting this in context, smoking causes about 30% of all cancer deaths, 17% of all heart disease deaths and over 80% of bronchitis and emphysema deaths

Prevalence and epidemiology

The number of smokers over the age of 16 in the UK is falling – from a high of 45% in 1974 to 24% (25% of men and 23% of women) in 2005, although the fall over the last decade has been small (28% in 1996 to 24% in 2005). Current UK Government targets are to reduce this figure to 21% or less by 2010, although this is unlikely to be achieved. Smoking is most common in those aged 20 to 34 (approx. 33%) and least common in people over 60 (14%). The latter lower figure is partially influenced by many smokers dying before reaching retirement age. In those under 16, 16% of boys and 25% of girls are regular smokers. To combat this problem the legal age limit to buy cigarettes in the UK rose to 18 from October 2007.

Compared to other EU countries, only Sweden has lower numbers of both men and women smokers. However, the percentage of women smokers in the UK is relatively high being ranked 7th out of 25 countries.

Recent legislation changes to ban smoking in public places (the first country was the Republic of Ireland in 2004, and are now joined by England, Scotland, Finland, Italy, Ireland, Norway, France and Malta) have been championed as having a potentially positive impact on smoking rates, for example, decreasing exposure to passive smoking and increasing quit rates. To establish any effect will take time but statistical data from Ireland have shown a fall in cigarette sales and surveys in Italy show a decrease in tobacco consumption.

Aetiology

Hundreds of compounds have been identified in tobacco smoke; however, only three compounds are of real clinical importance:

- tar-based products, which have carcinogenic properties
- carbon monoxide, which reduces the oxygen-carrying capacity of the red blood cells
- nicotine, which produces dependence by activation of dopaminergic systems

Tolerance to the effects of nicotine is rapid. Once plasma nicotine levels fall below a threshold, patients begin to suffer nicotine withdrawal symptoms and will crave another cigarette. Treatment is therefore based on maintaining plasma nicotine just above this threshold.

Evidence base for over-the-counter medication

Nicotine replacement therapy (NRT) has established itself as an effective treatment option. Numerous well-designed clinical trials and a Cochrane review (Silagy et al 2004) of such trials have shown NRT increases the success rate by one and a half to two times compared to placebo regardless of which NRT delivery system is used. It is not possible to say if one delivery system is better than another because comparative trials between delivery systems have not been conducted. Personal choice will therefore be the determining factor in which is chosen as being most suitable. In addition, the effectiveness of NRT is affected by the level of additional support provided to the smoker, and many Primary Care Trusts (PCTs) now offer smoking cessation services through the pharmacy.

It is clear then that NRT has efficacy over the short term but this effect appears to decrease over time. Etter et al (2006) showed that at least a third of quitters began to smoke again after NRT or placebo, and NRT rather than placebo would have to be used in 12 patients to induce one more patient to quit smoking at 12 months.

Brief advice (up to 5 minutes) to smokers to encourage them to make an attempt to quit is effective in promoting smoking cessation. Results involving GPs show that about 40% of smokers will make some attempt to quit, but only 1 to 3% (more than controls) will stop smoking for at least 6 months. Although the overall efficacy of brief advice is small, if sufficiently offered (i.e. by pharmacists), the reduction in rates of smoking in the general population could be substantial.

It should be noted that relapse is a normal part of the quitting process, and occurs on average three to four times. If a smoker has made repeated attempts to stop and failed, or has experienced severe withdrawal, or has requested more intensive help, then referral to a specialist smoking cessation service should be considered.

Practical prescribing and product selection

Prescribing information relating to medicines for NRT reviewed in the section 'Evidence base for over-the-counter medication' is discussed and summarised in Table 10.3.

Prior to instigation of any treatment it is important that the patient does want to stop smoking. Work has shown that motivation is a major determinant for successful smoking cessation and interventions based on the transtheoretical model of change put forward by Prochaska and colleagues have proved effective (Fig. 10.1). The model identifies six stages, progress through

Table 10.3
Practical prescribing: Summary of medicines used as nicotine replacement therapy

Name of medicine	Use in children	Likely side effects	Drug interactions of note	Patients in whom care should be exercised	Pregnancy and breast-feeding
Nicorette	>12 years	GI disturbances	None	Patients with heart disease	OK
Nicotinell NiQuitinCQ	>18 years	GI disturbances	None	Patients with heart disease	Manufacturers of Nicotinell liquorice gum advise it not to be used in pregnancy

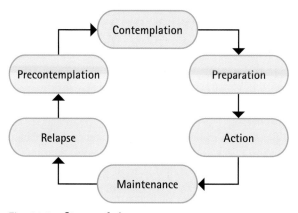

Fig. 10.1 Stages of change

which is cyclical and patients need varying types of support and advice at each stage.

Most patients who ask directly for NRT will be at the preparation stage of the model and ready to enter the action stage. However, a small number of patients may well be buying NRT to please others and are actually in the precontemplation stage and do not want to stop smoking.

NRT is formulated as gum, lozenges, patches, nasal spray, inhalator and sublingual tablets, therefore there should be a treatment option to suit all patients. When first deregulated, product licence restrictions did not allow OTC sale to certain patient groups such as those with heart disease, diabetes or who were pregnant. However, in 2006, the Department of Health decided to lift the restrictions on NRT in these patient groups and people over the age of 12 (although some manufacturers still state use in those over 18 years). The recommendation, according to the Department of Health, was based on strong evidence that it is 'far more harmful' for these groups to continue smoking than to use NRT. Side effects with NRT are rare and are either normally limited to gastrointestinal problems associated with accidental ingestion of nicotine when chewing gum or local skin irritation and vivid dreams associated with patches.

Headache, nausea and diarrhoea have also been reported. Intermittent forms of NRT are preferable during pregnancy although a patch may be appropriate if nausea and/or vomiting are a problem. NRT also appears not to have any significant interactions with other medicines.

Nicorette

Nicorette is available as gum (2 and 4 mg), inhalation cartridge (10 mg), microtab (2 mg), nasal spray (10 mg) and patch (5, 10 and 15 mg).

Gum

Nicorette gum is available as either fruit or mint flavours (unflavoured gum leaves a bitter taste in the mouth). The gum should be chewed slowly until the taste becomes strong; it should then be rested between the cheek and gum until the taste fades. The Nicorette gum can then be re-chewed. Each piece of gum lasts approximately 30 minutes. A maximum of 15 pieces of gum can be chewed in any 24-hour period.

Inhalation cartridge

The inhalator can be particularly helpful to those smokers who still feel they need to continue the hand-to-mouth movement. Each cartridge is inserted into the inhalator and air is drawn into the mouth through the mouthpiece. Deep drawing or short sucking can be used as required by the individual. Each cartridge lasts about 20 minutes. Cessation of smoking is planned to take 3 months. For the first 2 months patients should use between 6 and 12 cartridges a day. During weeks 8 to 10 the aim is to reduce the number of cartridges used by half and after the final 2 weeks the number of cartridges used should be zero. A maximum of 12 cartridges per day can be used.

Microtabs

Microtabs are delivered sublingually and patients who smoke less than 20 cigarettes a day should use one tablet per hour (doubled for heavy smokers), increased to two tablets per hour if the patient fails to stop smoking with the one tablet per hour regimen or for those whose nicotine withdrawal symptoms remain so strong they believe they will relapse. Most patients require between 8 and 24 tablets a day, although the maximum is 40 tablets in 24 hours. Treatment should be stopped when daily consumption is down to one or two tablets a day.

Spray
At the start of treatment one spray should be put into each nostril, twice an hour, to treat cravings. The maximum daily limit is 64 sprays; equivalent to two sprays in each nostril every hour for 16 hours.

Patches
Nicorette patches are usually applied in the morning and removed at bedtime (a 16-hour patch). Patients who smoke more than 20 cigarettes a day should start on the highest strength patch (15 mg) for 8 weeks before stepping down to the 10 mg patch for a further 2 weeks. The lowest strength patch (5 mg) should be finally worn for another 2 weeks.

Nicotinell

Nicotinell is available as gum (2 or 4 mg), patches (7, 14 and 21 mg) and lozenges (1 mg).

Nicotinell gum
Nicotinell gum is flavoured and available as fruit, mint or liquorice. The dosage and administration of Nicotinell gum is the same as that for Nicorette gum, except that a maximum of 25 pieces can be chewed in any 24-hour period.

Patches
Nicotinell patches are suitable for those smokers who must have a cigarette as soon as they wake up. The patches are worn continuously and changed every 24 hours; thus, when the patient awakes nicotine levels will be above the threshold of nicotine withdrawal (see Hints and Tips Box 10.3). People who smoke more than 20 cigarettes a day should use the highest strength patch

(TTS 30 patch, 21 mg) for 3 to 4 weeks, after which the strength of the patch should be reduced to the middle strength (TTS 20 patch, 14 mg) for a further 3 to 4 weeks before finally using the lowest patch (TTS 10 patch, 7 mg). If the patient smokes less than 20 cigarettes a day then they should start on the middle strength patch.

Lozenges
Patients should be instructed to suck one lozenge every 1 to 2 hours when they have the urge to smoke. The usual dosage is 8 to 12 lozenges per day, with a maximum of 25 lozenges in 24 hours. Lozenges are mint flavoured and should be sucked until the taste becomes strong and then placed between gum and cheek (similar to the nicotine gum) until the taste fades, when sucking can recommence. Each lozenge takes approximately 30 minutes to dissolve completely.

NiQuitinCQ

NiQuitinCQ is available as gum (2 or 4 mg), patches (7, 14 and 21 mg) and lozenges (2 and 4 mg).

Patches
Patients who smoke more than 10 cigarettes a day should use the 21 mg patch (Step 1) for 6 weeks, followed by the 14 mg patch (Step 2) for 2 weeks and finally the 7 mg patch (Step 3) for the last 2 weeks. If the person smokes less than 10 cigarettes each day the patient should start on Step 2 for 6 weeks followed by Step 3 for a final 2 weeks.

Lozenges
The low strength lozenge (2 mg) is aimed at those who smoke more than 30 minutes after waking and the higher strength (4 mg) for those who smoke within 30 minutes of waking. Like NiQuitinCQ patches the dose of lozenges are marketed as Steps.

Step 1 × 6 weeks	1 lozenge every 1 to 2 hours
Step 2 × 3 weeks	1 lozenge every 2 to 4 hours
Step 3 × 3 weeks	1 lozenge every 4 to 8 hours

HINTS AND TIPS BOX 10.3: NICOTINE REPLACEMENT THERAPY

Application of patches	Patches should be applied to non-hairy skin on the hip, chest or upper arm. The next patch should be placed on a different site to avoid skin irritation
16- or 24-hour patches?	A 16-hour patch will be suitable for most patients; however, if a patient requires a cigarette within the first 20 to 30 minutes after waking then a 24-hour patch should be given
	If sleep disturbances are experienced with the 24-hour patches the patient can switch to a 16-hour patch or alternatively remove the 24-hour patch when they go to bed

After this programme patients can use one to two lozenges a day over the next 12 weeks when strongly tempted to smoke.

Gum

Like lozenges, the lower strength is used for those smokers who smoke more than 30 minutes after waking and the higher strength for those who smoke within 30 minutes of waking. Like Nicorette and Nicotinell the 'chew and rest' technique is used. The dose is marketed as Steps.

Step 1 (up to 3 months)   8 to 12 pieces of gum per day
Step 2   Reduce to 1 to 2 pieces per day
Step 3   Occasional use if urge to smoke

Further reading

Etter J, Stapleton JA. Nicotine replacement therapy for long-term smoking cessation: a meta-analysis. Tobacco Control 2006;15:280–5.
Hajek P. Treatments for smokers. Addiction 1994;89:1543–9.
Silagy C, Lancaster T, Stead L, et al. Nicotine replacement therapy for smoking cessation. Cochrane Database of Systematic Reviews 2004, issue 3.

Web sites

Department of health information: http://www.gosmokefree.co.uk/
NHS Stop Smoking Service: Call 0800 169 0 169 or text 'give up' and your postcode to 88088.
Action on Smoking and Health (ASH): http://www.ash.org/
QUIT: http://www.quit.org.uk/
Company site giving general advice on smoking cessation: http://www.nicotinell.com/intl/firstmoment.php

Malaria prophylaxis

Background

Malaria is a parasitic disease spread by the female anopheles mosquito. Four species of the protozoan *Plasmodium* produce malaria in humans: *P. vivax, P. ovale, P. malariae* and *P. falciparum*. *P. falciparum* is the most virulent form of malaria and is responsible for the majority of deaths associated with malaria infection. It acts by altering the surface of red blood cells making them adhere to blood vessel walls leading to sequestration. Clinically, patients suffer from chills, nausea, vomiting and headache. This is followed by fever, which concludes with sweating. This cycle repeats every 2 to 3 days.

Prevalence and epidemiology

Malaria is a leading cause of death in areas of the world where the infection is endemic, with an estimated 300 million cases each year resulting in over 1 million deaths.

However, malaria is not only confined to endemic malarial areas and the number of cases reported in Western countries, for example the UK, is on the increase as more and more people travel to countries where malaria is common. There are between 1500 and 2000 cases reported in the UK each year. In 2005, there were 1754 cases that resulted in 11 deaths. Figures for that year show that *P. falciparum* accounted for 76% of cases (1338), *P. vivax* 15% (258), *P. ovale* 7% (116) and just 2% (29) for *P. malariae*.

The risk of contracting malaria varies greatly and depends on the area visited, the time of year and altitude (parasite maturation cannot take place above 2000 m) and how many infectious bites are received. In general, risk tends to be higher in more remote areas than in urban/tourist areas, after rainy or monsoon seasons and at low altitude. It is therefore possible to have a different risk of contracting malaria within the same country, for example, visiting the Southern lowlands of Ethiopia after the rainy season would pose a very high risk whereas trekking in the Simien mountains in the north of the country during the dry season would pose minimal risk.

Aetiology

Malarial parasites are transmitted to humans when an infected female anopheles mosquito bites its host. Once in the human host, the parasites (which at this stage of their life-cycle are known as sporozoites) are transported via the bloodstream to the liver. In the liver they divide and multiply (they are now known as merozoites). After 5 to 16 days the liver cells rupture, to release up to 400 000 merozoites, which invade the human host's erythrocytes. The merozoites reproduce asexually in the erythrocytes before causing them to rupture and release yet more merozoites into the bloodstream to invade yet more erythrocytes. Any mosquito that bites an infected person at this stage will ingest the parasites and the cycle will begin again. It is worth noting that *P. vivax* and *P. ovale* parasites can remain dormant in the liver, which explains why malarial symptoms can manifest months after return from an infected region.

Evidence base for over-the-counter medication

Effective bite prevention should be the first line of defence against malarial infection. Total avoidance of being bitten is not practical and patients must ensure that protective measures from being bitten are always taken.

Insect repellents containing *N,N*-diethyl-*m*-toluamide (DEET) in high concentrations are recommended (see Hints and Tips Box 10.4). In controlled laboratory studies DEET provides the longest protection compared to other products. Evidence for other insect repellents suggests

HINTS AND TIPS BOX 10.4: MALARIA

Application of DEET	The concentration of DEET in commercial products varies widely. Products with concentrations in excess of 50% can cause skin irritation and occasionally skin blistering. It is advisable that these are patch tested first before widespread application The higher the concentration of DEET, the greater the length of protection: • 50% DEET provides protection for up to 12 hours • 30% DEET provides protection for up to 6 hours • 20% DEET provides protection for 1 to 3 hours Note – reapplication is necessary after swimming or sweating DEET can damage certain plastics, for example, sunglasses. It is important to emphasise to the patient that they wash their hands after applying DEET Make sure exposed areas such as feet and ankles are adequately protected DEET reduces the effectiveness of sunblock but sunblock does not affect the effectiveness of DEET
Illness on return from malarial region	Patients should be told to report cold or flu-like symptoms to their GP for 3 months after returning from holiday. However, symptoms of malaria can take up to a year to manifest themselves because the liver can harbour a reservoir of parasites
Electronic mosquito repellents	These products are designed to repel female mosquitoes by emitting high-pitched sounds almost inaudible to the human ear. There is no evidence in field studies to support any repelling effects
Alternative remedies	There is currently no evidence supporting the use of vitamin B1, garlic, tee tree oil or Marmite – they should not be recommended

they have comparable efficacy to low concentrations of DEET but have shorter duration of protection than DEET (Fradin et al 2002). Current guidelines from the advisory committee for malaria prevention (http://www.hpa.org.uk/publications/PublicationDisplay.asp?PublicationID=87&TandC=true) recommend that all people use a product containing 50% DEET (except those under the age of 2 months).

Besides applying DEET, other preventative measures to reduce the chance of being bitten include wearing long loose-fitting sleeved shirts and trousers, especially between dawn and dusk. Protection of ankles appears to be particularly important. Hotel windows should be checked to make sure they have adequate screening and ideally the bed should have a mosquito net. Mosquito nets do reduce the incidence of being bitten and subsequent contraction of malaria, although those impregnated with insecticides are the gold standard and are more effective than non-impregnated nets (Lengeler 2004). If the person is travelling to more remote areas they should purchase their own mosquito net that has been impregnated with an insecticide. There are a number of travel centres and specialist outdoor shops where such products can be bought, including insecticide-impregnated clothes.

Doors and windows should remain closed during the evening and night and mosquito coils or plug-in dispensers should be used.

Chemoprophylaxis

In addition to taking precautions to avoid being bitten, travellers should also take antimalarial medication. Chloroquine and proguanil are licensed for pharmacy sale when used for prophylaxis of malaria and have proven efficacy but drug resistance to these two medicines, e.g. chloroquine-resistant *P. falciparum* is now widespread, and limits their usefulness.

It is important to check current guidelines for the destination the person is travelling to or through. Two easily available UK reference sources in which recommendations can be found are the *British National Formulary* and *MIMS*. In addition, a number of organisations produce reference material (e.g. The National Pharmacy Association's vaccination updates). In most instances, *MIMS* would be a first-line reference source as the guidelines are updated monthly (compared to the *British National Formulary*'s biannual publication) and are more likely to be still up to date. For those who are travelling to very high-risk areas (usually sub-Saharan Africa or South East Asia) or for long periods of time it might be better to refer them to a specialist centre.

Practical prescribing and product selection

Prescribing information relating to medicines for malaria reviewed in the section 'Evidence base for over-the-

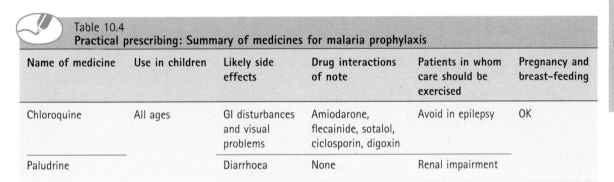

Table 10.4
Practical prescribing: Summary of medicines for malaria prophylaxis

Name of medicine	Use in children	Likely side effects	Drug interactions of note	Patients in whom care should be exercised	Pregnancy and breast-feeding
Chloroquine	All ages	GI disturbances and visual problems	Amiodarone, flecainide, sotalol, ciclosporin, digoxin	Avoid in epilepsy	OK
Paludrine		Diarrhoea	None	Renal impairment	

counter medication' is discussed and summarised in Table 10.4; useful tips relating to patients travelling to regions where malaria is endemic are given in Hints and Tips Box 10.4.

Medicine regimens

Antimalarials need to be taken at least 1 week before departure, during the stay in the malaria endemic region and for 4 weeks on leaving the area. Taking the medication prior to departure allows the patient to know whether they are going to experience side effects and, if they do, still have enough time to obtain a different antimalarial before departure. It also helps to establish a medicine-taking routine that will, hopefully, help with compliance. Medicine taking for a further 4 weeks after leaving the region ensures that any possible infection that could have been contracted during the final days of the stay does not develop into malaria.

Chloroquine (e.g. Avloclor, Nivaquine)

Chloroquine, as a single agent, is now almost obsolete against *P. falciparum* but still remains effective against the other forms of malaria.

Adults and children over 13 should take 300 mg of chloroquine base each week; this is equivalent to two tablets. Chloroquine can be given to children of all ages and is based on a milligram per kilogram basis. A syrup formulation of Nivaquine is available (50 mg of base/5 mL) and should be recommended for children because an accurate dose can be given according to their weight.

Chloroquine is associated with a number of side effects including nausea, vomiting, headaches and visual disturbances. Most patient groups, including pregnant women, can take chloroquine, although it is contraindicated in epilepsy because it might lower the seizure threshold and tonic–clonic seizures have been reported with prophylactic doses. Patients with psoriasis might notice a worsening of their condition. Chloroquine should be avoided in patients taking amiodarone, flecainide and sotalol because there is a risk of QT prolongation and ventricular arrhythmia. It should also be avoided with ciclosporin (increased

risk of toxicity) and possibly digoxin (increases digoxin levels?).

Proguanil (Paludrine)

Proguanil is always used in combination with chloroquine unless the patient is contraindicated from taking chloroquine. Adults and children over the age of 13 should take 200 mg (two tablets) daily. Like chloroquine, it can be given to children of all ages and the dose ideally should be on a milligram per kilogram basis. To aid compliance a travel pack suitable for adults on a 2-week holiday is available that combines 14 chloroquine tablets with 98 proguanil tablets. Side effects associated with proguanil are usually mild and include diarrhoea. Patients with known mild renal impairment should take 100 mg daily and the dose should be further reduced if renal impairment is moderate or severe.

Further reading

Enayati AA, Hemingway J, Garner P. Electronic mosquito repellents for preventing mosquito bites and malaria infection. Cochrane Database of Systematic Reviews 2007, issue 2.

Fradin MS, Day JF. Comparative efficacy of insect repellents against mosquito bites. New Engl J Med 2002;347:13–18.

Lengeler C. Insecticide-treated bed nets and curtains for preventing malaria. Cochrane Database of Systematic Reviews 2004, issue 2.

Web sites

Health protection agency information on malaria: http://www.hpa.org.uk/infections/topics_az/malaria/guidelines.htm

Prodigy guidance: http://www.cks.library.nhs.uk/malaria_prophylaxis

The National Travel Health Network and Centre: http://wwwnathnac.org

Malaria Reference Laboratory: http://www.malaria-reference.co.uk

Liverpool School of Tropical Medicine: http://www.liv.ac.uk/lstm

Bites and stings

Background

A whole host of animals (and plants) have the capacity to cause injury to the skin, and depending on the severity can result in systemic symptoms. The majority of cases are caused by insects and are of nuisance value.

Prevalence and epidemiology

The prevalence of bites and stings is largely unknown. Most people self-treat and never seek advice. Biting and stinging insects are generally more common in warmer climates and in warmer months, with summer being the peak time.

Aetiology

Stinging insects are broadly defined as those that use some sort of venom as a defence mechanism or to imobilise their prey. Examples include bees, wasps and ants. The venom is usually 'injected' using a stinger and includes proteins and substances that help break down cells and increase the penetration of the venom, e.g. phospholipase A and hyaluronidase. People can develop allergic reactions to these substances and, unlike with most biting insects, can occasionally suffer significant reactions, including anaphylaxis, to stings. The severity of the reaction depends on the quantity of the venom injected and the person's predisposition to hypersensitivity.

Biting insects are those that feed off the blood supply of humans and other creatures. They include mosquitoes, ticks and fleas. Apart from having some sort of apparatus to draw the blood, these insects usually secrete anticoagulant-like substances to facilitate feeding. It is these anticoagulant substances that people will react to. However, it is only after repeated bites that sensitivity occurs.

Clinical features of bites and stings

Itching papules, which can be intense, is the hallmark symptom of insect bites. Weals, bulla and pain can occur, especially in sensitised individuals. Lesions are often localised and grouped together and occur on exposed areas, e.g. hands, ankles and face. Scratching can cause excoriation, which might lead to secondary infection. In contrast, stings are associated with intense burning pain. Erythema and oedema follow but usually subside within a few hours. If systemic symptoms are experienced, they occur within minutes of the sting.

Evidence base for over-the-counter medication

Avoiding bites and stings in the first place is obviously important. This means using an effective insect repellant and avoiding times and places when insects are about. DEET is the most effective insect repellant and is found in most commercial preparations. For avoidance measures and more information on DEET see pages 303–304.

Before OTC treatment is offered, the severity of symptoms should be assessed, because small local reactions can be managed primarily with topical products whereas large local reactions will generally require systemic treatment. Patients with systemic symptoms should be referred.

Topical OTC treatments for bites and stings include local anaesthetics, corticosteroids and antihistamines. For local anaesthetics, there is a lack of clinical data to support their use for stings and bites, either alone or in combination with antihistamines. However, their use in practice is well established and is appropriate on theoretical grounds. Hydrocortisone, like lidocaine, has a lack of clinical data for bites and stings, but its use could be justified on theoretical grounds. Crotamiton is also marketed for conditions associated with itching. Prodigy guidance (Dec 2007) recommends crotamiton for local reactions to control itching, but there is a lack of evidence to support this and is based on expert opinion.

Stingose is a 20% aluminium acetate solution marketed for the treatment of bites and stings. The proposed mechanism of action is that aluminium ions cause denaturing of the proteins and bind polysaccharides in bites and stings resulting in inactivation of the venom. There are no randomised comparative or placebo controlled trials. However, a large case series of over 1000 patients found it to be effective in treating a range of marine, plant and animal bites and stings in over 99% of cases (Henderson et al 1980).

Antihistamines (both topical and systemic) have been used for their antipruritic properties. There are limited studies in the treatment of insect bites and stings. Some studies with systemic antihistamines have shown efficacy of the less sedating antihistamines for mosquito bites (Foëx et al 2006).

Practical prescribing and product selection

Prescribing information relating to products for bites and stings reviewed in the section 'Evidence base for over-the-counter medication' is discussed and summarised in Table 10.5.

Local anaesthetics (e.g. benzocaine (Lanacane), lidocaine (Dermidex))

Local anaesthetics can be used in adults and children over 3 years (Solarcaine spray, benzocaine 2.85%) and are in general applied three times a day. They are safe to use in pregnancy and are generally well tolerated. Local anaesthetics are known to be skin sensitisers and can produce contact dermatitis.

Table 10.5
Practical prescribing: Summary of medicines used for insect bites and stings

Name of medicine	Use in children	Likely side effects	Drug interactions of note	Patients in whom care should be exercised	Pregnancy and breast-feeding
Benzocaine					
Lanacane	>12 years	Can cause sensitisation reactions	None	None	OK
Solarcane	>3 years				
Lidocaine					
Dermidex	>4 years	Can cause sensitisation reactions	None	None	OK
Hydrocortisone	>10 years	None	None	None	OK
Crotamiton	>3 years	None	None	None	OK
Chlorphenamine	>1 year	Dry mouth, sedation and constipation	Increased sedation with alcohol, opioid analgesics, anxiolytics, hypnotics and antidepressants	Glaucoma, prostate enlargement	Standard references state OK, although some manufacturers advise avoidance

Local anaesthetic/antihistamine combination (Wasp-Eze spray)

This product contains benzocaine 1% and mepyramine 0.5%. It can be used on people over the age of 2 years. The dose is one spray onto the affected area of skin for 2 to 3 seconds. This dose can be repeated after 15 minutes if required.

Hydrocortisone (e.g. Dermacort)

Hydrocortisone is applied once or twice a day to the affected areas. It can be used in adults and children over 10 years of age. It can be used for a maximum of 7 days.

Antihistamines (e.g. chlorphenamine)

Chlorphenamine, as all antihistamines, are associated with sedation. They interact with other sedating medication, resulting in potentiation of the sedative properties of the interacting medicines. They also possess antimuscarinic side effects, which commonly result in dry mouth and possibly constipation. It is these antimuscarinic properties that mean patients with glaucoma and prostate enlargement should ideally avoid their use, because it could lead to increased intraocular pressure and precipitation of urinary retention.

Chlorphenamine (Piriton)

Chlorphenamine can be given from the age of 1 year. Children up to the age of 2 should take 2.5 mL of syrup (1 mg) twice a day. For children aged between 2 and 5 the dose is 2.5 mL (1 mg) three or four times a day and

those over the age of 6 should take 5 mL (2 mg) three or four times a day. Adults should take 4 mg (one tablet) three or four times a day.

Crotamiton (Eurax)

Adults and children over 3 years of age should apply crotamiton two or three times a day. A combination product containing hydrocortisone is available (Eurax HC) but is best avoided if possible. This is to decrease the exposure of patients to unnecessary corticosteroids and their potential adverse effects.

Aluminium acetate (Stingose)

Aluminium acetate is safe to use at any age and comes in a spray and gel. It should be applied as soon as possible after the sting, and is unlikely to be effective if used more than 30 minutes after the sting or bite. It has no significant side effects. However, some local skin reactions are possible. It is safe to use in pregnancy.

Further reading

Foëx BA, Lee C. Oral antihistamines for insect bites. Emerg Med J 2006;23:721–2.

Henderson D, Easton RG. Stingose: a new and effective treatment for bites and stings. Med J Aust 1980;2:143–50.

Web sites

Prodigy guidance: http://cks.library.nhs.uk/insect_bites_and_stings

Coronary heart disease

Background

Coronary heart disease (CHD) is the biggest preventable cause of mortality in the UK. More than 1.4 million people suffer from angina and 275 000 people have a heart attack annually; consequently, reducing deaths from CHD is a key government priority. In 2000, the UK government launched the national service framework (NSF) for CHD. This 10-year programme consists of 12 standards that cover the whole spectrum of CHD, from its prevention and diagnosis to treatment and rehabilitation. The UK government has set ambitious targets to reduce the death rate from CHD, stroke and related diseases in people under 75 by at least 40% by 2010. However, the NSF for CHD has prioritised interventions to those at greatest risk of CHD – all patients who have had an event (secondary prevention) and those who have a high risk of developing CHD (primary prevention). High risk is defined as a 10-year CHD event risk greater than 30%. The UK government has indicated that as resources permit this value should be lowered to 15%, although in 2008 this has yet to occur. Standard intervention for CHD includes: smoking cessation, reducing modifiable risk factors, controlling blood pressure to agreed targets and use of medication (especially statins for both primary and secondary prevention).

In 2004 simvastatin was reclassified to pharmacy sale. The deregulation of simvastatin represented an important milestone for pharmacists because it was the first medicine to become available that treats a chronic rather than acute condition. The intention of the reclassification was to target the moderate risk group (i.e. those the government have excluded – people with a 10 to 15% chance of developing CHD in the next 10 years).

Prevalence and epidemiology

In the UK, 5% of the population suffer from CHD (3 million people). Figures for 2002 show that 22% of all male deaths were due to CHD and 9% from stroke, and for women the figures were 17% and 13% respectively. Despite these alarming figures, CHD is in decline in the UK. For example, in people aged under 65 the number of deaths has fallen from approximately 80 deaths per 100 000 in 1980 to approximately 30 deaths per 100 000 in 2000. Much of this fall can be attributed to modifying risk factors (e.g. stopping smoking) and drug intervention. However, within the population there are major health inequalities. For example, people from lower social classes are more likely to suffer from CHD – working men in social class V (unskilled occupations) are 50% more likely to die from CHD than men in the population as a whole. People from some ethnic backgrounds have a much higher risk for developing CHD. In the UK, people of South Asian descent have a 40% greater risk of CHD than white people. Geography also plays a part with people from southern England having lower death rates than northern England and Scotland.

While mortality from CHD is falling rapidly, morbidity is not, and in older age groups has risen by over a third in the past 10 years.

Aetiology

Atherosclerosis of the coronary arteries is responsible for CHD. This usually begins before adulthood and is a complex process. Exactly how atherosclerosis begins or what causes it is not known. Current thinking is that the innermost layer of the artery (endothelium) becomes damaged. Over time, fats, cholesterol, platelets, cellular debris and calcium are deposited in the artery wall. Collagen is synthesised and makes a fibrous cap around damaged tissue known as a plaque. This narrows the coronary artery and the reduced supply of oxygen to the heart muscle causes coronary ischaemia. This can present as angina, myocardial infarction, unstable angina or sudden death.

Evidence base for over-the-counter medication

No specific clinical trials have been conducted in the population since simvastatin was granted an OTC licence. However, based on evidence from clinical trials, simvastatin is considered likely to confer benefits in terms of reducing CHD events. It has been shown to lower low-density lipoprotein (LDL) cholesterol by about 27% in practice.

Practical prescribing and product selection

The pharmacist has an important role in getting people to understand the risk factors associated with CHD and what they can do to reduce their risk. Standards 1 and 2 of the NSF for CHD pay particular attention to how the NHS and other organisations can reduce CHD risks in the population. The main advice to tell people is summarised in Table 10.6.

Recommendation of simvastatin (Zocor Heart-Pro) is not based on the person's cholesterol measurements but on their risk factors. OTC sale of Simvastatin can be made to:

- all men aged between 55 and 70 years
- men aged between 45 and 55, and women aged over 55, who have one or more of the following risk factors: family history of CHD, smoker, overweight or of South Asian family origin.

To assist in the assessment of a person's suitability the company have produced a questionnaire for people to

Table 10.6
Lifestyle measures to prevent CHD

Measure	
Smoking cessation	• Stopping smoking has been shown in several large cohort studies to decrease associated risks. For CHD, the risk of coronary events declines in 2 to 3 years to that of people who have never smoked. The risk of stroke declines more slowly
Exercise	• People who are moderately physically active have a 30 to 50% lower risk of CHD than people who are sedentary • Moderate-to-high physical activity also reduces the risk of stroke. It helps control weight, blood pressure and diabetes; protects against osteoporosis; and increases well-being. • Offer advice on gradually increasing exercise, if appropriate; about 60% of men and 70% of women in the UK are considered to be sedentary • Brisk walking for half an hour (or more) per day reduces the relative risk of CHD by about 20% • It is not necessary to participate in sport or weight training activities to achieve exercise targets: brisk walking, climbing stairs and heavy housework are all moderate-intensity physical activities
Dietary management – Up to 30% of all deaths from CHD have been attributed to unhealthy diets	• Replace saturated and *trans*-fats with unsaturated fats (especially monounsaturated and non-hydrogenated polyunsaturated fat). • Increase consumption of omega-3 fatty acids from fish oil or plant sources • Consume a diet high in fruits, vegetables, nuts and whole grains and low in refined grains • Replace butter with olive oil and monounsaturated margarine (e.g. rapeseed- or olive oil-based) • Eat less red meat (replace beef, lamb and pork with poultry). If eating red meat, use lean cuts. Remove the skin from poultry • Eat more fish, including at least one portion of oily fish per week, e.g. mackerel, herring, kipper, pilchard, sardine, salmon or trout • Eat more bread (especially wholegrain bread) • Eat more root vegetables and green vegetables • Eat fruit every day • Eat fewer commercial bakery and deep-fried foods (these contain high levels of *trans*-fats and sugar) • Aim to eat five portions of fruit and vegetables every day • Tinned and frozen fruit and vegetables are as good as fresh vegetables • Reduce salt intake
Weight control – Excess weight is associated with raised blood pressure, raised blood cholesterol, type 2 diabetes and low levels of physical activity, all of which increase the risk of CHD	• Encourage all obese and overweight* people to lose weight, aiming towards a body mass index (BMI) of less than 25 • Even if a BMI less than 25 cannot be achieved, a reduction in 5 to 10% of initial bodyweight still has significant health benefits • The risk of CHD is two to three times greater in overweight women than in lean women • The risks are further increased when fat is concentrated mainly in the abdomen (central obesity) • Frequent fluctuations in weight are also associated with an increased risk of CHD. Weight-management programmes must therefore aim to maintain weight loss, not just to achieve initial weight loss

table continues

Table 10.6   continued

Measure	
Alcohol consumption – Men should limit their alcohol consumption to a maximum of 21 units per week (i.e. a maximum of 3 units per day). For women, the maximum is 14 units per week (i.e. a maximum of 2 units per day). In the UK 26% of men already drink more than 21 units per week and 15% of women drink more than 14 units per week	• Up to 2 units of alcohol per day is associated with a 20% relative risk reduction of CHD and all types of alcohol have been associated with lowering the risk of CHD; the effect is not solely confined to red wine • The pattern of drinking is also important. Consumption of alcohol on at least 3 to 4 days per week has been found to be inversely associated with the risk of myocardial infarction in men. Conversely, binge drinking is associated with increased mortality and fatal myocardial infarction • There is not enough information available to justify encouraging those who do not drink alcohol to start doing so. Moderate drinking is likely to have most benefits in people who are at highest risk of CHD, i.e. middle-aged and elderly people. In younger people (who are at low risk of CHD) the risks of alcohol-related problems, such as accidents, may outweigh the potential benefits. There are also concerns that moderate drinking may increase the risk of breast cancer in young women (less than 50 years) For more information on units see: http://www.at-bristol.org.uk/Alcoholandyou/Facts/units.html

*Overweight BMI >25; obesity >30

complete. The dose is one tablet per day, preferably in the evening. It has very few side effects (even at high doses), which are classed as rare ($>1/10\,000$, $<1/1000$), and include GI upset (e.g. abdominal pain, flatulence, nausea and vomiting) and CNS effects such as dizziness, blurred vision and headache. Simvastatin can also cause reversible myositis (unexplained generalised muscle pain, tenderness or weakness not associated with flu, exercise or recent strain or injury) and if suspected treatment should be discontinued. It can interact with other fibrates, azole antifungals, ciclosporin, nefazadone and macrolide antibiotics (increased risk of myopathy). It also can affect warfarin levels and should not be given with grapefruit juice (grapefruit juice inhibits cytochrome P450 3A4 and increases simvastatin levels).

Simvastatin is not intended for those who are known to have existing CHD, diabetes, history of stroke or peripheral vascular disease, familial hypercholesterolaemia or hypertension. These people should be referred to their GP.

Web sites
UK Department of Health information on CHD:
http://www.dh.gov.uk/en/Policyandguidance/
Healthandsocialcaretopics/Coronaryheartdisease/index.
htm

Potential medicines for reclassification

Orlistat

The licence holders of orlistat (GSK) have applied for a European-wide OTC licence for orlistat. Currently, orlistat is available in Australia and the US, and it seems unlikely that the application for OTC use in Europe will not go ahead. The projected launch of this product is the first quarter of 2009.

Obestiy is a growing epidemic, particularly in Western countries. As a consequence the risk of diseases such as diabetes and cardiovascular disease are also increasing, resulting in a situation where the current and future generations could have a shorter life span than their parents. Although a number of measures of obesity have been proposed, the internationally accepted measure is the body mass index (BMI). This is calculated as the weight (kg) divided by height squared (m^2). The usual cut off for being classified as overweight is $25\ kg/m^2$ and for obesity it is $30\ kg/m^2$.

Evidence base for over-the-counter medication

Diet and exercise are still considered the first-line treatment for obesity. Orlistat inhibits pancreatic and gastric lipase, which reduces the absorption of fat from the gut. Clinical trials have shown that orlistat produces a modest weight loss of approximately 5 to 10% of body weight (Hill et al 1999). The best results with orlistat are seen in the short term (6 to 12 months); long-term results rely heavily on lifestyle changes. Orlistat is likely to be indicated for those patients with a BMI > 30 kg/m², or with a BMI > 27 kg/m² where other co-morbidities exist such as diabetes, hypercholesterolemia and hypertension. The recommended dose will be one capsule with each main meal. Patients should be realistic about the weight loss that can be achieved. Side effects are largely gastrointestinal and include faecal urgency and incontinence, oily evacuation and spotting, flatus and abdominal pain. These can be minimised by restricting fat intake to less than 20 g per meal. Supplementation with fat-soluble vitamins (A, D, E and K) is recommended, and this should be taken at least 2 hours before an orlistat dose or at bedtime. Because of the effect on vitamin K levels, patients on warfarin should have their international normalised ratio (INR) checked regularly. Also, orlistat may decrease ciclosporin levels and requires close monitoring.

Further reading

Hill J, Hauptman J, Anderson J. Orlistat, a lipase inhibitor, for weight maintenance after conventional dieting: a 1-y study. Am J Clin Nutr 1999;69:1108–16.

Lindgarde F. The effect of orlistat on body weight and coronary heart disease risk profile in obese patients: the Swedish Multimorbidity Study. J Intern Med 2000;248:245–54.

National Prescribing Service 2004 Orlistat (Xenical) over-the-counter for obesity. NPS Radar. Available online (cited Feb 2007): http://www.npsradar.org.au/npsradar/content/orlistat.pdf (accessed 17 Jan 2007).

Trimethoprim

An application from Alpharma to reclassify trimethoprim is currently being considered. Current UK guidelines (Prodigy 2007) recommend empirical treatment with trimethoprim or nitrofurantoin for uncomplicated cystitis in women. Three-day courses of trimethoprim have been shown to be as effective as 5- and 7-day courses and associated with fewer side effects. The application for reclassification follows this UK guidance. If approved trimethoprim (traded as Cysticlear) will be licensed for women aged 16 to 70 who have had a previous diagnosis of cystitis made by a medical practitioner. The dose is one tablet (200 mg) twice a day for 3 days. Cysticlear will have a number of restrictions placed on its supply and 'cystitis customer questionnaires' have been produced by the manufacturer to ensure appropriate sales are made. (Note: nitrofurantoin is also now in the process of deregulation (ARM 51) and will have similar indications to trimethoprim.)

Diclofenac potassium

Diclofenac is currently available OTC in the UK as a topical formulation (Voltarol Emulgel P) but in November 2007, Novartis Consumer Health UK Ltd applied to the Medicines and Healthcare Products Regulatory Authority (MHRA) (ARM 49) to reclassify diclofenac potassium (traded under the name of Voltarol Pain-eze tablets). Diclofenac potassium is already available as an OTC medication in many countries and this application mirrors its use in other countries. If approved, it will be indicated for the short-term relief of headache, dental pain, period pain, rheumatic and muscular pain, backache and the symptoms of colds and flu, including fever. The dose will be two tablets (25 mg) taken initially, followed by one (12.5 mg) or two tablets (25 mg) every 4–6 hours when needed, with a maximum daily dose limited to six tablets (75 mg). People aged under the age of 14 will not be allowed to take diclofenac and pack sizes will be limited to 18 tablets. (Note: diclofenac was granted OTC status in Summer 2008)

Azithromycin

Actavis UK Ltd applied to the MHRA in June 2007 (ARM 43) to reclassify azithromycin from POM control for the treatment of known or suspected asymptomatic *Chlamydia trachomatis* in people aged 16 years and over.

Chlamydia trachomatis is the most common sexually transmitted bacterial infection in the UK, and the incidence is increasing. In response to the growing problem, the Department of Health has introduced the National Chlamydia Screening Programme (NCSP), which saw national roll out in April 2006. Community pharmacy was included in this programme and supply of azithromycin has occurred via patient group directions. The reclassification of azithromycin will follow the NCSP model. In summary, patients are offered opportunistic chlamydia screening and informed of the result. Those with a positive result who are asymptomatic are assessed for suitability for pharmacy supply, and if they are, then they receive public health advice (chlamydia awareness information, risk of other STIs, safe sex information and partner notification information) and are supplied with azithromycin (two 500 mg tablets stat.).

Future applications

A number of medicines are currently being considered for reclassification that might well become pharmacy products during the lifespan of this edition. Table 10.7

Table 10.7
Possible future deregulated medicines from POM to P

Oral contraception	Low risk of side effects Fits in with government sexual health policies, especially those tackling teenage pregnancy PGD to undergo trials in community pharmacies in 2008
Salbutamol	Already OTC in some countries, e.g. Singapore, New Zealand
Doxycycline (and possibly others) for malaria prophylaxis	Given current resistance to proguanil and chloroquine deregulation seems likely
Topical antibiotics for impetigo (e.g. fusidic acid, mupirocin)	Strong support from a number of studies gaining GP opinion Condition easy to identify Low risk of side effects
Topical antibiotics (e.g. erythromycin) and azelaic acid for acne	Same reasons as indicated for impetigo
Antiretrovirals for influenza	Already established patient group directions (PGDs) through community pharmacy Fits in with government public health policy
Antihistamines	Desloratadine and fexofenadine available OTC in some countries, e.g. Australia
Steroid-based preparations	Likely that topical and inhaled steroid products will become increasingly available to treat allergic-type conditions
Metoclopramide	Low risk of side effects Available OTC in some countries already
NSAIDs	Naproxen was deregulated in April 2008 and Diclofenac in July 2008. Other NSAIDs that are likely to be reclassified include mefenamic acid
Insomnia ('Z' drugs)	Low risk of side effects

highlights some future candidates that are potential POM to P switches.

In addition, it is probable that some medicines used in chronic disease states will be deregulated. Currently, the medical profession is generally opposed to chronic disease states being managed by community pharmacists but this is at odds with government policy. In time, medicines for a wide range of conditions might be available OTC, with coronary heart disease and respiratory conditions being key areas.

Self-assessment questions

The following questions are intended to supplement the text. Two levels of questions are provided: multiple choice questions and case studies. The multiple choice questions are designed to test factual recall and the case studies allow knowledge to be applied to a practice setting.

Multiple choice questions

10.1 Which antihistamine used for motion sickness is subject to abuse?

a. Cinnarizine
b. Cyclizine
c. Promethazine
d. Meclozine
e. Hyoscine

10.2 What is the main side effect of Levonelle One Step?

a. Vomiting
b. Headache
c. Diarrhoea
d. Nausea
e. Dizziness

10.3 In which group of the population is smoking on the increase?

a. Middle-aged males
b. Middle-aged females
c. Teenage females
d. Teenage males
e. None of the above

10.4 Which patients should use 24-hour patches?

a. People who smoke more than 20 cigarettes a day
b. People who smoke more than 40 cigarettes a day
c. People who need a cigarette within 20 minutes of waking up
d. People who need a cigarette before they go to sleep
e. People who smoke cigars

10.5 Which dermatological condition can be worsened by taking chloroquine?

a. Psoriasis
b. Acne vulgaris
c. Eczema
d. Rosacea
e. Atopic dermatitis

10.6 How long after unprotected sex can EHC be given?

a. 24 hours
b. 48 hours
c. 72 hours
d. 96 hours
e. 120 hours

10.7 What is regarded as the most important smoking-related disease?

a. Lung cancer
b. Chronic obstructive pulmonary disease
c. Throat cancer
d. Motor neurone disease
e. Ischaemic heart disease

10.8 With which patient group should care be taken when recommending promethazine for motion sickness?

a. Glaucoma
b. Hypertension
c. Peptic ulceration
d. Diabetes mellitus
e. Parkinson's disease

Questions 10.9 to 10.11 concern the following NRT products:

A. Patch
B. Gum
C. Inhalator
D. Lozenge
E. Microtab

Select, from A to E, which of the above products

10.9 Is most suitable for patients in whom compliance may be an issue

10.10 Delivers constant levels of plasma nicotine

10.11 Is useful for those people who need to have their hands occupied

Questions 10.12 to 10.14 concern the following medicines:

A. Chloroquine
B. Proguanil
C. Hyoscine
D. Nicotine replacement therapy
E. Levonorgestrel

Select, from A to E, which of the above medicines

10.12 Causes diarrhoea *B*

10.13 Causes visual disturbances *A*

10.14 Causes dry mouth *c*

Questions 10.15 to 10.17: for each of these questions *one or more* of the responses is (are) correct. Decide which of the responses is (are) correct. Then choose:

A. If a, b and c are correct
B. If a and b only are correct
C. If b and c only are correct
D. If a only is correct
E. If c only is correct

Directions summarised

A	B	C	D	E
a, b and c	a and b only	b and c only	a only	c only

B **10.15** When using DEET, the following rule(s) should be followed:

　　a. It should be applied regularly
　　b. It should be kept away from plastic
　　c. It should never be applied to the face

A **10.16** *Plasmodium falciparum* is associated with:

　　a. High levels of drug resistance
　　b. The highest incidence of death compared to other forms of malaria
　　c. Widespread distribution on the African continent *Malariae → least common*

10.17 What side effects are commonly associated with chewing nicotine gum?

　　a. Hypotension
　　b. Taste disturbance
　　c. GI disturbances

Questions 10.18 to 10.20: these questions consist of a statement in the left-hand column followed by a statement in the right-hand column. You need to:

● decide whether the first statement is true or false
● decide whether the second statement is true or false

Then choose:

A. If both statements are true and the second statement is a correct explanation of the first statement
B. If both statements are true but the second statement is NOT a correct explanation of the first statement
C. If the first statement is true but the second statement is false
D. If the first statement is false but the second statement is true
E. If both statements are false

Directions summarised

	1st statement	2nd statement	
A	True	True	2nd statement is a correct explanation of the first
B	True	True	2nd statement is not a correct explanation of the first
C	True	False	
D	False	True	
E	False	False	

	First statement	Second statement
10.18 *A*	Antimalarials have to be taken before travel	Side effects may preclude patients from taking antimalarials
10.19	Malaria can be contracted months after return from an endemic area	The liver holds a reservoir of parasites that are hard to eradicate
10.20 *E*	Pregnancy is a contraindication for malaria prophylaxis	Infants cannot take antimalarials

Case study

CASE STUDY 10.1

Mr and Mrs J and their two children, Sammy aged 5 and Jessica aged 12, are going on their summer holidays. They want to know what travel sickness tablets they should take.

a. What information do you need to know before recommending a suitable product? For each question state your rationale

You need to know:

- *Who is affected by travel sickness: this may influence recommendation, especially if it affects one of the parents who might be driving.*
- *The length of the trip: this will influence which product will be the most appropriate. It is sensible to match up the length of journey with a medicine that has the same duration of action as the trip.*
- *Medication history: patients who are taking medication for glaucoma or prostate enlargement should avoid taking OTC medicines. Additionally, medicines with anticholinergic side effects will potentiate the side effects of OTC travel medication.*
- *Past medication for similar journeys: it is likely that the family have had to purchase such products in the past. It is worth finding out what they were and how well tolerated they were before potentially recommending the same product.*

You find out they are going to northern France by ferry. This is a 2-hour boat journey followed by a further 2-hour drive. Mr J gets seasick and neither of the children like boats or car journeys. Jessica also suffers from narcolepsy.

b. What would be the best drug regimen for the family? State your rationale.

It appears that the total journey time is relatively short and a hyoscine-based product would be the most suitable product for the two children and their father. Kwells Kids could be used by everyone; Mr J would have to take two tablets, Jessica one tablet and Sammy half a tablet. As Jessica has narcolepsy it is necessary to see if she takes any medication to help with the condition. If she does then checks would have to be made to ensure that Jessica could still take hyoscine.

c. What practical advice would you also offer the family?

Hyoscine will cause dry mouth and potential sedation. Sucking sweets can compensate dry mouth. Sedation might be a problem for Mr J because he has to drive after the ferry crossing. He should be told about the possible effects of hyoscine. He might choose not to take the medication, although no alternative is available that does not cause possible sedation.

The two children might experience less nausea if they are kept occupied by playing games.

CASE STUDY 10.2

Ms HS walks into the pharmacy on Saturday morning and asks to buy the morning after pill.

a. What questions do you need to ask?

You need to discover:

- *Her age*
- *How long ago she had unprotected sex*
- *Whether she used a form of contraception? If so, what form*
- *The date of her last period and was it different from normal*

You find out she is 18 and had sex last night. She normally takes Microgynon. Her period was about 3 weeks ago and was the same as previous periods.

b. What else do you need to know?

You also need to know about her pill taking compliance.

She says that she has not taken her last 2 days (Thursday and Friday) and doesn't know whether she should take today's tablet. She has three tablets left before the end of the packet.

c. What advice are you going to give her?

There is no need for EHC as she has forgotten to take her tablets at the end of the cycle. She should be told to continue taking the rest of her tablets but when the last tablet is taken she should not have a 7-day pill free period but go straight on to the next packet.
She is very anxious and doesn't feel confident in the advice you have given.

d. Could you supply EHC even though it is not necessary?

There is no reason why you could not supply Levonelle. If this would relieve the patient's anxiousness then supply would not be unreasonable.

Answers to multiple choice questions

1 = b	2 = d	3 = c	4 = c	5 = a	6 = c	7 = e	8 = a	9 = a	10 = a
11= c	12 = b	13 = a	14 = c	15 = b	16 = a	17 = e	18 = a	19 = a	20 = e.

Abbreviations

μg	microgram
ACE	angiotension converting enzyme
ADR	adverse drug reaction
CB	chronic bronchitis
CSM	Committee for Safety of Medicines
DEET	diethyl toluamide
DPH	diphenhydramine
EHC	emergency hormonal contraception
FDA	Food and Drug Administration (equivalent to the Medicines Control Authority in the UK)
GORD	gastro-oesophageal reflux disease
GP	general practitioner
GSL	general sales list
h	hour
IHS	International Headache Society
HMG-CoA	beta-hydroxy beta-methyl glutaryl coenzyme A
HPV	human papilloma virus
HSV	herpes simplex virus
IBS	irritable bowel syndrome
IgE	immunoglobulin E
INR	international normalised ratio
IUCD	intrauterine contraceptive device
KCS	keratoconjunctivitis sicca

L	litre
MAOI	monoamine oxidase inhibitor
MAU	minor aphthous ulcers
mEq	milliequivalent
mg	milligram
MI	myocardial infarction
mL	millilitre
mmol	millimole
NRT	Nicotine replacement therapy
NSAID	non-steroidal anti-inflammatory drug
ORT	oral rehydration therapy
OTC	over-the-counter
P	pharmacy
PD	primary dysmenorrhoea
PID	pelvic inflammatory disease
PMS	premenstrual syndrome
POM	prescription-only-medicine
PV	per vagina
SSRI	selective serotonin reuptake inhibitor
STD	sexually transmitted disease
TB	tuberculosis
TCA	tricyclic antidepressant
UTI	urinary tract infection
WHO	World Health Organization

Glossary of terms

Chapter 1

Atopy: A form of hypersensitivity characterised by a familial tendency.

Cervical lymphadenopathy: Enlargement of the cervical lymph nodes.

Agranulocytosis: Acute deficiency of neutrophil white blood cells leading to neutropenia.

Auroscopical examination: Examination of the ear drum by means of an apparatus that shines light onto the ear drum.

Haemoptysis: Coughing up blood.

Dyspnoea: Difficulty in breathing.

Malaise: General feeling of being unwell.

Gastro-oesophageal reflux: The back flow of gastric contents into the oesophagus.

Orthopnoea: Difficulty in breathing when lying down.

Pleurisy: Inflammation of the pleural membranes caused by the two pleural membranes adhering to one another.

Purulent: Term used to describe a material containing pus.

Rhinorrhoea: Watery nasal discharge.

Vascular engorgement: An area of tissue that has been excessively perfused with blood.

Vasodilatation: Increase in the diameter of the blood vessels.

Chapter 2

Chalazion: Also referred to as meibomian cyst.

Conjunctivitis medicamentosa: conjunctivitis caused by repeated administration of ocular eye drops, especially sympathomimetic agents. On withdrawal of the medicine the patient suffers from rebound redness of the eyes.

Glands of Zeiss and Moll: Both are located within the eyelid. The gland of Zeiss secretes sebum and the gland of Moll secretes sweat.

Hordeola: Commonly known as styes.

Limbal area: Area where the cornea meets the sclera.

Meibomianitis: Inflammation of the meibomian gland.

Photophobia: A dislike of bright lights.

Visual acuity: The ability to read text. For example, distance visual acuity is the person's ability to read letters across the room and near visual acuity is the person's ability to read letters close to.

Chapter 3

Conductive deafness: Sound waves are hindered from reaching the inner ear (e.g. by ear wax) resulting in distortion of sounds that impairs the understanding of words.

Effusion: Escape of fluid, e.g. exudates, from the ear.

FDA: Federal Drug Administration (equivalent to the MCA in the UK).

Laceration: A tear in the skin causing a wound.

Oedematous: Abnormal accumulation in intercellular spaces of the body.

Tinnitus: A noise in the ears likened to ringing or buzzing.

Chapter 4

ADRs: Adverse drug reactions.

Amenorrhoea: Absence or the stoppage of menstruation

Haematoma: A localised collection of blood, usually clotted, in an organ, space or tissue.

Myalgia: Muscular pain.

Paraesthesia: An abnormal sensation, for example, a burning or prickling sensation.

Pericranial: Area relating to around the skull.

Purpuric rash: Rash with a distinctive red/purple colouration caused by haemorrhage of small blood vessels in the skin.

Chapter 5

Anovulatory: Term used to describe women that do not ovulate.

Bacteriuria: Bacteria in the urine.

Dyspareunia: Difficult or painful sexual intercourse.

Dysuria: Painful or difficult urination.

Haematuria: Blood in the urine.

Menarche: Onset of menstruation.

Nocturia: Excessive urination at night.

Perianal: The area around the anus.

Perineal: The area around the perineum. The perineum describes the area between the vulva and anus.

Postmenopausal women: Women that have finished menstruating. The average age for women to be postmenopausal is 51.

Prostate gland: The gland that surrounds the neck of the bladder and urethra in men.

Pyelonephritis: Inflammation of the kidney due to bacterial infection.

Suprapubic: Area above the pubic region.

Chapter 6

Annular lesions: Skin lesions that are circular.

Diverticulitis: Inflammation of a diverticulum, which is a pouch or sac. It occurs normally after herniation.

Halitosis: Bad breath.

Suprapubic: Area above the pubis area of the abdomen.

Tenesmus: Cessation of incomplete bowel evacuation

Ureter: Tube connecting the kidney to the bladder.

Chapter 7

Atopy: Literally means 'strange disease'. The triad of atopic dermatitis, asthma and allergic rhinitis.

Comedone: A plug of oxidised sebaceous material obstructing the surface opening of a pilosebaceous follicle, commonly referred to as a blackhead.

Crust: The term given to dried exudate.

Erythema: Redness of the skin.

Intertrigo: Dermatitis on apposing areas of skin in flexural body sites, e.g. groin, axillae.

Macules: Flat stains or spots of altered skin colour.

Maculo-papular: Literally a papule developed on a macule, i.e. a mixture of the two types of lesion.

Nodule: A solid elevation whose greater part lies beneath the skin surface.

Papules: Raised palpable spots

Punctiform: Pinpoint-like lesions.

Pustule: A pus-filled lesion.

Vesicles: Small, raised, fluid-filled lesions or blisters.

Wheal: Areas of transient dermal oedema. Classically associated with urticaria and also following insect bites.

Chapter 8

Abduction: The term used to describe movement of a part away from the median plane of the body, for example, moving the leg straight out to the side.

Ankylosis: When the joint becomes stiff or fused in a particular position.

Arthropathy: Pathology in a joint.

Articular cartilage: Cartilage occurring in the joint.

Disc herniation: Abnormal protrusion of the nucleus pulposus of the disc, which may impinge on a nerve root.

Epicondylitis: Inflammation of the epicondyle, which is the protuberance above the condyle. The condyle refers to the rounded part at the end of the bone used for articulation with another bone.

Chapter 9

Erythrematous: Redness of the skin due to capillary vasodilation.

Intertriginous area: Skin eruption on apposed skin surfaces.

Lichenification: Thickening and hardening of the skin.

Chapter 10

Erythrocytes: Alternative name for red blood cells.

Melanocytes: Cells in the skin epidermis responsible for producing melanin.

Yuzpe method: The name given to the combined oestrogen and progestogen method of emergency contraception.

Index